Contact Dermatitis

Guest Editor

SUSAN NEDOROST, MD

DERMATOLOGIC CLINICS

www.derm.theclinics.com

Consulting Editor

BRUCE H. THIERS, MD

July 2009 • Volume 27 • Number 3

SAUNDERS an imprint of ELSEVIER, Inc.

W.B. SAUNDERS COMPANY
A Division of Elsevier Inc.

1600 John F. Kennedy Boulevard • Suite 1800 • Philadelphia, PA 19103-2899

http://www.theclinics.com

DERMATOLOGIC CLINICS Volume 27, Number 3
July 2009 ISSN 0733-8635, ISBN-13: 978-1-4377-1210-0, ISBN 10: 1-4377-1210-X

Editor: Carla Holloway
Developmental Editor: Donald Mumford

Dermatologic Clinics (ISSN 0733-8635) is published quarterly by Elsevier Inc., 360 Park Avenue South, New York, NY 10010-1710. Months of publication are January, April, July, and October. Business and editorial offices: 1600 John F. Kennedy Blvd., Suite 1800, Philadelphia, PA 19103-2899. Customer service office: 11830 Westline Drive, St. Louis, MO 63146. Periodicals postage paid at New York, NY, and additional mailing offices. Subscription prices are USD 274.00 per year for US individuals, USD 423.00 per year for US institutions, USD 321.00 per year for Canadian individuals, USD 506.00 per year for Canadian institutions, USD 376.00 per year for international individuals, USD 506.00 per year for international institutions, USD 131.00 per year for US students/residents, and USD 189.00 per year for Canadian and international students/residents. International air speed delivery is included in all *Clinics* subscription prices. All prices are subject to change without notice. **POSTMASTER:** Send address changes to *Dermatologic Clinics*, Elsevier Journals Customer Service, 11830 Westline Drive, St. Louis, MO 63146. **Customer Service: 1-800-654-2452 (US and Canada). From outside of the US and Canada, call 1-314-453-7041. Fax: 1-314-453-5170. For print support, E-mail: JournalsCustomer Service-usa@elsevier.com. For online support, E-mail: JournalsOnlineSupport-usa@elsevier.com.**

Reprints. For copies of 100 or more, of articles in this publication, please contact the Commercial Reprints Department, Elsevier Inc., 360 Park Avenue South, New York, New York 10010-1710. Tel.: (212) 633-3813; Fax: (212) 462-1935; E-mail: reprints@elsevier.com.

The *Dermatologic Clinics* is covered in *MEDLINE/PubMed (Index Medicus)*, *Current Contents/Clinical Medicine*, *Excerpta Medica*, *Chemical Abstracts*, and *ISI/BIOMED*.

Printed and bound by CPI Group (UK) Ltd, Croydon, CR0 4YY
Transferred to Digital Print 2011

Contributors

GUEST EDITOR

SUSAN NEDOROST, MD
Associate Professor of Dermatology; and
Associate Professor of Environmental Health
Sciences, University Hospitals Case Medical
Center, Cleveland, Ohio

AUTHORS

TINA BHUTANI, MD
Resident Physician, Department of Internal
Medicine, University of California, San Diego,
California

DAVID S. BROOKSTEIN, ScD
Dean of Engineering and Research, Pennsylvania
Advanced Textile Research and Innovation
Center, Philadelphia University, Philadelphia,
Pennsylvania

LAUREN Y. CAO, BS, MD/MS
Clinical Research Scholars Program (CRSP)
Student, Case Western Reserve University School
of Medicine, Cleveland, Ohio

MARI PAZ CASTANEDO-TARDAN, MD
Post-Doctoral Research Fellow, Section of
Dermatology, Dartmouth-Hitchcock Medical
Center, Lebanon, New Hampshire

SHANE C. CLARK, BA
Department of Internal Medicine, Division of
Dermatology, Ohio State University College
of Medicine, Columbus, Ohio

MARK D.P. DAVIS, MD
Consultant, Department of Dermatology, Mayo
Clinic; and Professor of Dermatology, College
of Medicine, Mayo Clinic, Rochester, Minnesota

AN GOOSSENS, RPharm, PhD
Professor, Department of Dermatology, University
Hospital St.Raphaël, Katholieke Universiteit
Leuven, Leuven, Belgium

DANIEL J. HOGAN, MD
Clinical Professor of Medicine (Dermatology),
NOVA Southeastern University,
Largo, Florida

SHARON E. JACOB, MD
Assistant Professor of Medicine and Pediatrics
(Dermatology), Rady Children's Hospital-
University of California; and Veterans
Administration Hospital–San Diego,
San Diego, California

HEATHER P. LAMPEL, MD, MPH
Dermatology Resident Physician, Department
of Dermatology, University of California, Irvine,
California

JOHNATHAN J. LEDET, MD
Louisiana State University Health Sciences
Center, Shreveport, Los Angeles

LISA E. MAIER, MD
Assistant Professor of Dermatology, Department
of Dermatology, University of Michigan; and
Veterans Administration Medical Center, Ann
Arbor, Michigan

MATTHEW MOLENDA, MD
Dermatology Resident, Ohio State University,
Columbus, Ohio

SUSAN NEDOROST, MD
Associate Professor of Dermatology; and
Associate Professor of Environmental Health
Sciences, University Hospitals Case Medical
Center, Cleveland, Ohio

STEVEN A. NELSON, MD
Department of Dermatology, Mayo Clinic Arizona, Scottsdale, Arizona

RAJIV I. NIJHAWAN, MD
Intern, St. Luke's Roosevelt Hospital, New York, New York

DENIS SASSEVILLE, MD, FRCPC
Associate Professor, Department of Medicine, McGill University; and Director, Division of Dermatology, McGill University Health Centre, Royal Victoria Hospital, Montreal, Quebec, Canada

MARY C. SMITH, RN, MSN
Clinical Nurse Manager, Department of Dermatology, University Hospitals Case Medical Center, Cleveland, Ohio

APRA SOOD, MD
Associate Staff, Department of Dermatology, Dermatology-Plastic Surgery Institute, Cleveland Clinic Foundation, Cleveland, Ohio

JAMES S. TAYLOR, MD
Consultant Dermatologist, Department of Dermatology, Dermatology-Plastic Surgery Institute, Cleveland Clinic Foundation, Cleveland, Ohio

NIELS K. VEIEN, MD, PhD
Dermatology Clinic, Aalborg, Denmark

JAMES A. YIANNIAS, MD
Associate Professor of Dermatology, Mayo School of Graduate Medical Education, Department of Dermatology, Mayo Clinic Arizona, Scottsdale, Arizona

MATTHEW J. ZIRWAS, MD
Assistant Professor, Division of Dermatology, Ohio State University, Columbus, Ohio

KATHRYN A. ZUG, MD
Associate Professor of Medicine (Dermatology), Dartmouth-Hitchcock Medical Center, Lebanon, New Hampshire

Contents

The diagnosis of a contact allergy requires several important and essential steps, because the failure to recognize a contact allergy can occur in any of the various stages of the contact allergy investigation. If the results of the skin tests are negative for a patient for whom a diagnosis of allergic contact dermatitis has been proposed, one has to go back to the beginning, that is, with a thoroughgoing anamnesis of the patient (perhaps with a visit to his or her environment). The assumed allergens must be retested (perhaps in another concentration, with another vehicle, or with another testing method), and additional allergens must be tested. The patient can also be asked to keep a journal, in the hope that a correlation can be discerned between exposure to a substance and the occurrence of the skin problems. Once an allergen has been identified, it is the dermatologist's task to provide specific advice about the products that have to be avoided, or about the products that can safely be used, because subjects sensitive to specific ingredients must avoid products containing them.

Plastic resin systems have an increasingly diverse array of applications but also induce health hazards, the most common of which are allergic and irritant contact dermatitis. Contact urticaria, pigmentary changes, and photoallergic contact dermatitis may occasionally occur. Other health effects, especially respiratory and neurologic signs and symptoms, have also been reported. These resin systems include epoxies, the most frequent synthetic resin systems to cause contact dermatitis, (meth)acrylics, polyurethanes, phenol-formaldehydes, polyesters, amino resins (melamine-formaldehydes, urea-formaldehydes), polyvinyls, polystyrenes, polyolefins, polyamides and polycarbonates. Contact dermatitis usually occurs as a result of exposure to the monomers and additives in the occupational setting, although reports from consumers, using the raw materials or end products periodically surface. Resin- and additive-induced direct contact dermatitis usually presents on the hands, fingers, and forearms, while facial, eyelid, and neck involvement may occur through indirect contact, eg, via the hands, or from airborne exposure. Patch testing with commercially available materials, and in some cases the patient's own resins, is important for diagnosis. Industrial hygiene prevention techniques are essential to reduce contact dermatitis when handling these resin systems.

Hand dermatitis is a common disease of the skin resulting in significantly decreased quality of life. Allergic contact dermatitis is a frequent cause of hand dermatitis. Recent studies have revealed that biocides used as preservatives are frequent allergens affecting the hands. This article reviews common biocides implicated in hand dermatitis.

Certain patterns of dermatitis, such as those affecting the face, eyelids, lips, and neck, should raise the suspicion of a cosmetic-related contact allergy. Patch testing with a broad screening series, supplemented by a patient's own personal care products, should be considered when evaluating patients with suspected cosmetic dermatitis. Once the offending allergen is identified, an avoidance regimen should be established to avoid further exposure.

The anatomic distribution of dermatitis affecting the hands and feet can provide clues to the likelihood that a contact allergen is provoking the dermatitis. Dermatitis presenting on the hands or feet, but not both, is more likely because of allergic contact dermatitis, whereas dermatitis affecting both the hands and feet is more likely a result of a systemic cause. Exceptions are reviewed in this article. When allergic contact dermatitis affects only the hands and feet, rubber chemicals and chromates are the most common allergens. Pattern recognition can assist with choice of patch test allergens, counseling regarding routes of exposure, and selection of alternative contactants.

Allergic contact dermatitis to topical medicaments occurs often. Common medicaments associated with allergic contact dermatitis include topically applied antibiotics, antihistamines, nonsteroidal antiinflammatory drugs, anesthetics, and corticosteroids. In cases of suspected allergic contact dermatitis, medicaments that the patient is using should be included when patch testing. Body sites susceptible to allergic contact dermatitis to topical medicaments include scalp, face, anogenital area, and lower extremities.

Exposure to plants is very common, through leisure or professional activity. In addition, plant products and botanic extracts are increasingly present in the environment. Cutaneous adverse reactions to plants and their derivatives occur fairly frequently, and establishing the correct diagnosis is not always easy. The astute clinician relies on a detailed history and a careful skin examination to substantiate his opinion. This article reviews the characteristic clinical patterns of phyto- and phytophotodermatitis and some less common presentations.

From as early as 1869, textile dyes and subsequently finishes have been reported to cause various manifestations of contact dermatitis, from mild to severe and debilitating. The European Union, through Directive (2002/61/EC) to restrict the marketing and use of certain dangerous substances and preparations (azo colorants) in textile and leather products, has taken the worldwide lead in restricting some dyes as a result of their carcinogenic nature. Given the recent discovery of the new route to contact dermatitis, it is important to continue to be vigilant for new and unexpected sources of allergens from textile, apparel, and furniture items.

Patient education plays an important role in empowering patients who have allergic contact dermatitis. Having the knowledge about a disease process does not guarantee healthy behaviors. Through careful assessment of educational needs, awareness of stages of change that adults go through, and use of resources available to members of the American Contact Dermatology Society, nurses can provide patient education that completes the patch testing process.

Patch testing can be particularly rewarding when skin-care product allergens are identified. Careful determination of relevance, followed by careful education regarding allergen avoidance, can result in dramatic clinical improvement. Several common clinical scenarios are reviewed with a focus on pragmatic solutions to heighten positive patient outcomes.

The terminology of eruptive, symmetric, vesicular, and/or bullous dermatitis on the palms and/or palmar aspects or sides of the fingers includes the terms *pompholyx*, *dyshidrosis*, and *dyshidrotic eczema*. This article presents the case for a standard, broad definition of this condition and reviews the epidemiology, clinical features, etiology, and treatment of acute and recurrent vesicular hand dermatitis with special emphasis on endogenous causes.

Systemic contact dermatitis (SCD) describes a cutaneous eruption in response to systemic exposure to an allergen. The exact pathologic mechanism remains uncertain. The broad spectrum of presentations that are often nonspecific can make it difficult for the clinician to suspect this disease, but it is an important diagnosis to consider in cases of recalcitrant, widespread, or recurrent dermatitis, in which patch testing often reveals allergy to nickel or balsam of Peru. Diagnosis and appropriate management can be life-altering for affected patients. This article on SCD provides an overview of the disease with descriptions of common allergens and some insight into the possible mechanism of action seen in SCD.

Contact dermatitis is the most common occupational skin disorder, responsible for up to 30% of all cases of occupational disease in industrialized nations.

Epidemiologic data suggest that contact dermatitis accounts for 90% to 95% of all cases of occupational skin disease, imposing considerable social and economic implications. Occupational contact dermatitis is broadly classified into allergic and irritant subtypes. Irritant contact dermatitis is widely quoted in the literature to account for 80% of occupational contact dermatitis cases, with allergic cases held responsible for the remaining 20%.

Contact dermatitis is a serious public health and dermatologic concern. The prevalence of contact dermatitis in the United States was estimated to be 13.6 per 1000 population according to the National Health and Nutritional Examination Survey using physical examinations by dermatologists of a selected sample of Americans. The American Medical Care Survey estimated that for all American physicians dermatitis is the second most common dermatologic diagnosis proffered. It is essential that government, industry, and dermatologists work together to enhance regulatory methods to control and prevent contact allergy epidemics. Increased knowledge and awareness of occupational skin diseases by dermatologists and other health care professionals will assist in achieving national public health goals. This article reviews governmental regulations-some helpful for patients and workers and some not helpful for dermatologists in their quest to assist patients with contact dermatitis.

Dermatologic Clinics

THE CLINICS ARE NOW AVAILABLE ONLINE!

Access your subscription at:
www.theclinics.com

Preface

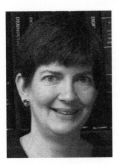

Susan Nedorost, MD
Guest Editor

Diagnosis and treatment of allergic contact dermatitis is one of the most gratifying patient interactions in dermatology. Successful identification of an allergen and subsequent allergen avoidance patient education can lead to cure without side effects of drugs, additional procedures, or need for frequent physician visits. Often patients return to the workforce. Quality of life improves.

Helping patients with contact dermatitis requires knowledge. Dermatologists are obligated to stay current regarding new sensitizers introduced into industry or personal care products. In this issue, Dr. Goossens, a pharmacist who has made great contributions to the understanding of sensitizers, writes about recognition of new allergens and cross-reactions.

The pattern of dermatitis is important in estimating the clinical likelihood of allergic contact dermatitis and determining whether to patch test and which allergens to test. Related allergens are discussed in this volume whenever possible in the context of common patterns of presentation. Thus "sticky problems" from resins and adhesives are noted by Drs. Cao, Sood, and Taylor to often present with hand involvement and also ectopic facial and neck dermatitis. Drs. Castanedo-Tardan and Zug discuss allergens in hair products that often present with a "run-off pattern" on neck and chest. Glove and shoe components can cause hand/foot dermatitis that may mimic endogenous dermatoses; Dr. Maier and colleagues discuss hands with generalized dermatitis as seen in patients allergic to biocides and preservatives. Medicament allergy can lead to unusual shapes or localization of dermatitis depending on how the patient applies their topical products, as discussed by Dr. Davis. Photoexposed and textile patterns suggest the need for specialized photoallergen and textile patch test series, respectively. Dr. Sasseville, a world expert on plant dermatitis, provides a beautifully illustrated article. Dr. Brookstein is a textile scientist who contributes an article on textile pattern dermatitis.

Interpretation of patch test results and patient education are the most critical and underrecognized aspects of the allergic contact dermatitis evaluation process. Drs. Nelson and Yiannias, who have created an important tool to teach patients about acceptable personal care products free of their allergens, write about determining relevance of positive patch tests and avoidance strategies. Ms. Smith discusses patient education from the perspective of a clinical nurse specialist. This includes assessments that physicians rarely record, such as the physician's credibility with the patient, the patient's willingness to change behaviors (in this case to avoid allergens), and the patient's level of literacy. She also discusses the use of return demonstrations in the patch test clinic to allow patients to practice reading ingredient labels.

Increasingly, dermatologists recognize the role of systemic allergen in exposure in chronic vesicular hand dermatitis and generalized systemic contact dermatitis. Drs. Veien and Jacob and their colleagues cover these cutting-edge topics.

Finally, systems issues directly affect patients with occupational allergic contact dermatitis, and these patients need to interact with the Bureau of Workers' Compensation and other

Dermatol Clin 27 (2009) xi–xii
doi:10.1016/j.det.2009.05.015

derm.theclinics.com

government agencies. Drs. Clark and Zirwas discuss management of occupational dermatitis. Governments, especially in Europe, have increasingly instituted public health regulations to decrease allergic contact dermatitis. Drs. Ledet and Hogan point out the irony that in the United States, patch tests themselves are sometimes more regulated than consumer or worker exposures to sensitizers.

Diagnosis and treatment of contact dermatitis is gratifying and intellectually stimulating. I hope that you enjoy this issue on current best practices and that it helps you to help patients.

Susan Nedorost, MD
University Hospitals Case Medical Center
11100 Euclid Avenue, Mailstop 5028
Cleveland, OH 44106, USA

E-mail address:
stn@case.edu (S. Nedorost)

Recognizing and Testing Allergens

An Goossens, RPharm, PhD

KEYWORDS

- Allergic contact dermatitis • Clinical symptoms
- Diagnosis • Patch testing • Relevance • Test technique

The diagnosis of an allergic contact dermatitis is made on the basis of a clinical examination, in which much attention is given to the nature and the location of the lesions, the recording of a thorough anamnesis, the consideration of all possible etiologic factors, and the administration of patch tests, whereby the determination of the relevance of the positive results obtained is critical. Basic knowledge of the chemicals contacted is essential, not only to make the correct diagnosis, but also to understand cross-reaction patterns. Moreover, not only low–molecular weight compounds, but also proteinous substances, such as in the case of "protein contact dermatitis," need to be taken into account as potential causes of the patient's dermatitis. The failure to recognize this diagnosis can occur in any of the various stages of the contact-allergy investigation.

DETECTION OF THE ALLERGEN(S)

The causal allergens can be detected by:[1]

- experience and motivation of the investigator
- knowledge of materials, chemicals, and chemistry
- careful history taking
- the way of exposure
- the clinical symptoms
- the localization of the lesions
- coincidence
- the use of an expert system
- the performance of skin tests:
  - patch testing (series, own products + ingredients, extracts, etc)
  - other skin tests (repeat open application test (ROAT), usage tests, prick test, etc)
- determining the relevance for the positive reactions found
- chemical analysis

EXPERIENCE AND MOTIVATION

It is evident that the more experience the investigator has, the more accurately allergens can be identified. Furthermore, his knowledge needs to be based on good training, keeping up with the literature, attending courses and meetings, and the use of relevant websites. Last but not least, his motivation is very important because one needs to be eager to detect the allergen(s), thereby acting in a "Sherlock Holmes" style.

KNOWLEDGE OF MATERIALS, CHEMICALS, AND CHEMISTRY

Knowledge of the chemical ingredients, along with their synonyms, is important to identify the allergens present in products that the patients are in contact with.[2] Moreover, the chemical relationship between molecules will help to understand cross-reactivity patterns. Hence, an allergen might be found that by itself is not relevant to the patient's dermatitis but that cross-reacts to the actual culprit.

HISTORY OF THE PATIENT

An extensive and standardized anamnesis is essential, and it should cover all possible etiologic factors, such as profession, leisure-time activities, use of topical pharmaceutical products and cosmetics, the type of clothing and shoes, contact with plants, and so on.

Department of Dermatology, University Hospital St.-Raphaël, Katholieke Universiteit Leuven, Kapucijnenvoer 33, B-3000 Leuven, Belgium
E-mail address: an.goossens@uz.kuleuven.ac.be

Dermatol Clin 27 (2009) 219–226
doi:10.1016/j.det.2009.05.004

In case of an occupation-induced dermatitis, besides information obtained from the occupational physician and the data sheets or any other information on the products and materials the patients are in contact with, a factory visit is, in most cases, very instructive.

The patients can themselves provide many indications about the possible allergens, but they often need to be convinced that the allergenic product may not have been introduced recently into their environment. Moreover, because allergic contact dermatitis represents a delayed-type sensitivity reaction, it can take several days before the clinical symptoms and signs appear after the contact. This is also related to the concentration of the allergen present: the less concentrated it is, the more time it takes before the allergic reaction appears. This has been clearly shown in studies involving fragrance chemicals, for example, isoeugenol in deodorants.[3]

WAY OF EXPOSURE

There are several ways the allergen may contact the skin:

- intentional application to the skin, eg, with cosmetics;
- contact with allergenic or allergen-contaminated surfaces, eg, handgrips or tools;
- transfer of an allergen from the hands to the face or other more sensitive sites, which gives rise to an "ectopic" contact dermatitis, for example, with nail polish or plants;
- products used by the patient's partner or other persons in his/her environment, which is referred to as "connubial" or "consort" dermatitis, or dermatitis "by proxy," for example, cosmetics;
- airborne contact with allergenic gasses or vapors, droplets, or powders (dust), which gives rise to an "airborne" dermatitis;
- eczematous reactions spreading outside the area in contact with the allergen, often in the form of small papules, which can be explained by hematogenous dissemination of the allergen;
- after previous sensitization of the skin, systemic exposure to the allergen (or to a cross-reacting substance), for example, in drugs or food, may produce a flare-up of the eczema at the previous contact sites or a diffuse or, sometimes, generalized eczema. In this context, the term "endogenous" or "systemic contact dermatitis-type reaction" is often used.

- photoallergic contact dermatitis, the result of exposure to a chemical associated with sunlight exposure giving rise to a photoallergen, for example, with nonsteroidal antiinflammatory drugs (NSAIDs), particularly ketoprofen and sunscreen agents.

CLINICAL SYMPTOMS

The skin symptoms of a contact allergy manifest themselves classically in the form of eczema that, by themselves , can be very polymorphic. However, a contact allergic reaction can also produce noneczematous lesions.[4,5] In this way, follicular and dermal lesions can determine the clinical picture to a greater or lesser degree. In addition, other forms of expression are known, such as erythema-multiforme-like lesions or urticarial papular plaques (examples of such allergens are tropical woods); lichen planus-like and lichenoid eruptions (eg, color developers in photography); granulomatous and pustular reactions (metals); lymphomatoid contact dermatitis (eg, with metals and textile dyes); pigmentation disturbances, both hyperpigmentation and hypopigmentation (leukoderma); and finally, psoriasis, by way of the Köbner phenomenon, is also a possibility.

LOCALIZATION OF THE LESIONS

The localization of the lesions can be an important starting point in the identification of the causal allergen because a contact dermatitis generally starts at, and in many cases is even restricted to, the contact site. The skin reactions, however, can also only occur on more sensitive sites, such as the eyelids, where the skin is thin and thus where substances can penetrate more easily; they are sometimes the only sites affected when a facial cream or even a hair dye is the allergen source. So, too, the backs of the hands rather than the palms are more affected by a contact allergy to gloves, whereas in the case of a textile dermatitis, only friction and transpiration sites are often involved in the eczematous reaction.

This does not, of course, preclude other possibilities, and one needs to stay alert, for example, a dermatitis located on the feet might suggest a shoe dermatitis; on the other hand, a topical pharmaceutical product (antimycotic or corticosteroid preparation) that had been applied on that area and that had contaminated the shoe, might be the culprit.

COINCIDENCE

It may happen that allergens are identified purely by coincidence. Certain products or chemicals, when tested routinely or periodically in all patients investigated, for example, in the frame of a specific study, may reveal to be the actual cause of the dermatitis. In this way, in a small study in which several shower gels were tested for irritancy, the authors were able to show that alkylglucosides, being mild detergents and present in many products intended to be used for sensitive or intolerant skin, were responsible for the dermatitis of the hands of 1 of the patients investigated.

USE OF AN EXPERT SYSTEM

In 1990, the author's group developed an expert system "EXPCA," which is a complete package for the contact allergy clinic. The software comprises modules for patient management (retrieving files and printing): administrative data, localizations of the lesions, atopic history, test readings, diagnoses, causal factors, and so on. Based on data collected from 19,100 subjects tested since 1978, it was found that support during the anamnesis provides information about the potential causal factors and sensitization sources, thereby suggesting allergens to be tested. The patient data are analyzed statistically. This system has also proven to be of great value for the residents in their dermatology training.

SKIN TESTING

As far as skin testing is concerned, the allergen itself, the test method, test concentration and vehicle used, the time of reading, and, finally, the determination of relevance need to be taken into account.[1]

The Allergen

First of all, only an allergen that is tested can be detected.

Secondly, one should NEVER test completely unknown products.

Testing with a baseline standard series is essential; however, patch tests with additional series and the products supplied by the patient, along with their ingredients, are equally important. To form an idea of the yield of tests with the European baseline series standard series in contact-allergy examinations, the patch-test results of 4 European centers were compared several years ago. It turned out that the proportion of contact-allergic reactions diagnosed with the European standard series "only" varied between 37% and 73% and for other allergens "only" between 5% and 23%. This indicates that a standard series is far from diagnosing 80% of all contact allergies, because this percentage completely depends on which materials are being tested to detect allergens (testing with a standard series only would even provide detection in 100% of the cases).Therefore, testing with additional series and ingredients of products supplied by the patient are absolutely necessary.[6,7]

It happens that the cited allergen is not by itself the cause of the allergic reaction but an impurity in it. This is the case, for example, for cetyl alcohol (pharmaceutical quality), which contains an unidentified impurity, so patch tests with analytical quality cetyl alcohol give a "false" negative reaction. Allergenic impurities occur much more in industrial products, for example, allylglycidylether, a reactive epoxy thinner, was found as a contaminant in a fixation additive in silicon and polyurethane resins. Allergenic degradation products can also be formed during storage, primarily by oxidation, as in the case of terpenes, such as limonene and linalool.[8] This has immediate implications for the patch-test material, and thus the usefulness of stability checks.

Test Methods

Patch test

The patch test remains, at present, the most reliable method to identify a contact allergy. It is a biologic test, so the results can be erroneously negative or positive. The causes of a false-negative reaction are legion:[9,10] the sensitization level of the patient may have been too low; the tests may have been administered in a refractory phase; the test concentration and/or the amount of the substance may have been insufficient; the wrong test substance may have been used; the vehicle may not have released a sufficient amount of the allergen (the biologic availability was too low); the occlusion might have been insufficient; the test site might have been inappropriate; the reading may have been made too soon; or the reaction might have been suppressed immunologically by exposure to sunlight, local application of corticosteroid, or systemic administration of corticosteroids or immunomodulators, which can suppress the immunologic response. This list is certainly not exhaustive.

In the case of photoallergic contact dermatitis, photopatch tests are indicated. When patch testing with a particular product is negative in a patient who has an obvious dermatitis from the product, other skin-testing methods, such as open or semi-open tests and use tests and/or ROATs, may be recommended.

Photopatch tests

In case of photoallergic reactions, photopatch tests need to be performed; the allergens are tested in duplicate on the back and irradiated with ultraviolet (UV) light (most often UV-A 5 J/cm^2).

In Europe, a consensus has been reached concerning the test method.[11] With regard to the nature of the photoallergens, in the 1960s, antibacterials, such as salicylanilides, and in the 80s, certain fragrance ingredients, such as musk ambrette, were concerned; nowadays, sunscreen agents and NSAIDs are the most important culprits in this regard. A large European study, including photopatch tests, with a large set of sunscreen agents and NSAIDs is underway.

Open and semiopen (or semiocclusive) tests

Open or semiopen tests are indicated if the product causes irritation under occlusion. Highly acidic or alkaline products are not tested, unless they are buffered.[12]

These tests are useful modifications when testing products that have a certain irritation potential. The actual condition in which the product is used or the way in which the product is in contact with the skin needs to be taken into account; the rule could be that, when direct skin contact or contamination may occur during handling of the product (eg, paints, soluble oils, soaps, etc), an open or semi-open test could be performed. One should never test completely unknown or caustic products.

With an *open test*, the substance is applied uncovered on the upper arm or upper back, twice a day, during at least 2 days (without washing the test site).

The *semi-open test*[1,7] consists of the direct application on the skin, with a cotton Q-tip, of a minute amount (1–2 μL) of a liquid on a skin surface of about 1 cm^2. After complete evaporation of the liquid (the excess can be removed with a paper filter or another Q-tip), the *completely dry* test site is covered with acrylic tape. Diluted products (eg, 1%–2% aqueous) can also be tested this way. The reading of the skin test is performed 2 and 4 days later (sometimes later still), as with regular patch testing.

With regard to the *conditions of use*, this test method is based not on scientific research but on a longstanding expertise. The performance of the semiopen test depends mainly on the nature of the products that the patient brings, and it has the following purposes:

- Dispose of a practical and rapid method in case multiple "own" products need to be tested.

- Avoid false-positive or irritant reactions by patch testing potentially irritating products; this does not mean that a semiopen test cannot give rise to an irritant response. This explains why some basic knowledge about the nature of the product is absolutely necessary: corrosive products and products with a pH less than 3 or greater than 11 should never be tested. In the latter case, buffered products can be tested, and the potential allergenic ingredients can be tested individually.
- Avoid false-negative reactions which results by testing too diluted products, for example, in case of a contact allergy to a fragrance ingredient or a preservative in a shampoo. However, in case of a negative semiopen test, the existence of a contact allergy might not be discounted either: it is indeed possible that the allergen is present in too low of a concentration to produce a positive test. This also points to the importance of testing with all ingredients separately, in an appropriate concentration and vehicle, in case a contact allergy is really suspected.

Numerous products with a (slight) irritant potential can be tested using the semiopen test method, provided that the results are interpreted carefully and confirmed by testing with diluted products and with the individual ingredients. Examples include topical pharmaceutical products, such as antiseptic agents; products that contain solvents such as propylene glycol in high concentrations; creams based on the emulsifier sodium laurylsulphate; or cosmetic products containing emulsifiers, solvents, or other substances with an irritant potential, such as mascara (**Fig. 1**), nail lacquers, hair dyes, shampoos, permanent-wave solutions, liquid soaps, and peelings. For household and industrial products, after having verified that the

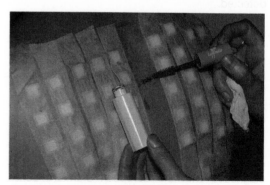

Fig. 1. Semiopen test with mascara.

pH is not too low or too high, or that a corrosive material is not involved, the semiopen test can be used for testing products such as paints, resins, varnish, glue, ink, wax, soluble oils, and so on.

Use tests and/or repeated open application tests

Patch tests are vastly different from normal use conditions; therefore tests can be completed by provocative use testing of sensitized subjects. For example, when dermatitis occurs after repeated exposure or after the use of products such as cosmetics on sensitive skin areas, such as the face, eyelids, or neck, and there is a negative patch-test result, use tests and/or ROATs are recommended. The intention is to approximate as nearly as possible the use situation.

With ROATs, about 0.1 mL of test material is applied twice daily to the flexor aspect of the forearm near the cubital fossa, to an area approximately 5 × 5 cm. The results are read after 1 week, but sometimes ROATs need to be performed up to 21 days, especially with low-concentrated allergens, to reveal an allergic reaction. The initial aspect of a positive ROAT is often follicular in nature (**Fig. 2**).

Prick tests

Prick tests are primarily used to detect allergens involved in the occurrence of type I immediate skin reactions, such as immunologic contact urticaria or the "contact urticaria syndrome," which may be caused by low–molecular weight allergens, such as chlorhexidine or bacitracin, or high–molecular weight proteins, such as those present in latex or food products. Moreover, prick testing is also used to diagnose "protein contact dermatitis," which is a form of contact dermatitis that affects mainly the hands and forearms in patients occupationally exposed to proteins.[13,14] Drops of allergen solutions are applied to the volar aspect of the forearm or the upper part of the back (approximately 3.5 cm apart to avoid overlapping of reactions at reading), after which they are pierced with a lancet. When proteins are the possible allergens, prick tests with fresh material or commercial reagents are the gold standard.[13]

Controls, both positive (histamine chlorohydrate to measure direct reactivity to histamine and codeine phosphate to verify the aptitude for mast cell degranulation) and negative (saline) need to be tested concomitantly.[10] Positive prick tests generally appear within 15 to 20 minutes and are characterized by a wheal and flare response; reactions greater than 3 mm and at least half of that produced by histamine are regarded as positive. Here again, false-negative reactions may occur. Interpretation of results need caution when reactions to positive controls are weak or negative, when the time interval between the test and reading is inadequate, or when patients are treated, for example, with antihistamines or oral corticosteroids. If there is a suspicion of any kind of serious extracutaneous symptoms, tests should be done with the necessary precautions, and resuscitation facilities should be adequately available.

Open testing (similar to the Skin Application Food Test or SAFT, which has only been mentioned in the diagnosis of food allergy in atopic children) or patch testing can be helpful, but they are generally negative, unless the substance is applied on damaged or eczematous skin (where it even may cause a vesicular reaction). Sometimes a rubbing test (gentle rubbing with the material) on intact or lesional skin might be indicated, if an open test is negative. Scratch and scratch-patch testing carry a higher risk for false-positive reactions, and the latter lacks sensitivity when compared with prick testing.

Test Concentration and Vehicle

Many of the low–molecular weight contact allergens are commercialized and thus have fixed concentrations and vehicles, but in other cases, adequate information can be obtained from the literature, such as De Groot[15] and Lecoz and Lepoittevin,[16] or from individual case reports in the literature. Because the sensitivity threshold of each patient is not the same, there is no optimal

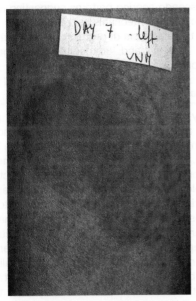

Fig. 2. Positive ROAT (often follicular) with fragrance component (7 day reading).

test concentration. For most allergens, higher concentrations elicit an allergic reaction more frequently than lower concentrations and also more easily cause irritant reactions. For corticosteroids, however, because of their intrinsic antiinflammatory properties, lower concentrations seem to be required.[17]

When new and not-previously-identified allergens are suspected, the conditions under which the product is used are taken into consideration to determine the patch test conditions. For example, when a pharmaceutical or cosmetic product produces a positive reaction, the potentially new allergenic ingredients should be obtained from the manufacturer, and the test concentration could be the same as in the product to start with (**Fig. 3**) provides an example of a positive patch test to isononyl isononanoate,[18] tested in the same concentration as in the causal cosmetic product. If the patch test is negative, the possibility of a false-negative test needs to be considered (for example, preservative agents need higher test concentrations than those present in the products), and upon information from the producer, higher (nonirritant) concentrations can be tested.

Sometimes dilution series are used to detect the sensitivity level of the patient and to determine the relevance with regard to the actual use situation. However, when the concentration of an allergen is too low in the final, solid product, as can be the case, for example, with rubber, shoes, textiles, paper, and plants, or when insufficient amounts are released in tests, extracts may have to be prepared[19,20] and patch tested.

The choice of the vehicle has an enormous influence on the biologic availability of an allergen. Petrolatum, in which most allergens are dispersed in a uniform way, is used most often for practical

reasons. When a contact allergy is assumed, and the tests are negative, another vehicle must be considered. One has, however, to take the solubility of the compound to be tested into account, which is not always done, according to certain reports published in the literature. For example, when a vehicle is used in which a poorly soluble or insoluble substance is "diluted" or dispersed, it will precipitate at the bottom of the container, resulting in testing of the supernatant not containing any substance, or in testing a substance for which the concentration cannot at all be determined. The influence of the vehicle on the outcome of patch tests has become clear, primarily for corticosteroids. Although petrolatum works well for tixocortol pivalate and budesonide, ethanol was the vehicle used to test all other corticosteroid molecules.[21,22] Because of their weak transepidermal penetration, hydrocortisone and cortisone acetate are exceptions to this rule and optimally require for their preparation, an equal mixture of ethanol and dimethyl sulfoxide.

Reading Time

Patch tests are read routinely after 2 and, sometimes, after 3 or 4 days and preferably also at day 6 or 7. Several articles have been published that demonstrate the importance of later readings, not only for corticosteroids, but also for other contact allergens.[23,24] With regard to photopatch tests,[11] readings should be recorded immediately postirradiation and 2 days postirradiation. Further readings on atleast 3 and 4 days postirradiation are desirable to enable detection of crescendo or decrescendo scoring patterns suggesting allergic and nonallergic mechanisms, respectively.

For the diagnosis of protein contact dermatitis, prick testing and immediate readings, as mentioned earlier, need to be performed.

Relevance

Allergy examination has reached a crucial phase when a positive reaction has been found, for, then the relevance of that reaction must be determined. Bruze[25] rightly pointed out that one may not conclude too quickly that a test reaction is not relevant, for such a determination depends primarily on the expertise of the investigator and the possibility of detecting the allergen in the environment of the patient. Sometimes, chemical relationship between molecules helps to understand cross-reactivity patterns. Therefore, an allergen might be found that by itself is not relevant to the patient's dermatitis but that cross-reacts to the actual culprit. This is the case, for example, for paraphenylenediamine that cross reacts with the

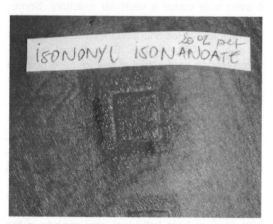

Fig. 3. Positive patch test to isononyl isononanoate tested in the same concentration (20%) as in the causal cosmetic product.

chemically related diaminodiphenylmethane, a marker to detect contact allergy to isocyanate- or polyurethane resins, or for tixocortol pivalate, which is a good marker for corticosteroids of the hydrocortisone type, and for budesonide, which is a marker for corticosteroids of the acetonide type and/or the labile esters, both detecting 90% of reactions to other corticosteoids (data to be published).

Chemical Analysis

In many cases, it is interesting to perform chemical analysis, not only to confirm the presence of a certain allergen in the materials contacted, and therefore to determine the relevance, but also for identification of the allergens. Gruvberger and colleagues[26] have extensively dealt with this subject.

SUMMARY

The diagnosis of a contact allergy represents several important and essential steps, because the failure to recognize a contact allergy can occur in any of the various stages of the contact allergy investigation.

If the results of the skin tests are negative for a patient for whom a diagnosis of allergic contact dermatitis has been proposed, one has to go back to the beginning, that is, with a thoroughgoing anamnesis of the patient (perhaps with a visit to his or her environment). The assumed allergens must be retested (perhaps in another concentration, with another vehicle, or with another testing method), and additional allergens must be tested. The patient can also be asked to keep a journal, in the hope that a correlation can be discerned between exposure to a substance and the occurrence of the skin problems.

Once an allergen has been identified, it is the dermatologist's task to provide specific advice about the products that have to be avoided, or about the products that can safely be used, because subjects sensitive to specific ingredients must avoid products containing them. Computer programs[27–29] are helpful in this regard. Patients reacting to ingredients may get lists of topical pharmaceutical products that contain the allergen(s) that need to be avoided. Moreover, although cosmetic labeling exists, providing the allergic patient with a limited list of cosmetics that can be used is most practical and effective.

REFERENCES

1. Goossens A. Minimizing the risks of missing a contact allergy. Dermatology 2001;202:186–9.
2. Lepoittevin JP, Basketter DA, Goossens A, et al. Allergic contact dermatitis. The molecular basis. Berlin: Springer-Verlag; 1998.
3. Andersen KE, Johansen JD, Bruze M, et al. The time-dose-response relationship for elicitation of contact dermatitis in isoeugenol allergic individuals. Toxicol Appl Pharmacol 2001;170:166–71.
4. Goon A, Goh CL. Non-eczematous contact reactions. In: Rycroft RJG, Menné T, Frosch PJ, editors. Textbook of contact dermatitis. Berlin: Springer-Verlag; 2006. p. 349–62.
5. Rietschel RL, Fowler JF. Noneczematous contact dermatitis. In: Rietschel RL, Fowler JF, editors. Fisher's contact dermatitis. 6th edition. Hamilton (ON): BC Decker; 2008. p. 88–109.
6. Dooms-Goossens A. Patch testing without a kit. In: Guin JD, editor. Practical contact dermatitis. A handbook for the practitioner. New York: McGraw-Hill Inc; 1995. p. 63–74.
7. Frosch PJ, Geier J, Uter W, et al. Patch testing with the patient's own products. In: Frosch PJ, Menné T, Lepoittevin JP, editors. Textbook of contact dermatitis. 4th edition. Berlin: Springer-Verlag; 2006. p. 929–41.
8. Sköld M, Hagvall L, Karlberg AT. Autoxidation of linalyl acetate, the main component of lavender oil, creates potent contact allergens. Contact Dermatitis 58:9–14.
9. Fregert S, Bandmann HJ. Patch testing. Berlin: Springer-Verlag; 1975. p. 24–27.
10. Lachapelle J-M, Maibach HI. Patch testing. Prick testing. A practical guide. Berlin: Springer; 2003.
11. Bruynzeel DP, Ferguson J, Andersen K, , et alThe European Task Force for Photopatch testing. Photopatch testing: a consensus methodology for Europe. J Eur Acad Dermatol Venereol 2004;18:679–82.
12. Bruze M. Use of buffer solutions for patch testing. Contact Dermatitis 1984;10:267–9.
13. Amaro C, Goossens A. Immunological occupational contact urticaria and contact dermatitis from proteins: a review. Contact Dermatitis 2008;58:757–67.
14. Levin C, Warshaw E. Protein contact dermatitis: allergens, pathogenesis, and management. Dermatitis 2008;19:241–51.
15. De Groot A. Patch testing 3rd edition. Test concentrations and vehicles for 4350 chemicals. Wapserveen, the Netherlands: A.C. de Groot; 2008.
16. Lecoz CJ, Lepoittevin J-P. Dictionary of contact allergens: chemical structures, sources and references. In: Frosch PJ, Menné T, Lepoittevin J-P, editors. Textbook of contact dermatitis. 4th edition. Berlin: Springer-Verlag; 2006. p. 943–1105.
17. Isaksson M, Bruze M, Björkner B, et al. The benefit of patch testing with a corticosteroid at a low concentration. Am J Contact Dermatitis 1999;10:31–3.

18. Goossens A, Verbruggen K, Cattaert N, et al. New cosmetic allergens: isononyl isononanoate and trioleyl phosphate. Contact Dermatitis 2008;59:320–1.

19. Bruze M, Trulsson L, Bendsöe N. Patch testing with ultrasonic bath extracts. Am J Contact Dermatitis 1992;3:1–5.

20. Karlberg A-T, Lidén C. Colophony (resin) in newspapers may contribute to hand eczema. Br J Dermatol 1992;126:161–5.

21. Wilkinson SM, Beck MH. Corticosteroid contact hypersensitivity: what vehicle and concentration? Contact Dermatitis 1996;34:305–8.

22. Isaksson M, Beck MH, Wilkinson SM. Comparative testing with budesonide in petrolatum and ethanol in a standard series. Contact Dermatitis 2002;47:123–4.

23. Geier J, Gefeller O, Weichmann K, et al. Patch test reactions at D4, D5, D6. Contact Dermatitis 1999; 40:119–26.

24. Jonker MJ, Bruynzeel DP. The outcome of an additional patch-test reading on days 6 or 7. Contact Dermatitis 2000;42:330–5.

25. Bruze M. What is a relevant contact allergy? Contact Dermatitis 1990;23:224–5.

26. Gruvberger B, Bruze M, Fregert S, et al. Allergens exposure assessment. In: Frosch PJ, Menné T, Lepoittevin J-P, editors. Textbook of contact dermatitis. 4th edition. Berlin: Springer-Verlag; 2006. p. 413–27.

27. Goossens A, Drieghe J. Computer applications in contact allergy. Contact Dermatitis 1998;38:51–2.

28. Yiannias JA. Facilitation of the management of allergic contact dermatitis via on-line tools. Dermatitis 2004;5:101.

29. Yiannias JA. What ACDS members asked for new functionality of the contact allergen replacement database and more. Dermatitis 2007;18:109.

Hand/Face/Neck Localized Pattern: Sticky Problems—Resins

Lauren Y. Cao, BS, MD/MS[a], Apra Sood, MD[b], James S. Taylor, MD[b],*

KEYWORDS

- Plastic • Resin • Epoxy • (Meth)acrylic
- Polyurethane • Phenol-formaldehyde
- Allergic contact dermatitis
- Irritant contact dermatitis

Plastics are a complex group of chemicals with continuously expanding uses in a wide range of industries. They are large polymers made from the combination of simple monomeric subunits. The production of plastics uses oil; 5% of the world's total oil production is applied to the synthesis of plastics.[1] Whereas plastics are synthetic polymeric end products, resins are low-, medium-, and high-molecular-weight (MW) intermediate synthetic compounds from which plastics are made.[1]

Most dermatologic and other health hazards occur during the production and manipulation of plastics rather than during the use of the final product by the consumer.[2] Dermatoses from synthetic plastic resin systems are caused mostly by epoxies, with fewer reactions to other resins (**Box 1**) and their additives.[2] Final plastic products which are completely cured are generally harmless to the skin unless machined (eg, by sawing, sanding, drilling, buffing), whereas dermatoses do arise from plastic components of low MW, such as monomers from uncured or incompletely cured resins, hardeners, reactive diluents, degradation products, and other additives.[1,2]

Contact dermatitis, irritant (ICD) or allergic (ACD), is the most frequent presentation after exposure to components of synthetic plastic resin systems.[2] It usually first appears on the hands and fingers in small patches, and may easily spread to other body areas (eg, face, eyelids, neck) by indirect contact (eg, via the hands).[2] Some resins and additives may be volatile, which means that exposure to their vapors or dusts may cause airborne dermatitis on exposed body areas.[2]

EPOXY RESINS

Epoxy resins are commonly used chemicals of which 75% to 90% are based on diglycidyl ether of the bisphenol A (DGEBA), formed from a combination of epichlorohydrin and bisphenol A.[1,3] When various proportions of epichlorohydrin and bisphenol A are used during manufacturing, different amounts of low- and high-MW epoxy resins are produced. Epoxy resin systems (ERSs) consist not only of uncured epoxy monomers but also additives and modifiers (**Box 2**). Carbon and glass fibers are sometimes impregnated with ERSs to increase the strength of materials in products such as those required in aircraft manufacturing.[1,4,5] However, DGEBA resins have low adherence to carbon fibers, resulting in the development of other epoxy compounds: tetraglycidyl-4,4'-methylenediaaniline (TGMDA), triglycidyl p-aminophenol (TGPAP),

[a] MD/MS Clinical Research Scholars Program, Case Western Reserve University School of Medicine, 2109 Adelbert Road, Cleveland, OH 44106, USA
[b] Department of Dermatology, Dermatology-Plastic Surgery Institute, Cleveland Clinic Foundation, A-61, 9500 Euclid Avenue, Cleveland, OH 44195, USA
* Corresponding author.
E-mail address: taylorj@ccf.org (J.S. Taylor).

Dermatol Clin 27 (2009) 227–249
doi:10.1016/j.det.2009.05.012

derm.theclinics.com

and o-diglycidyl phthalate.[1,4,5] Additionally, instead of bisphenol A, bisphenol F may be used to manufacture the 3 isomers of diglycidyl ether of bisphenol F (DGEBF), which may be mixed with DGEBA resins to increase physical (eg, heat) and chemical resistance.[6]

Epoxy resins have properties such as easy curing, low shrinkage, excellent adhesiveness, high physical strength and resistance, and great electrical resistance, which make them ideal candidates for diverse commercial applications.[7] World production of epoxy resins totals around 1 million tons annually, of which 40% to 50% are used in protective surface coatings and adhesives (eg, paints and lacquers; laminates; electric insulation and encapsulation; floor covering; molding; corrosion protection of metals; castings for metal tools; mending of cracks and fissures in concrete; and glues for metal, plastics, rubber, wood, glass, and ceramics).[1,2,8,9] Epoxy resins are also used in other products, such as electronic circuit boards, filling agents, printing inks, polyvinyl chloride products, and immersion oil for microscopes.[1,2,9,10]

The most frequent adverse cutaneous effects from ERSs are ACD and ICD, most of which arise in the occupational setting during production of epoxy resins or manipulation of finished epoxy products.[1–3,7,9–12] Nevertheless, there have been occasional reports of nonoccupational causes of epoxy resin contact dermatitis, such as from hobby glues and residues of unhardened resin on coated objects (eg, knee patches, bottle caps, film cassettes, metal packages) (**Fig. 1**).[13,14] A Finnish study revealed that ERS compounds (DGEBA, hardeners, reactive diluents) were the third most common cause (12.1%) of currently relevant occupational ACD, and accounted for 0.8% of occupational ICD cases.[15] Another Finnish study reported that ERS compounds were responsible for 7.7% of occupational skin disease: Of the 142 patients with ERS-induced occupational dermatoses, 135 (95%) had ACD, 5 (4%) had ICD, and 2 (1%) had contact urticaria.[16] Analyzing data from the Register of Occupational Skin Diseases in Northern Bavaria, Dickel and colleagues[8] found that epoxy resin was the second most common (67%) occupationally relevant sensitizer. A fourth study of a group of Norwegian industrial painters revealed an incidence rate of 4.5 per 1000 person years for ACD caused by ERS compounds.[17] The prevalence of ACD or sensitization to ERS chemicals has been reported for various occupations: ACD to ERS chemicals was found to be 45% in marble workers[18] and 18% in construction workers.[19] Sensitization to ERS chemicals upon patch testing

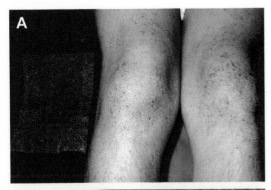

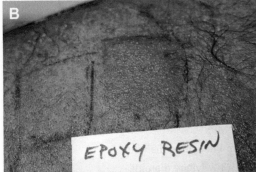

Fig. 1. Allergic contact dermatitis of the knees from epoxy resin which was demonstrated to be present in the knee patch of this boy's jeans (*A*). Patch testing with epoxy resin yielded a positive reaction (*B*).

was demonstrated to be 56% in aircraft manufacturing workers,[5] 27% in ski factory workers,[20] 21% in paint manufacturing workers,[21] and 20% in construction workers.[19] However, some of these studies did not include patch tests with ERS hardeners or reactive diluents, which means that the actual prevalence of sensitization to ERS chemicals may be even higher. Other occupations with common exposures and sensitizations to ERS compounds are outlined in **Box 3**.

ACD sensitization is generally caused by low-MW or short-chain chemicals.[7,23] Fregert and Thorgeirsson demonstrated that whereas all 34 of their epoxy resin-sensitized patients reacted to the MW 340 oligomer of DGEBA epoxy resin upon patch testing, none reacted when tested with the higher MW oligomers.[23] The sensitizing potential of epoxy resin decreases as the average MW increases.[23] However, other investigators have indicated that DGEBA epoxy resins with higher average MW are potential sensitizers, especially with simultaneous exposure to skin irritants such as organic solvents and amine hardeners.[16] Exposure to paints and their raw materials, surface coatings, and adhesives has been reported to be the most common cause of occupational

dermatoses induced by ERSs.[16] The most frequent causes of ERS-induced ACD are epoxy resins,[21,23,24] which together induced 93% of all ERS dermatoses in one study.[16] Approximately 60% to 80% of patients with ACD to epoxy resins

Box 3
Occupations with frequent exposures to epoxy resin system compounds
Adhesive and glue manufacturing
Aircraft manufacturing
Appliance finishing
Assembling
Automobile manufacturing
Boat manufacturing
Can coating
Cement work
Ceramics
Construction and building
Electric insulation
Electronics
Floor covering
Furniture building
Lacquering
Laminating
Laboratory work with microscope immersion oil
Machining
Marble work
Metal casting
Other plastic material (eg, polyvinyl chloride) manufacturing
Paint, lacquer, and varnish manufacturing
Painting
Printing ink manufacturing
Sculpting
Sporting equipment manufacturing (eg, tennis rackets, skis)
Soldering
Terrazzo work
Tile setting
Tunnel work
Varnishing
Wood processing
Data from Refs.[1,2,8–10,22]

are sensitized to DGEBA,[1] the most common cause of contact allergy to ERS compounds,[16] but other epoxy resins are also capable of sensitization (**Box 4**). Significant cross-reactivity has been noted between DGEBA and DGEBF owing to structural similarity.[25] According to Jolanki, hardeners are the second most common cause of contact allergy induced by ERS compounds (**Box 5**).[16] Jolanki identified reactive diluents as the fourth most common cause of ERS-induced ACD after DGEBA epoxy resins, hardeners, and non-DGEBA epoxy resins.[16] Reactive diluents noted to induce contact allergy are presented in **Box 6**. Cross-sensitization between reactive diluents has been reported to be common.[16] Other additives in ERSs, such as epoxy accelerators containing hexavalent chromate, are capable of causing ACD as well.[26,27]

ICD is a less common form of ERS-induced occupational contact dermatitis, and has been reported with high-MW DGEBA epoxy resins (average MW above 700), hardeners (eg, polyamines, methyl hexahydrophthalic anhydride [MHHPA]), and carbon or glass fiber fragments which are mixed with epoxy resins.[15,16,31] Rarely, contact urticaria has been noted with use of DGEBA resins and aliphatic polyamine and anhydride (eg, methylhexahydrophthalic anhydride, methyltetrahydrophthalic anhydride) hardeners,[24,32] and photoallergic contact dermatitis has been reported with heating of DGEBA resins, possibly owing to the bisphenol A component.[33] IgE-mediated occupational asthma induced by epoxy resins has additionally been reported.[34]

Because sensitization is usually observed in workers who handle uncured epoxy resins, the hands, forearms, face, and neck are predominantly affected by dermatitis, with the face and neck involved through indirect contact with hands or airborne exposure.[8,15,35] ICD presents with a similar pattern of distribution.[15,16,31] Airborne exposure resulting in ACD or ICD of the face,

eyelids, and neck is more likely to occur with hardeners and reactive diluents, which are more volatile than epoxy resins themselves.[36] Nevertheless, even in cured ERSs, up to 25% of epoxy resin monomers may be unhardened and capable of eliciting ACD in previously sensitized individuals, especially when cured at room temperature.[1] Moreover, when there are unexplained patch test reactions to epoxy resins, it is important to inquire about the occupations of family and friends, because the patient may have a connubial or consort dermatitis (ie, "epoxy-by-proxy").[37]

When ERS-induced ACD is suspected by the patient's history and cutaneous findings, patch testing with low-MW epoxy resin containing high amounts of DGEBA oligomer MW 340 (1% in petrolatum), as included in most standard series, is adequate in most cases to detect sensitization. When other components of ERSs, such as other epoxy resins, hardeners, and reactive diluents, are potential culprits, patch testing to these ERS chemicals with appropriate concentrations has been recommended (**Table 1**). In some cases, it

---

Box 5
Epoxy resin system hardeners reported to cause contact allergy

Aliphatic polyamines

    Diethylenetriamine (DETA)

    3-Dimethylaminopropylamine

    Ethylenediamine (EDA)

    Hexamethylenetetramine

    Triethylenetetramine (TETA)

    Trimethylhexamethylenediamine (TMDA)

Cycloapliphatic polyamines

    3,3'-Dimethyl-4,4-diaminodicyclohexylmethane

    Isophoronediamine (IPDA)

Aromatic amines

    4,4'-Diaminodiphenylmethane (MDA)

    2,4,6-tris-Dimethylaminomethyl phenol (tris-DMP)

    m-Phenylene diamine

    1,3-Xylylene diamine

Anhydrides

Dicyanodiamide

Triglycidyl isocyanurate

Data from Refs.[16,22,29]

Box 4
Types of epoxy resins

Diglycidyl ether of the bisphenol A (DGEBA)

Diglycidyl ether of the bisphenol F (DGEBF)

Brominated

Cycloaliphatic

Heterocyclic dimethyl hydantoin

Phenol novolak

Data from Refs.[6,16,22,28]

Box 6
Epoxy resin system reactive diluents reported to cause contact allergy

Allyl glycidyl ether (AGE)

1,4-Butane-diol diglycidyl ether (BDDGE)

n-Butyl glycidyl ether (BGE)

Cresyl glycidyl ether (CGE)

ortho-Cresyl glycidyl ether (ortho-CGE)

Cyclohexanedimethanol glycidyl ether

Diethyleneglycol diglycidyl ether

p-Fluorphenyl glycidyl ether

Glycidyl ester of synthetic fatty acids

Glycidyl ether of aliphatic alcohols

1,6-Hexanediol diglycidyl ether (HDDGE)

α-Naphthyl glycidyl ether

Neopentyl glycol diglycidyl ether (NPGDGE)

Phenyl glycidyl ether (PGE)

m-Xylene diamine

Data from Refs.[16,18,20,22,30]

may be necessary to patch test with an appropriate dilution of the patient's own resin, products obtained from the patient's work environment, or samples acquired directly from the manufacturer. Workers found to be sensitized to ERS components should be instructed to employ a no-touch technique and to try to avoid as much exposure as possible; and in some cases, they may need to change jobs. Immediate transfer of workers sensitized to epoxy resins may prevent aggravation of their contact dermatitis and broadening of sensitizations to other ERS components such as hardeners and reactive diluents.[19] To reduce the sensitization potential of DGEBA epoxy resins, the use of low-MW 340 and MW 624 oligomers should be kept at a minimum and their concentrations should be specified on product labels.[22,23] Hardeners should not contain remains of aliphatic polyamines, and reactive diluents should be high (>1000) MW.[22]

(METH)ACRYLIC RESINS

(Meth)acrylic resins are formed by various combinations of the monomers acrylic acid and its esters, methacrylic acid and its esters, cyanoacrylic acid and its esters, acrylamides and acrylonitrile, during which initiators, accelerators, catalysts, electron beams, ultraviolet (UV) light, or visible light are used to speed up the process.[1]

(Meth)acrylic resins have a diverse array of uses (**Box 7**). Various groups of (meth)acrylics include mono(meth)acrylics, which have 1 functional acrylic group; multifunctional (meth)acrylics, which have 2 or more reactive acrylic groups; epoxy (meth)acrylics (eg, 2,2-bis[4-(2-hydroxy-3-methacryloxypropoxy)phenyl]propane [BIS-GMA]), which are derived from reacting epoxy resins or glycidyl derivatives with acrylic acid; urethane (meth)acrylics, which combine aromatic or aliphatic isocyanates with acrylic acid; and polyester (meth)acrylics.[1] **Table 2** lists the (meth)acrylics which are commonly used in artificial nails, dental materials, UV cured inks, coatings, paints and lacquers, and anaerobic adhesives, along with their recommended patch test concentrations.

There have been numerous animal reports on the sensitization potentials of various (meth)acrylics. Guinea pig studies have revealed that the addition of a methyl group to the alpha-carbon atom of acrylic groups appears to decrease their sensitization potential. Monoacrylics are strong sensitizers, whereas monomethacrylics are weak to moderate sensitizers.[1,39,47,48] Likewise, whereas di- and tri-acrylics are potent sensitizers, the multifunctional methacrylics are weak or nonsensitizers.[49] Of the epoxy (meth)acrylics, 2,2-bis-(4-(2-hydroxy-3-acryloxy-propoxy)phenyl) propane (epoxy diacrylate), 2,2-bis-(4-(2-methacryloxyethoxy)phenyl)propane (BIS-EMA) and 2,2-bis-(4-(methacryloxy)phenyl)propane (BIS-MA) have been demonstrated to be strong sensitizers, whereas the linear fraction of BIS-GMA and its isomers and 2,2-bis-(4-(3-methacryloxypropoxy)phenyl)propane (BIS-PMA) have little or no sensitizing capacity.[50] Sensitization appears to be caused by the entire epoxy (meth)acrylic molecule, although free epoxy resin oligomer MW 340 may also sensitize.[51] Aliphatic urethane (meth)acrylics appear to be more potent sensitizers than aromatic ones, and aliphatic urethane methacrylics seem to have lower contact allergenicity than corresponding aliphatic urethane acrylics.[52] However, the author cautioned that whether these generalizations apply to all aliphatic and aromatic urethane (meth)acrylics merits further investigation.[52] The whole polyester (meth)acrylic structure appears to be a contact allergen, although polyester and (meth)acrylate have also been shown to be moderate sensitizers.[53]

Although (meth)acrylic-induced asthma and rhinoconjunctivitis have been reported,[54] the principal health problems from (meth)acrylic resins are cutaneous diseases (eg, contact dermatitis), and these occur both occupationally[55] and in consumers using end products.[39,43]

Table 1
Recommended patch test concentrations for epoxy resin system chemicals

Epoxy Resin System Chemicals	Patch Test Concentration (% in Petrolatum)
Epoxy resins	
Diglycidyl ether of the bisphenol A (DGEBA)	1
Diglycidyl ether of the bisphenol F (DGEBF)	1
Amine hardeners	
4,4'-Diaminodiphenylmethane (MDA)	0.5
Diethylenetriamine (DETA)	1
Ethylenediamine (EDA)	1
Hexamethylenetetramine	1–2
Isophoronediamine (IPDA)	0.5
Triethylenetetramine (TETA)	0.5
Reactive diluents	
Allyl glycidyl ether (AGE)	0.25
1,4-Butane-diol diglycidyl ether (BDDGE)	0.25
n-Butyl glycidyl ether (BGE)	0.25
Ortho-Cresyl glycidyl ether (ortho-CGE)	0.25
Glycidyl ester of synthetic fatty acids	0.25
Glycidyl ether of aliphatic alcohols	0.25
1,6-Hexanediol diglycidyl ether (HDDGE)	0.25
Neopentyl glycol diglycidyl ether (NPGDGE)	0.25
Phenyl glycidyl ether (PGE)	0.25
Other chemicals	
Bisphenol A	1
Epichlorohydrin	0.1–0.3
2,2-Bis[4-(2-hydroxy-3-methacryloxypropoxy)phenyl]propane (BIS-GMA)	2
2,2-Bis[4-(methacryloxy)phenyl]-propane (BIS-MA)	2

Data from Rietschel RL, Fowler JF. Plastics, adhesives and synthetic resins. In: Rietschel RL, Fowler JF, editors. Fisher's contact dermatitis, 6th edition. Hamilton (ON): BC Decker Inc; 2008. p. 542–65. and de Groot AC, Frosch PJ. Patch test concentrations and vehicles for testing contact allergens. In: Frosch PJ, Menné T, Lepoittevin JP, editors. Contact dermatitis, 4th edition. Berlin: Springer Verlag; 2006. p. 907–28.

Mono(meth)acrylics and multifunctional (meth)acrylics have frequently been noted to cause sensitizations and ACD. Because of cross-reactivity, sensitized persons will often have contact allergic reactions to many other (meth)acrylic compounds.[56–58] Other less frequent presentations include paronychia, nail dystrophy, onycholysis (**Fig. 2**), and paresthesias.[59–62] Contact allergy from artificial nails has been reported with methyl methacrylate, which was banned from use in the United States in 1974.[39] Since then, other monomethacrylics have been used in nails, such as ethyl methacrylate, butyl methacrylate, and methacrylic acid, which may be even stronger sensitizers.[39,62] 2-Hydroxyethyl methacrylate (2-HEMA) and 2-hydroxypropyl methacrylate (2-HPMA) are other common mono(meth)acrylic contact allergens in artificial nails.[60,63] Dimethacrylics, such as ethylene glycol dimethacrylate (EGDMA) and triethylene glycol dimethacrylate (TREGDMA), are among the most common multifunctional (meth)acrylic allergens found in artificial nails.[39,60,63] ACD from artificial nails usually involves the hands and fingers, with dermatitis being the most common presentation.[60] It was shown in one study that involvement of dorsal hands, fingers, forearms, face, and neck through direct contact in beauticians owing to occupational exposures was more frequent than in consumers.[60] Workers and consumers should be educated to use no-touch techniques before the mono(meth)acrylics in the artificial nails are polymerized.[39]

Because most composite materials used in dentistry today contain resins based on

Beauty products

Artificial nails, nail polishes, hair sprays, fragrances, dentifrices, insecticides

Construction materials

Adhesives, paints, sealers and stoppers, concrete additives

Medical uses

Dentures and other dental materials, artificial eye lens implants, orthopedic prostheses, heart valves, artificial joints, contact lenses, eyeglasses, hearing aids, adhesive plasters, wound sprays, infusion systems, splints

Printing uses

Ultraviolet cured inks, photopolymer and flexographic printing plates

Textiles

Synthetic fibers, finishes (eg, on leather)

Utensils

Synthetic rubbers, acrylic glass (Plexiglas), veneers

Other uses

Ultraviolet cured coatings, paints, glues, plastic foams, molecular sieves, gel electrophoresis, low temperature embedding media for electron microscopy, lubricant additives, aircraft windows, highway reflectors, glass, mineral sedimentation, water purification, soil improvers, synthesis of other plastics

Data from Refs.[1,2,22,46]

primarily presents as ACD on the first 3 fingers and may induce onycholysis.[66]

Among those working with photoprepolymer printing plates and UV cured inks, coatings, paints, and lacquers, 2-HEMA and 2-HPMA are common causes of contact allergy.[41,42] Contact allergy to multifunctional di- and tri-acrylics (eg, pentaerythritol triacrylate [PETA], trimethylol propane triacrylate [TMPTA], 1,6-hexanediol diacrylate [HDDA]) has been reported to be especially prevalent in those exposed to UV cured inks and coatings.[43]

Epoxy (meth)acrylics are rather unusual sensitizers in humans.[56,67] Likewise, few reports on contact allergy from urethane (meth)acrylics have been published.[68,69]

When patch testing with (meth)acrylic compounds, use of petrolatum as the test vehicle in a plastic test chamber is recommended, because false negatives have occurred from acetone and alcohol vehicles and aluminum chambers owing to induction of rapid polymerization of (meth)acrylic monomers.[70] In general, methacrylic monomers should be patch tested at 2% in petrolatum, and acrylic monomers should be tested at 0.1% in petrolatum to avoid patch test sensitizations.[1,38]

ICD has been reported with various (meth)acrylic use.[43,47,64,71,72] A study among dental technicians reported that whereas fingertips were primarily involved in ACD, ICD occurred mostly on dorsa of the fingers (especially of the dominant hand).[64] Studies in guinea pigs have revealed diacrylics to be strong irritants, monoacrylics to be weak to moderate irritants, and mono- or di-methacrylics to have little or no sensitizing potential.[1,47]

POLYURETHANE RESINS

Polyurethanes are generally formed from reacting isocyanates with polyhydroxy compounds (eg, polyesters, polyethers, water, amines), in the presence of appropriate catalysts and additives (Box 8).[1,2] Isocyanates are low-MW aromatic, aliphatic, or cycloaliphatic compounds with a highly reactive –N=C=O functional group.[1,73] Aromatic diisocyanates, especially diphenylmethane diisocyante (MDI) and toluene diisocyanate (TDI), are most commonly used. Industrial applications include acting as rubber substitutes in the manufacturing of foam used for mattresses, cushions, dashboards, packages, insulation, and Spandex; use in coatings, paints, lacquers, adhesives, binders, castings, elastomers, and fibers; and use in industries such as construction, furniture production, automobile manufacturing, electronics, shoe manufacturing, and health

methacrylics,[50,52] contact allergy to mono- and multifunctional methacrylics (eg, 2-HEMA, methyl methacrylate, EGDMA, TREGDMA) is often seen in dental personnel and patients.[40,63] One study reported that screening for (meth)acrylic contact allergy with 2-HEMA alone picked up 96.7% of (meth)acrylic-allergic dental patients and 100% of (meth)acrylic-allergic dental personnel, and the addition of bis-GMA increased the detection rate of (meth)acrylic-allergic dental patients to 100%.[40] Fingertip dermatitis is common among dental personnel.[64]

Additionally, mono- and multifunctional methacrylics (eg, 2-HEMA, 2-HMPA, EGDMA, TREGDMA, tetrahydrofurfuryl methacrylate) frequently cause contact allergy in those working with anaerobic acrylic adhesives and sealants (Fig. 3),[44,63,65] which

Table 2
Commonly used (meth)acrylic monomers in selected commercial products and their recommended patch test concentrations

Commercial Use	Commonly Used (Meth)Acrylic Monomers	Patch Test Concentration (% in Petrolatum)
Artificial nails	Butyl methacrylate	2
	Diethylene glycol dimethacrylate (DEGDMA)	2
	Ethyl acrylate	0.1
	Ethylcyanoacrylate (ECA)	5
	Ethylene glycol dimethacrylate (EGDMA)	2
	Ethyl methacrylate	2
	2-Hydroxyethyl acrylate (2-HEA)	0.1
	2-Hydroxyethyl methacrylate (2-HEMA)	2
	Isobutyl methacrylate	2
	Methyl acrylate	0.1
	Methacrylic acid	1
	Methyl methacrylate	2
	Tetrahydrofurfuryl methacrylate (THFMA)	2
	Triethylene glycol diacrylate (TREGDA)	0.1
	Triethylene glycol dimethacrylate (TREGDMA)	2
	Trimethylol propane trimethacrylate (TMPTMA)	2
	Tripropylene glycol acrylate	0.1
	Tripropylene glycol diacrylate (TPGDA)	0.1
	Urethane methacrylate	2

Dental materials		
	Benzaldehyde glycol methacrylate	2
	Biphenyl dimethacrylate	2
	2,2-Bis[4-(2-hydroxy-3-methacryloxypropoxy)phenyl]propane (BIS-GMA)	2
	2,2-Bis[4-(2-methacryloxyethoxy)-phenyl]-propane (BIS-EMA)	1
	2,2-Bis[4-(methacryloxy)phenyl]-propane (BIS-MA)	2
	2,2-Bis[4-(3-methacryloxypropoxy)phenyl]-propane (BIS-PMA)	N/A
	1,4-Butanediol dimethacrylate (BUDMA)	2
	1,3-Butyleneglycol diacrylate	0.1
	Butyl methacrylate	2
	1,10-Decanediol dimethacrylate	2
	Diethylene glycol dimethacrylate DEGDMA)	2
	2-(Dimethylamino)ethyl methacrylate	2
	3,6-Dioxaoctamethylene dimethacrylate	2
	1,12-Dodecanediol dimethacrylate	2
	Epoxy methacrylates	2
	Ethylene glycol dimethacrylate (EGDMA)	2
	Ethyl methacrylate	2
	Glycerol phosphate dimethacrylate	2
	1,6-Hexanediol diacrylate (HDDA)	0.1
	2-Hydroxyethyl methacrylate (2-HEMA)	2
	Methyl methacrylate	2
	Phenylsalicylate glycidyl methacrylate	2
	Tetrahydrofurfuryl methacrylate (THFMA)	2
	n-Tolylglycine-glycidylmethacrylate	2
	Triethylene glycol dimethacrylate (TREGDMA)	2
	Trimethylol propane trimethacrylate (TMPTMA)	2
	Urethane dimethacrylate	2

(continued on next page)

Table 2
(continued)

Commercial Use	Commonly Used (Meth)Acrylic Monomers	Patch Test Concentration (% in Petrolatum)
Ultraviolet cured inks, coatings, paints, and lacquers	Butyl acrylate	0.1
	Diethylene glycol diacrylate (DEGDA)	0.1
	Dipropolene glycol diacrylae (DPGDA)	0.1
	Epoxy acrylates	0.5
	2-Ethyl-hexyl acrylate (2-EHA)	0.1
	1,6-Hexanediol diacrylate (HDDA)	0.1
	2-Hydroxyethyl acrylate (2-HEA)	0.1
	2-Hydroxyethyl methacrylate (2-HEMA)	2
	2-Hydroxypropyl acrylate (2-HPA)	0.1
	2-Hydroxypropyl methacrylate (2-HPMA)	2
	Pentaerythritol triacrylate (PETA)	0.1
	Polyester acrylates	0.1
	Trimethylol propane triacrylate (TMPTA)	0.1
	Tripropylene glycol diacrylate (TPGDA)	0.1
	Tripropylene glycol triacrylate (TPGTA)	0.1
	Urethane acrylates	0.1
Anaerobic adhesives	Diethylene glycol diacrylate (DEGDA)	0.1
	Epoxy diacrylate	0.5
	Ethylcyanoacrylate (ECA)	5
	Ethylene glycol dimethacrylate (EGDMA)	2
	2-Hydroxyethyl methacrylate (2-HEMA)	2
	2-Hydroxypropyl methacrylate (2-HPMA)	2
	Methyl methacrylate	2
	Polyethylene glycol dimethacrylate (PEGDMA)	2
	Tetraethylene glycol dimethacrylate (TETEGDMA)	2
	Tetrahydrofurfuryl methacrylate (THFMA)	2
	Triethylene glycol diacrylate (TREGDA)	0.1
	Triethylene glycol dimethacrylate (TREGDMA)	2

N/A, not available.
Data from Refs.[1,38–45]

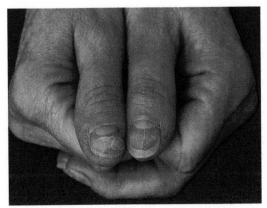

Fig. 2. Patient with onycholysis caused by acrylic nails.

care.[1,2,74] However, because aromatic diisocyanates undergo oxidative discoloration when exposed to light and moisture, aliphatic diisocyanates (eg, 1,6-hexamethylene diisocyanate [HDI], isophorone diisocyanate [IPDI]) are used instead in these applications, and are often found in paints, lacquers, and coatings.[1] In industry, these diisocyanates are often made into higher MW polyisocyanates to reduce their volatility.[1,75] Other examples of diisocyanates used industrially are shown in **Box 9**.

Although isocyanates in polyurethane resins primarily cause respiratory and other mucosal

diseases, such as asthma, rhinitis, conjunctivitis, bronchial hyperreactivity, hypersensitive pneumonitis, extrinsic allergic alveolitis, and chronic obstructive lung diseases,[76,77] they may also induce ICD, ACD, and contact urticaria, which typically present on the hands and face.[1,73] Isocyanates appear to induce more ICD than ACD, and have been reported as mild to strong irritants.[1,78–81] Amine accelerators used in polyurethanes, such as diaminodiphenyl methane

---

Box 8
Polyurethane resin system additives

Antioxidants

Biocides

Blowing agents (eg, pentane, carbon dioxide, water)

Coloring agents

Cross-linking agents

Fillers

Fire retardants

Hardening catalysts (eg, tertiary amines, tin)

Initiators

Metallic compounds

Plasticizers

Ultraviolet light absorbers

Data from Bjorkner B, Ponten A, Zimerson E, Frick M. Plastic materials. In: Frosch PJ, Menné T, Lepoittevin JP, editors. Contact dermatitis, 4th edition. Berlin: Springer Verlag; 2006. p. 583–621.

Box 9
Commonly used diisocyanates in industry

Diphenylmethane diisocyanate (MDI)

Toluene diisocyanate (TDI)

1,6-Hexamethylene diisocyanate (HDI)

Isophorone diisocyanate (IPDI)

Dicyclohexylmethane diisocyanate (DMDI)

Naphthalene diisocyanate (NDI)

Trimethyl hexamethylene diisocyanate (TMDI)

Triphenylmethane triisocyanate (TPMTI)

Data from Bjorkner B, Ponten A, Zimerson E, Frick M. Plastic materials. In: Frosch PJ, Menné T, Lepoittevin JP, editors. Contact dermatitis, 4th edition. Berlin: Springer Verlag; 2006. p. 583–621; and Estlander T, Keskinen H, Jolanki R, et al. Occupational dermatitis from exposure to polyurethane chemicals. Contact Dermatitis 1992;27(3):161–5.

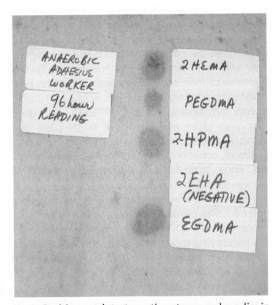

Fig. 3. Positive patch test reactions to several acrylics in an anaerobic adhesive worker. *Abbreviations:* 2-HEMA, 2-hydroxyethyl methacrylate; PEGDMA, polyethyleneglycol dimethacrylate; 2-HPMA, 2-hydroxypropyl methacrylate; 2-EHA, 2-ethylhexyl acrylate (negative); EGDMA, ethyleneglycol dimethacrylate.

(MDA), triethylenediamine and triethylamine, are also skin irritants.[1] Diisocyanates, including MDI, TDI, HDI, and dicyclohexylmethane diisocyanate (DMDI) have been shown to be strong contact sensitizers in mice, with cross-reactions occurring between aromatic and aliphatic diisocyanates.[82–84] There have also been reports of contact sensitizations and ACD from isocyanates in humans, mostly occupational cases[73,74,81,85–90] but some in consumers,[91–94] although these reports have been few and sporadic considering isocyanates' ubiquitous uses; this is likely because of extensive worker protections from the harmful effects of polyurethanes on the respiratory and other mucosal systems.[1] Contact sensitizations and ACD have been noted with MDI, TDI, HDI, IPDI, DMDI, and trimethyl hexamethylene diisocyanate (TMDI).[73,74,81,85–92] Many studies have reported simultaneous positive reactions to MDI and MDA (an aromatic diamine used as a hardener in epoxy and polyurethane resins, as an antioxidant in rubber production, and in insecticides and germicides).[73,74,85,86,88–90,95] Fregert first noted the simultaneous reactions to MDI and MDA, and attributed this to cross-reaction.[90,95] Another explanation was proposed by Rothe[96] in 1976: MDA may be the allergen and is formed from hydrolysis of MDI when MDI contacts the skin.[90] Indeed, later reports confirm that positive patch test reactions can occur only to MDA, and not to the isocyanates with which patients had come in contact.[90,97] MDA may also co-react with numerous other substances such as para-phenylenediamine, cobalt, fragrance mix, paraben mix, and benzocaine.[98] Furthermore, rare instances of isocyanates inducing contact urticaria have been reported.[99,100]

Although fully cured polyurethane products generally do not cause dermatitis, there are other circumstances where skin problems arise. Firstly, isocyanate products which are not fully cured represent a source of skin exposure.[101] Bello and colleagues[101] demonstrated that curing is a slower process than expected—unbound isocyanate species were detected on painted surfaces for a few days to a month. Hence, recently cured isocyanate products are another potential cause of dermatitis. Moreover, release of free isocyanates may occur during heating of cured isocyanate products, such as during machining, cutting, grinding, or sanding such products.[102,103]

When contact allergy to polyurethane resins is suspected, patients should be tested with relatively fresh preparations of common diisocyanates—4,4'-MDI and 2,4-TDI at 1.5% to 2% in petrolatum, HDI, IPDI, and 4,4'-DMDI. They should also be patch tested to MDA 0.25% in petrolatum (although some true positives may be missed, active sensitization with MDA 0.5% in petrolatum has been reported).[73,104,105] A late reading at day 7 may be needed to detect positive reactions to isocyanates (eg, MDI), and patients should be instructed to report reactions that appear after day 7.[90,104] Amines of isocyanates (eg, MDA) appear to serve as good markers for detecting isocyanate sensitization.[86] Although Estlander and colleagues[73] had suggested that MDI and TDI test preparations may be used for over a year because preparations which were 5.5 and 15.5 months old had elicited positive patch test reactions, Frick and colleagues[106] performed chemical analyses which showed that commercially available patch test preparations of MDI contained concentrations lower than those stated on labels, even before expiry dates, risking false negative reactions during patch testing. Hence, patch testing with the patient's own fresh occupational or consumer products, diluted as necessary, is sometimes needed for detecting polyurethane resin contact allergies which may be missed by standard patch testing.[90,106]

PHENOL-FORMALDEHYDE RESINS

Phenol-formaldehyde resins (PFRs) are formed by the combination of phenols (eg, phenol, bisphenol A, p-tert-butylphenol) and aldehydes (especially formaldehyde, but also acetaldehyde, glyoxal).[1] These resins were the first plastics to be made on a large scale in the United States and were often used as casting compounds.[2,8] However, their use has declined over the years: Today, because of their adhesive power, durability, heat resistance, and elasticity, PFRs and p-tert-butylphenol-formaldehyde resin (PTBFR) are used mainly as glues and adhesives in the paint and varnish, decorative laminate, rubber, building, plywood, construction, automobile, aircraft, boating, shoe, artificial nail, leather, and electronic (for insulation) industries.[8,107,108]

The adverse effects of handling PFRs are mostly cutaneous (ie, contact dermatitis), of which a higher proportion is ACD than ICD, which may occur on the hands and face (from occupational exposure) or feet (from shoes).[109,110] These generally occur in the occupational setting,[8,111] although non-occupationally-induced dermatitis may develop as a result of hobby work or exposure to unpolymerized monomers or dimers left in the finished products (eg, shoes, clothing, watch band, adhesive label, athletic tape) (**Figs. 4** and **5**).[107,110–113]

Most reports of contact dermatitis are because of PTBFR sensitization. In an analysis of patch

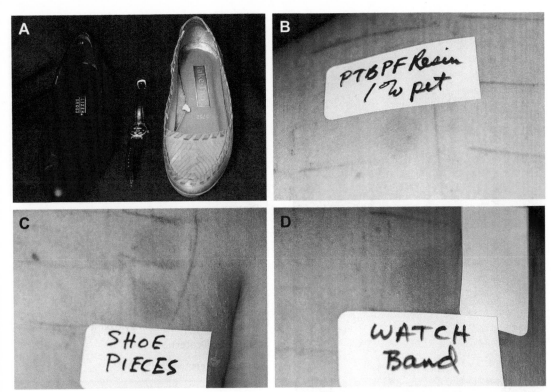

Fig. 4. Shoe and watch band allergy in a patient with foot and wrist dermatitis (*A*). Patient had positive patch test reactions to the adhesive *p-tert*-butylphenol-formaldehyde resin (PTBFR) (*B*) and to thin pieces of 2 shoes (*C*) and a watch band (*D*) which likely contained PTBFR.

test results with the plastics and glues series, Tarvainen found that PTBFR was the most common contact allergen.[111] Similar reports of sensitizations and ACD induced by PTBFR have been made.[107,108,110,114–118] As noted by Foussereau and colleagues,[117] occupational contact allergies to PTBFR represent 71% of cases, and footwear and clothing allergies to PTBFR account for the other 29%. Positive reactions may be caused by the resin itself (especially when unhardened or incompletely hardened), or less frequently by *p-tert*-butylphenol and formaldehyde.[2,108,117–119] A number of substances in PTBFR have been found to be contact allergens from human and guinea pig studies (**Box 10**). Guinea pigs sensitized to 2,6-dimethylol *p-tert*-butylphenol (2,6-MMPTBP) showed cross-reactions to 2-methylol *p-tert*-butylphenol (2-MPTBP) and *p-tert*-butylcatechol.[120] The strong sensitizer *p-tert*-butylcatechol has been noted to be present in PTBFR, but also is used as a stabilizer in the production of other plastic monomers.[1,121] Human and guinea pig studies have demonstrated cross-reactions between *p-tert*-butylcatechol when tested with *p-tert*-butylphenol.[121,122]

Although there are fewer reports on ACD induced by other PFRs,[126,127,128] allergens in these resins have been noted as well (**Box 11**). Monomers have weaker allergenic potentials than dimers.[108] Of the dimers, the 4,41-dihydroxydiphenyl methanes have been shown in guinea pigs to be the most potent contact allergens.[108] Potential cross-reacting substances to the simple methylol phenol monomers include *o*-cresol, *p*-cresol, salicylaldehyde, 2,4-dimethyl phenol and 2,6-dimethyl phenol.[129] Bruze and Zimerson also demonstrated that *o*-cresol is a sensitizer which is present in PFRs.[130]

Patch testing with PTBFR at 10% in petrolatum, which is included in most standard series, should be supplemented with other PFRs to which the patient has likely been exposed given the history, or with the patient's own products, because there is no single screening agent for detecting contact allergies to the numerous available PFRs.[22,116] Contact allergy to *p-tert*-butylcatechol should be suspected in patients who react to PTBFR on patch testing but have no clinically relevant exposure.[1,121]

PFRs have been reported to cause ICD, depigmentation, and chemical burns as well.[116,131,132]

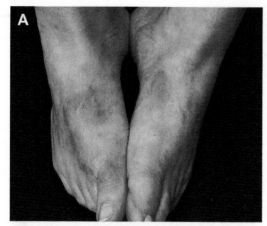

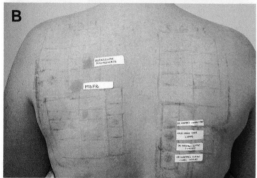

Fig. 5. Shoe dermatitis (*A*) in a patient with positive patch test reactions to PTBFR, potassium dichromate, and shoe pieces (*B*).

Phenols and aldehydes (eg, formaldehyde) are skin irritants, and concentrated phenol may cause chemical burns.[1] PTBFR in the adhesive material of bindis has been noted to cause contact depigmentation.[133,134]

OTHER SELECTED RESINS

Polyester resins are divided into saturated and unsaturated polyesters. Saturated polyesters are made from combining dicarboxylic acids (eg, phthalic acid, maleic acid) primarily in their anhydride forms with polyalcohols (eg, glycerol), and they are often used in the manufacturing of other plastics or water-based paints and coatings.[1,2] Unsaturated polyesters are produced through esterifications of organic acids or their anhydrides (eg, maleic anhydride, phthalic anhydride, fumaric acid) and diols (eg, diethylene glycol), and they are frequently used in coatings, finishes, varnishes, lacquers, cements, fiberglass mouldings, and glues for industries such as automobile manufacturing, boating, and construction.[1,2,135]

Box 10
Contact allergens in *p-tert*-butylphenol-formaldehyde resins

Monomers

  5-*tert*-butyl-2-hydroxy-3-hydroxymethyl-benzaldehyde

  4-*tert*-butyl-2-hydroxymethyl-6-methoxy-methyl-phenol

  2,6-dimethylol   *p-tert*-butylphenol   (2,6-MMPTBP)

  2-methylol *p-tert*-butylphenol (2-MPTBP)

Dimers

  5,5′-di-*tert*-butyl-2,2′-dihydroxy-3,3′-hydroxymethl-dibenzyl ether

  5,5′-di-*tert*-butyl-2,2′-dihydroxy-3-dihydroxymethyl-dibenzyl ether

Linear trimer

  4-tert-butyl-2,6-bis-(5-tert-butyl-2-hydroxy-3-hydroxymethyl-benzyloxymethyl)-phenol

p-tert-butylcatechol

Data from Refs.[1,115,118,120,122–125].

Box 11
Contact allergens in other phenol-formaldehyde resins

Monomers

  2-methylol phenol

  4-methylol phenol

  3-methylol phenol

  2,3-dimethylol phenol

  2,6-dimethylol phenol

  2,4,6-trimethylol phenol

Dimers

  4,4-dihydroxy-3-(hydroxymethyl)-diphenyl methane

  4,4-dihydroxy-3,5-di-(hydroxymethyl)-diphenyl methane

  4,41-dihydroxy-3,31-di-(hydroxymethyl)-diphenyl methane

o-Cresol

Data from Bruze M. Contact sensitizers in resins based on phenol and formaldehyde. Acta Derm Venereol Suppl (Stockh) 1985;119:1–83; and Bruze M, Zimerson E. Contact allergy to o-cresol—a sensitizer in phenol-formaldehyde resin. Am J Contact Dermat 2002;13(4):198–200.

Despite frequent contact with skin, polyester resins themselves rarely cause ACD and ICD.[2] When ACD is caused by polyester resins, mostly by unsaturated polyester resins (eg, diethyleneglycol maleate monomer or fumaric acid in the resins) and extremely rarely by saturated polyester resins, involved body areas are mostly the hands and areas associated with airborne exposure (wrists, face, eyelids, neck).[136–141] This occurs mostly in the occupational setting[136–140] and occasionally in consumers.[141] ICD occurs more frequently than ACD from exposure to polyester resin systems, and may be caused by additives such as styrene, organic peroxides, acetone, and fiberglass fillers, or resin components, including polybasic acids (eg, phthalic anhydride) and polybasic alcohols (eg, propylene glycol).[2,135,142,143] Chemical burns may also be caused by styrene and organic peroxide additives.[135] Likewise, ACD occurs more often from additives, auxiliary agents,

and catalysts such as cobalt octoate than from polyester resins themselves.[2,22,144] Other additives, such as benzoyl peroxide, methyl ethyl ketone peroxide, and cobalt naphthenate appear to be less of a problem today than in the 1950s,[135,142] although a few case reports of ACD caused by these additives have been made recently.[145,146] **Table 3** lists recommended patch test concentrations and vehicles for various polyester resin system chemicals.

Amino resins are formed from reactions between an aldehyde and a compound with 1 or more amino groups.[1] These include melamine-formaldehyde and urea-formaldehyde resins, used commonly as laminating and bonding agents in wood and furniture industries; in products such as foam insulations, buttons, and tableware; and to improve wet strength of paper and shrinkage- and crease-resistance of textiles.[1] Finished products containing amino resins generally do not

Table 3
Recommended patch test concentrations and vehicles for polyester resin system chemicals

Polyester Resin System Chemicals	Patch Test Concentration(s) and Vehicle(s)
Unsaturated polyester resin	10% acet
Activators/accelerators	
Cobalt naphthenate	5% pet
Cobalt octoate	5% pet
Diethylaniline	10% alc
Cross-linking agents	
Methyl methacrylate	2% pet
α-Methylstyrene	1% pet
Styrene (vinyl benzene)	1% olive oil
Vinyl toluene	1% olive oil
Inhibitors	
Hydroquinone	1% pet
Quinone	5% pet
p-tert-butylcatechol	1% acet[22]; 0.25% pet, or 1% pet[38]
Organic peroxide catalysts	
Benzoyl peroxide	1% pet
Cumene hydroperoxide	0.5% pet
Cyclohexanone peroxide	0.5% pet
Methyl ethyl ketone peroxide	0.5% pet
Ultraviolet light absorbers	
Benzophenone	5% pet
Benzotriazoles	1% pet

Abbreviations: acet, acetone; pet, petrolatum; alc, alcohol.
Data from Rietschel RL, Fowler JF. Plastics, adhesives and synthetic resins. In: Rietschel RL, Fowler JF, editors. Fisher's contact dermatitis, 6th edition. Hamilton (ON): BC Decker Inc; 2008. p. 542–65; and de Groot AC, Frosch PJ. Patch test concentrations and vehicles for testing contact allergens. In: Frosch PJ, Menné T, Lepoittevin JP, editors. Contact dermatitis, 4th edition. Berlin: Springer Verlag; 2006. p. 907–28.

sensitize, but uncured substances may sensitize on occasion.[1] Contact allergy to amino resins can be occupational or nonoccupational and is often combined with formaldehyde allergy, having been reported from textiles, shin pads, facial tissues, fiberboards, foam insulation, composite, orthopedic casts, and gypsum molds.[147–158] ICD from amino resins is mainly caused by the formaldehyde that can be released.[1] ICD has also been reported in manufacturers of fiberboards with urea-formaldehyde resin.[159] Additionally, airborne skin irritation of the face, ears, and neck has been noted from dust during the production of urea-formaldehyde insulating foam.[160] Even though the amount of formaldehyde released from amino resins has been on the decline (the percentage of high-formaldehyde-releasing textile resins has decreased in the United States from 55% in 1980 to 27% in 1990), ACD or ICD induced by formaldehyde released from amino resins

remains a problem.[1,147,161,162] Patients should be advised to wash all new clothes before wearing them, because the potential for formaldehyde release from resins decreases with the number of washes with alkaline wash powders.[163] Patients should also be instructed not to use chlorine bleaches, which increase formaldehyde release.[163]

Polyvinyl resins are produced from the polymerization of vinyl group monomers (eg, vinyl chloride), during which numerous additives, such as antioxidants, stabilizers, initiators, plasticizers, pigments, and flame retardants are used.[1] Polyvinyl chloride (PVC) is the most used plastic after polyethylene, partly because of its low price.[1] The addition of a small amount (<5%) of plasticizer produces a hard PVC, whereas the addition of 30% to 50% plasticizer produces a soft PVC. Soft PVC is used in the production of shoes, cables, gloves, hoses, and films.[164] Because of

Table 4
Recommended patch test concentrations and vehicles for polyvinyl resin system chemicals

Polyvinyl Resin System Chemicals	Patch Test Concentration and Vehicle
Polyvinyl resins	10% aq
Aldehydes	
Glyoxal (dialdehyde)	1% aq
Antioxidants	
Bisphenol A	1% pet
Biocides	
Benzisothiazolinone	0.1% pet
Pyridine derivatives	N/A
Inhibitors	
Bisphenol A	1% pet
Organic pigments	N/A
Plasticizers	
Dibutyl phthalate	5% pet
Diethyl phthalate	5% pet
Dioctyl phthalate	5% pet
Epoxy resin	1% pet
Stabilizers	
Dibutyl tin dilaurate	0.5% pet
Dibutyl tin maleate	0.5% pet
Diphenylthiourea	1% pet
Epoxy resin	1% pet
Ultraviolet light absorbers	
Benzophenones	5% pet
Resorcinol monobenzoate	1% pet

Abbreviations: aq, aqueous; pet, petrolatum; N/A, not available.
Data from Refs.[22,38,164–173]

its toughness and rigidity, hard PVC is used in agricultural products, sewage systems, drinking water pipes, furniture, window frames, dishes, and packages.[1] In the final PVC product, there are free monomers and additives which may cause sensitizations and ACD.[165–174] **Table 4** gives recommended patch test concentrations and vehicles for polyvinyl resin system chemicals which have been reported to induce contact sensitization. ICD has been noted to occur with plasticizers and stabilizers (eg, dibutyl thiomalate, dibutyl sebacate, dioctyl phthalate),[1,166,175] but it may also be caused by exposure to PVC powder in hot and humid environments.[176] Contact urticaria caused by PVC components (eg, phthalates) has also been reported.[174,177]

Polystyrene resins are formed from the polymerization of styrene monomers using peroxide as an initiator.[1] Stabilizers (eg, benzophenones, organic nickel) are usually added to improve light stability.[1] Polystyrene resins are used in such products as packaging and insulation material, disposable tableware, electrical appliances, toys, handles, and pipes.[1] Contact allergy to styrene is rare but has been reported.[178–180] Although styrene has generally been considered a mild irritant,[1] it has occasionally been reported to cause chemical burns.[135]

Other resins, such as polyolefins (eg, polyethylene, polypropylene), polyamides, and polycarbonates, very rarely cause ACD and ICD.[1]

SUMMARY

Plastic resin systems have an increasingly diverse array of applications and also induce health hazards, the most common of which are ACD and ICD, and less commonly contact urticaria, pigmentary changes, and photoallergic contact dermatitis. Other health hazards, especially in the occupational setting, include asthma, rhinoconjunctivitis, and paresthesias ([meth]acrylics). These resin systems include epoxies (the most frequent synthetic resin system to cause contact dermatitis), (meth)acrylics, polyurethanes, phenol-formaldehydes, polyesters, amino resins (melamine-formaldehydes, urea-formaldehydes), polyvinyls, polystyrenes, polyolefins, polyamides, and polycarbonates. Contact dermatitis usually occurs as a result of exposure to the monomers and additives in the occupational setting, although reports from consumers using the raw materials or end products periodically surface. Resin- and additive-induced direct contact dermatitis usually presents on the hands, fingers, and forearms, whereas facial, eyelid, and neck involvement may occur through indirect contact (eg, via the hands), or from airborne exposure.

To prevent irritation, sensitization, or both from resins and additives, workers should be educated and informed of the risks before handling these compounds, and taught no-touch techniques. All workers should minimize skin contact with these chemicals, using such protective measures as working in isolated and well-ventilated areas; regularly cleansing hands and contaminated equipment; and using appropriate chemical protective clothing, especially gloves which fit well, are frequently changed, have low sensitization potentials, and are technically adequate and not easily torn or penetrated. Only thicker PVC gloves, nitrile gloves, or the Silver Shield/4-H gloves (North Safety Products, Cranston, Rhode Island), made of 5 layers of polyethylene-ethylene-vinylalcohol copolymer-polyethylene, provide sufficient protection, because most resins can penetrate thinner PVC, polyethylene, and rubber gloves.[15,21,135,181–184] However, some investigators have noted that polyethylene gloves do provide protection against methyl methacrylate diffusion.[1] Contaminated skin should be washed thoroughly with soap and water, and contaminated clothing and gloves should be removed immediately. Workers should also protect inflamed or injured skin from resin or additive exposure and should minimize simultaneous exposure to irritants such as organic solvents, because skin irritation increases the risk of sensitization.[15,181]

REFERENCES

1. Bjorkner B, Ponten A, Zimerson E, et al. Plastic materials. In: Frosch PJ, Menné T, Lepoittevin JP, editors. Contact dermatitis. 4th edition. Berlin: Springer Verlag; 2006. p. 583–621.

2. Taylor JS. Occupational dermatoses. In: Alderman MH, Hanley MJ, editors. Clinical medicine for the occupational physician. New York: Marcel Dekker, Inc; 1982. p. 299–344.

3. Amado A, Taylor JS. Contact allergy to epoxy resins. Contact Dermatitis 2008;58(3):186–7.

4. Kanerva L, Jolanki R, Estlander T, et al. Airborne occupational allergic contact dermatitis from triglycidyl-p-aminophenol and tetraglycidyl-4,4'-methylene dianiline in preimpregnated epoxy products in the aircraft industry. Dermatology 2000;201(1):29–33.

5. Burrows D, Fregert S, Campbell H, et al. Contact dermatitis from the epoxy resins tetraglycidyl-4,4'-methylene dianiline and o-diglycidyl phthalate in composite material. Contact Dermatitis 1984;11(2):80–2.

6. Ponten A, Zimerson E, Bruze M. Contact allergy to the isomers of diglycidyl ether of bisphenol F. Acta Derm Venereol 2004;84(1):12–7.

7. Bray PG. Epoxy resins. Occup Med 1999;14(4): 743–58.

8. Dickel H, Kuss O, Schmidt A, et al. Occupational relevance of positive standard patch-test results in employed persons with an initial report of an occupational skin disease. Int Arch Occup Environ Health 2002;75(6):423–34.

9. Flyvholm MA. Contact allergens in registered chemical products. Contact Dermatitis 1991;25(1): 49–56.

10. Hughes R, Taylor JS. Surveillance of allergic contact dermatitis: epoxy resin and microscopic immersion oil. J Am Acad Dermatol 2002;47(6): 965–6.

11. Rietschel RL, Mathias CG, Taylor JS, et al. A preliminary report of the occupation of patients evaluated in patch test clinics. Am J Contact Dermat 2001; 12(2):72–6.

12. Amado A, Taylor JS. Contact dermatitis in the bowling pro shop. Dermatitis 2008;19(6):334–8.

13. Taylor JS, Bergfeld WF, Guin JD. Contact dermatitis to knee patch adhesive in boys' jeans: a nonoccupational cause of epoxy resin sensitivity. Cleve Clin Q 1983;50(2):123–7.

14. Fregert S. Epoxy dermatitis from the non-working environment. Br J Dermatol 1981;105(Suppl 21):63–4.

15. Jolanki R, Kanerva L, Estlander T, et al. Occupational dermatoses from epoxy resin compounds. Contact Dermatitis 1990;23(3):172–83.

16. Jolanki R. Occupational skin diseases from epoxy compounds. Epoxy resin compounds, epoxy acrylates and 2,3-epoxypropyl trimethyl ammonium chloride. Acta Derm Venereol Suppl (Stockh) 1991;159:1–80.

17. Romyhr O, Nyfors A, Leira HL, et al. Allergic contact dermatitis caused by epoxy resin systems in industrial painters. Contact Dermatitis 2006; 55(3):167–72.

18. Angelini G, Rigano L, Foti C, et al. Occupational sensitization to epoxy resin and reactive diluents in marble workers. Contact Dermatitis 1996;35(1):11–6.

19. van Putten PB, Coenraads PJ, Nater JP. Hand dermatoses and contact allergic reactions in construction workers exposed to epoxy resins. Contact Dermatitis 1984;10(3):146–50.

20. Jolanki R, Tarvainen K, Tatar T, et al. Occupational dermatoses from exposure to epoxy resin compounds in a ski factory. Contact Dermatitis 1996;34(6):390–6.

21. Omer SA, al-Tawil NG. Contact sensitivity among workers in a paint factory. Contact Dermatitis 1994;30(1):55–7.

22. Rietschel RL, Fowler JF. Plastics, adhesives and synthetic resins. In: Rietschel RL, Fowler JF, editors. Fisher's contact dermatitis. 6th edition. Hamilton (ON): BC Decker Inc.; 2008. p. 542–65.

23. Fregert S, Thorgeirsson A. Patch testing with low molecular oligomers of epoxy resins in humans. Contact Dermatitis 1977;3(6):301–3.

24. Jolanki R, Estlander T, Kanerva L. Occupational contact dermatitis and contact urticaria caused by epoxy resins. Acta Derm Venereol Suppl (Stockh) 1987;134:90–4.

25. Lee HN, Pokorny CD, Law S, et al. Cross-reactivity among epoxy acrylates and bisphenol F epoxy resins in patients with bisphenol A epoxy resin sensitivity. Am J Contact Dermat 2002;13(3): 108–15.

26. Handley J, Burrows D. Dermatitis from hexavalent chromate in the accelerator of an epoxy sealant (PR1422) used in the aircraft industry. Contact Dermatitis 1994;30(4):193–6.

27. Kiec-Swierczynska M. Allergy to epoxy compounds over a decade. Contact Dermatitis 1995;32(3):180.

28. Maibach HI, Mathias CT. Allergic contact dermatitis from cycloaliphatic epoxide in jet aviation hydraulic fluid. Contact Dermatitis 2001;45(1):56.

29. Kanerva L, Estlander T, Jolanki R. Occupational allergic contact dermatitis caused by 2,4,6-tris-(dimethylaminomethyl)phenol, and review of sensitizing epoxy resin hardeners. Int J Dermatol 1996; 35(12):852–6.

30. de Groot AC. Occupational contact allergy to alpha-naphthyl glycidyl ether. Contact Dermatitis 1994;30(4):253–4.

31. Eedy DJ. Carbon-fibre-induced airborne irritant contact dermatitis. Contact Dermatitis 1996;35(6): 362–3.

32. Tarvainen K, Jolanki R, Estlander T, et al. Immunologic contact urticaria due to airborne methylhexahydrophthalic anhydride and methyltetrahydrophthalic anhydride. Contact Dermatitis 1995;32(4):201–9.

33. Allen H, Kaidbey K. Persistent photosensitivity following occupational exposure to epoxy resin. Arch Dermatol 1979;115(11):1307–10.

34. Hannu T, Frilander H, Kauppi P, et al. IgE-mediated occupational asthma from epoxy resin. Int Arch Allergy Immunol 2009;148(1):41–4.

35. Huygens S, Goossens A. An update on airborne contact dermatitis. Contact Dermatitis 2001;44(1):1–6.

36. Dahlquist I, Fregert S. Allergic contact dermatitis from volatile epoxy hardeners and reactive diluents. Contact Dermatitis 1979;5(6):406–7.

37. Lyon CC, Beck MH. Epoxy-by-proxy dermatitis. Contact Dermatitis 2000;42(5):306.

38. de Groot AC, Frosch PJ. Patch test concentrations and vehicles for testing contact allergens. In: Frosch PJ, Menné T, Lepoittevin JP, editors. Contact dermatitis. 4th edition. Berlin: Springer Verlag; 2006. p. 907–28.

39. Kanerva L, Lauerma A, Estlander T, et al. Occupational allergic contact dermatitis caused by photobonded sculptured nails and a review of (meth)acrylates in nail cosmetics. Am J Contact Dermat 1996;7(2):109–15.

40. Goon AT, Isaksson M, Zimerson E, et al. Contact allergy to (meth)acrylates in the dental series in southern Sweden: simultaneous positive patch test reaction patterns and possible screening allergens. Contact Dermatitis 2006;55(4):219–26.

41. Malten KE, Bende WJ. 2-Hydroxy-ethyl-methacrylate and di- and tetraethylene glycol dimethacrylate: contact sensitizers in a photoprepolymer printing plate procedure. Contact Dermatitis 1979; 5(4):214–20.

42. Bjorkner B. Contact allergy to 2-hydroxypropyl methacrylate (2-HPMA) in an ultraviolet curable ink. Acta Derm Venereol 1984;64(3):264–7.

43. Nethercott JR. Skin problems associated with multifunctional acrylic monomers in ultraviolet curing inks. Br J Dermatol 1978;98(5):541–52.

44. Ranchoff RE, Taylor JS. Contact dermatitis to anaerobic sealants. J Am Acad Dermatol 1985; 13(6):1015–20.

45. de Groot AC. Patch testing: test concentrations and vehicles for 3700 chemicals. 2nd edition. Amsterdam: Elsevier; 1994.

46. Tobler M, Wuthrich B, Freiburghaus AU. Contact dermatitis from acrylate and methacrylate compounds in Lowicryl embedding media for electron microscopy. Contact Dermatitis 1990;23(2): 96–102.

47. Cavelier C, Jelen G, Herve-Bazin B, et al. Irritation and allergy to acrylates and methacrylates. Part I: common monoacrylates and monomethacrylates. Ann Dermatol Venereol 1981;108(6–7):549–56.

48. Parker D, Turk JL. Contact sensitivity to acrylate compounds in guinea pigs. Contact Dermatitis 1983;9(1):55–60.

49. Bjorkner B. The sensitizing capacity of multifunctional acrylates in the guinea pig. Contact Dermatitis 1984;11(4):236–46.

50. Bjorkner B, Niklasson B, Persson K. The sensitizing potential of di-(meth)acrylates based on bisphenol A or epoxy resin in the guinea pig. Contact Dermatitis 1984;10(5):286–304.

51. Bjorkner B. Sensitization capacity of acrylated prepolymers in ultraviolet curing inks tested in the guinea pig. Acta Derm Venereol 1981;61(1):7–10.

52. Bjorkner B. Sensitizing potential of urethane (meth)acrylates in the guinea pig. Contact Dermatitis 1984;11(2):115–9.

53. Bjorkner B. Sensitization capacity of polyester methacrylate in ultraviolet curing inks tested in the guinea pig. Acta Derm Venereol 1982;62(2):153–4.

54. Lindstrom M, Alanko K, Keskinen H, et al. Dentist's occupational asthma, rhinoconjunctivitis, and allergic contact dermatitis from methacrylates. Allergy 2002;57(6):543–5.

55. Sanchez-Perez J, Gonzalez-Arriba A, Goiriz R, et al. Occupational allergic contact dermatitis to acrylates and methacrylates. Contact Dermatitis 2008;58(4):252–4.

56. Kanerva L, Jolanki R, Estlander T. 10 years of patch testing with the (meth)acrylate series. Contact Dermatitis 1997;37(6):255–8.

57. Kanerva L. Cross-reactions of multifunctional methacrylates and acrylates. Acta Odontol Scand 2001; 59(5):320–9.

58. Rustemeyer T, de Groot J, von Blomberg BM, et al. Cross-reactivity patterns of contact-sensitizing methacrylates. Toxicol Appl Pharmacol 1998; 148(1):83–90.

59. Mowad CM, Ferringer T. Allergic contact dermatitis from acrylates in artificial nails. Dermatitis 2004; 15(1):51–3.

60. Lazarov A. Sensitization to acrylates is a common adverse reaction to artificial fingernails. J Eur Acad Dermatol Venereol 2007;21(2):169–74.

61. Sadoh DR, Sharief MK, Howard RS. Occupational exposure to methyl methacrylate monomer induces generalised neuropathy in a dental technician. Br Dent J 1999;186(8):380–1.

62. Fisher AA, Baran RL. Adverse reactions to acrylate sculptured nail with particular reference to prolonged paresthesia. Am J Contact Dermat 1991;2: 38–42.

63. Sood A, Taylor JS. Acrylic reactions: a review of 56 cases. Contact Dermatitis 2003;48(6):346–7.

64. Rustemeyer T, Frosch PJ. Occupational skin diseases in dental laboratory technicians. (I). Clinical picture and causative factors. Contact Dermatitis 1996;34(2):125–33.

65. Aalto-Korte K, Alanko K, Kuuliala O, et al. Occupational methacrylate and acrylate allergy from glues. Contact Dermatitis 2008;58(6):340–6.

66. Corazza M, Bacilieri S, Virgili A. Anaerobic sealants: still a problem today. Eur J Dermatol 2000; 10(6):468–9.

67. Nethercott JR. Allergic contact dermatitis due to an epoxy acrylate. Br J Dermatol 1981;104(6): 697–703.

68. Nethercott JR, Jakubovic HR, Pilger C, et al. Allergic contact dermatitis due to urethane acrylate in ultraviolet cured inks. Br J Ind Med 1983;40(3): 241–50.

69. Dutree-Meulenberg RO, Naafs B, van Joost T, et al. Contact dermatitis caused by urethane acrylates in a hearing aid. Contact Dermatitis 1991;24(2): 143–5.

70. Bjorkner B, Niklasson B. Influence of the vehicle on elicitation of contact allergic reactions to acrylic compounds in the guinea pig. Contact Dermatitis 1984;11(5):268–78.

71. Estlander T, Rajaniemi R, Jolanki R. Hand dermatitis in dental technicians. Contact Dermatitis 1984;10(4):201–5.

72. Alanko K, Susitaival P, Jolanki R, et al. Occupational skin diseases among dental nurses. Contact Dermatitis 2004;50(2):77–82.

73. Estlander T, Keskinen H, Jolanki R, et al. Occupational dermatitis from exposure to polyurethane chemicals. Contact Dermatitis 1992;27(3):161–5.

74. Liippo J, Lammintausta K. Contact sensitization to 4,4'-diaminodiphenylmethane and to isocyanates among general dermatology patients. Contact Dermatitis 2008;59(2):109–14.

75. Bello D, Herrick CA, Smith TJ, et al. Skin exposure to isocyanates: reasons for concern. Environ Health Perspect 2007;115(3):328–35.

76. Baur X, Marek W, Ammon J, et al. Respiratory and other hazards of isocyanates. Int Arch Occup Environ Health 1994;66(3):141–52.

77. Littorin M, Truedsson L, Welinder H, et al. Acute respiratory disorder, rhinoconjunctivitis and fever associated with the pyrolysis of polyurethane derived from diphenylmethane diisocyanate. Scand J Work Environ Health 1994;20(3):216–22.

78. Larsen TH, Gregersen P, Jemec GB. Skin irritation and exposure to diisocyanates in orthopedic nurses working with soft casts. Am J Contact Dermat 2001;12(4):211–4.

79. Daftarian HS, Lushniak BD, Reh CM, et al. Evaluation of self-reported skin problems among workers exposed to toluene diisocyanate (TDI) at a foam manufacturing facility. J Occup Environ Med 2002;44(12):1197–202.

80. Duprat P, Gradiski D, Marignac B. The irritant and allergenic action of two isocyanates: toluene diisocyanate (TDI) and diphenylmethane diisocyanate (MDI). Eur J Toxicol Environ Hyg 1976;9(1):43–53.

81. White IR, Stewart JR, Rycroft RJ. Allergic contact dermatitis from an organic di-isocyanate. Contact Dermatitis 1983;9(4):300–3.

82. Thorne PS, Hillebrand JA, Lewis GR, et al. Contact sensitivity by diisocyanates: potencies and cross-reactivities. Toxicol Appl Pharmacol 1987;87(1):155–65.

83. Tanaka K, Takeoka A, Nishimura F, et al. Contact sensitivity induced in mice by methylene bisphenyl diisocyanate. Contact Dermatitis 1987;17(4):199–204.

84. Yasuda K, Nozawa G, Goto T, et al. Experimental studies on TDI dermatitis in mice. J Toxicol Sci 1980;5(1):11–21.

85. Militello G, Sasseville D, Ditre C, et al. Allergic contact dermatitis from isocyanates among sculptors. Dermatitis 2004;15(3):150–3.

86. Frick M, Isaksson M, Bjorkner B, et al. Occupational allergic contact dermatitis in a company manufacturing boards coated with isocyanate lacquer. Contact Dermatitis 2003;48(5):255–60.

87. Kerre S. Allergic contact dermatitis to DMDI in an office application. Contact Dermatitis 2008;58(5):313–4.

88. Frick M, Bjorkner B, Hamnerius N, et al. Allergic contact dermatitis from dicyclohexylmethane-4,4'-diisocyanate. Contact Dermatitis 2003;48(6):305–9.

89. Hannu T, Estlander T, Jolanki R. Allergic contact dermatitis due to MDI and MDA from accidental occupational exposure. Contact Dermatitis 2005;52(2):108–9.

90. Goossens A, Detienne T, Bruze M. Occupational allergic contact dermatitis caused by isocyanates. Contact Dermatitis 2002;47(5):304–8.

91. Belsito DV. Common shoe allergens undetected by commercial patch-testing kits: dithiodimorpholine and isocyanates. Am J Contact Dermat 2003;14(2):95–6.

92. Morgan CJ, Haworth AE. Allergic contact dermatitis from 1,6-hexamethylene diisocyanate in a domestic setting. Contact Dermatitis 2003;48(4):224.

93. Alomar A. Contact dermatitis from a fashion watch. Contact Dermatitis 1986;15:44–5.

94. Vilaplana J, Romaguera C, Grimalt F. Allergic contact dermatitis from aliphatic isocyanate on spectacle frames. Contact Dermatitis 1987;16(2):113.

95. Fregert S. Allergic contact reaction to diphenyl-4,4'-diisocyanate. Contact Dermatitis Newsletter 1967;2:17.

96. Rothe A. Zur Frage arbeitsbedingter Hautschadigungen durch Polyurethanchemikalien [Occupational dermatoses due to polyurethane drugs]. Berufsdermatosen 1976;24:7–24 [in German].

97. Tait CP, Delaney TA. Reactions causing reactions: allergic contact dermatitis to an isocyanate metabolite but not to the parent compound. Australas J Dermatol 1999;40(2):116–7.

98. Fortina AB, Piaserico S, Larese F, et al. Diaminodiphenylmethane (DDM): frequency of sensitization, clinical relevance and concomitant positive reactions. Contact Dermatitis 2001;44(5):283–8.

99. Kanerva L, Estlander T, Jolanki R, et al. Occupational urticaria from welding polyurethane. J Am Acad Dermatol 1991;24(5 Pt 2):825–6.

100. Valks R, Conde-Salazar L, Barrantes OL. Occupational allergic contact urticaria and asthma from diphenylmethane-4,4'-diisocyanate. Contact Dermatitis 2003;49(3):166–7.

101. Bello D, Sparer J, Redlich CA, et al. Slow curing of aliphatic polyisocyanate paints in automotive refinishing: a potential source for skin exposure. J Occup Environ Hyg 2007;4(6):406–11.

102. Boutin M, Dufresne A, Ostiguy C, et al. Determination of airborne isocyanates generated during the thermal degradation of car paint in body repair shops. Ann Occup Hyg 2006;50(4):385–93.

103. Littorin M, Welinder H, Skarping G, et al. Exposure and nasal inflammation in workers heating polyurethane. Int Arch Occup Environ Health 2002;75(7):468–74.

104. Frick-Engfeldt M, Isaksson M, Zimerson E, et al. How to optimize patch testing with diphenylmethane diisocyanate. Contact Dermatitis 2007; 57(3):138–51.

105. Aalto-Korte K, Alanko K, Kuuliala O, et al. Late reactions in patch tests: a 4-year review from a clinic of occupational dermatology. Contact Dermatitis 2007;56(2):81–6.

106. Frick M, Zimerson E, Karlsson D, et al. Poor correlation between stated and found concentrations of diphenylmethane-4,4'-diisocyanate (4,4'-MDI) in petrolatum patch-test preparations. Contact Dermatitis 2004;51(2):73–8.

107. Nagashima C, Tomitaka-Yagami A, Matsunaga K. Contact dermatitis due to para-tertiary-butylphenol-formaldehyde resin in a wetsuit. Contact Dermatitis 2003;49(5):267–8.

108. Bruze M. Contact sensitizers in resins based on phenol and formaldehyde. Acta Derm Venereol Suppl (Stockh) 1985;119:1–83.

109. Massone L, Anonide A, Borghi S, et al. Sensitization to para-tertiary-butylphenolformaldehyde resin. Int J Dermatol 1996;35(3):177–80.

110. Oztas P, Polat M, Cinar L, et al. Shoe dermatitis from para-tertiary butylphenol formaldehyde. Contact Dermatitis 2007;56(5):294–5.

111. Tarvainen K. Analysis of patients with allergic patch test reactions to a plastics and glues series. Contact Dermatitis 1995;32(6):346–51.

112. Dahlquist I. Contact allergy to paratertiary butylphenol formaldehyde resin in an adhesive label. Contact Dermatitis 1984;10(1):54.

113. Shono M, Ezoe K, Kaniwa MA, et al. Allergic contact dermatitis from para-tertiary-butylphenol-formaldehyde resin (PTBP-FR) in athletic tape and leather adhesive. Contact Dermatitis 1991; 24(4):281–8.

114. Avenel-Audran M, Goossens A, Zimerson E, et al. Contact dermatitis from electrocardiograph-monitoring electrodes: role of p-tert-butylphenol-formaldehyde resin. Contact Dermatitis 2003;48(2):108–11.

115. Barros MA, Baptista A, Correia TM, et al. Patch testing in children: a study of 562 schoolchildren. Contact Dermatitis 1991;25(3):156–9.

116. Bruze M, Fregert S, Zimerson E. Contact allergy to phenol-formaldehyde resins. Contact Dermatitis 1985;12(2):81–6.

117. Foussereau J, Cavelier C, Selig D. Occupational eczema from para-tertiary-butylphenol formaldehyde resins: a review of the sensitizing resins. Contact Dermatitis 1976;2(5):254–8.

118. Hayakawa R, Ogino Y, Suzuki M, et al. Allergic contact dermatitis from para-tertiary-butylphenol-formaldehyde resin (PTBP-F-R). Contact Dermatitis 1994;30(3):187–8.

119. Zimerson E, Bruze M. Contact allergy to the monomers in p-tert-butylphenol-formaldehyde resin. Contact Dermatitis 2002;47(3):147–53.

120. Zimerson E, Bruze M. Contact allergy to the monomers of p-tert-butylphenol-formaldehyde resin in the guinea pig. Contact Dermatitis 1998;39(5): 222–6.

121. Zimerson E, Bruze M, Goossens A. Simultaneous p-tert-butylphenol-formaldehyde resin and p-tert-butylcatechol contact allergies in man and sensitizing capacities of p-tert-butylphenol and p-tert-butylcatechol in guinea pigs. Occup Environ Med 1999;41(1):23–8.

122. Zimerson E, Bruze M. Demonstration of the contact sensitizer p-tert-butylcatechol in p-tert-butylphenol formaldehyde resin. Am J Contact Dermat 1999; 10(1):2–6.

123. Zimerson E, Bruze M. Sensitizing capacity of some trimers in p-tert-butylphenol-formaldehyde resin. Contact Dermatitis 2002;47(1):40–6.

124. Zimerson E, Bruze M. Contact allergy to 5,5'-di-tert-butyl-2,2'-dihydroxy-(hydroxymethyl)-dibenzyl ethers, sensitizers, in p-tert-butylphenol-formaldehyde resin. Contact Dermatitis 2000;43(1):20–6.

125. Zimerson E, Bruze M. Low-molecular-weight contact allergens in p-tert-butylphenol-formaldehyde resin. Am J Contact Dermat 2002;13(4):190–7.

126. Zimerson E, Bruze M. Sensitizing capacity of two monomeric aldehyde components in p-tert-butylphenol-formaldehyde resin. Acta Derm Venereol 2002;82(6):418–22.

127. Owen CM, Beck MH. Occupational allergic contact dermatitis from phenol-formaldehyde resins. Contact Dermatitis 2001;45(5):294–5.

128. Rademaker M. Contact dermatitis to phenol-formaldehyde resin in two plywood factory workers. Australas J Dermatol 2002;43(3):224–5.

129. Bruze M, Zimerson E. Cross-reaction patterns in patients with contact allergy to simple methylol phenols. Contact Dermatitis 1997;37(2):82–6.

130. Bruze M, Zimerson E. Contact allergy to o-cresol—a sensitizer in phenol-formaldehyde resin. Am J Contact Dermat 2002;13(4):198–200.

131. Fregert S. Irritant dermatitis from phenol-formaldehyde resin powder. Contact Dermatitis 1980;6(7): 493.

132. Bruze M, Almgren G. Occupational dermatoses in workers exposed to resins based on phenol and formaldehyde. Contact Dermatitis 1988;19(4): 272–7.

133. Mathur AK, Srivastava AK, Singh A, et al. Contact depigmentation by adhesive material of bindi. Contact Dermatitis 1991;24(4):310–1.

134. Bajaj AK, Gupta SC, Chatterjee AK. Contact depigmentation from free para-teriary-butylphenol in bindi adhesive. Contact Dermatitis 1990;22(2): 99–102.

135. Bourne LB, Milner FJ. Polyester resin hazards. Br J Ind Med 1963;20:100–9.

136. Tarvainen K, Jolanki R, Estlander T. Occupational contact allergy to unsaturated polyester resin cements. Contact Dermatitis 1993;28(4):220–4.

137. Kanerva L, Estlander T, Alanko K, et al. Occupational allergic contact dermatitis from unsaturated polyester resin in a car repair putty. Int J Dermatol 1999;38(6):447–52.

138. Pfaffli P, Jolanki R, Estlander T, et al. Identification of sensitizing diethyleneglycol maleate in a two-component polyester cement. Contact Dermatitis 2002;46(3):170–3.

139. Minamoto K, Nagano M, Yonemitsu K, et al. Allergic contact dermatitis from unsaturated polyester resin consisting of maleic anhydride, phthalic anhydride, ethylene glycol and dicyclopentadiene. Contact Dermatitis 2002;46(1):62–3.

140. Liden C, Lofstrom A, Storgards-Hatam K. Contact allergy to unsaturated polyester in a boatbuilder. Contact Dermatitis 1984;11(4):262–4.

141. MacFarlane AW, Curley RK, King CM. Contact sensitivity to unsaturated polyester resin in a limb prosthesis. Contact Dermatitis 1986; 15(5):301–3.

142. Malten KE. Recently reported causes of contact dermatitis due to synthetic resins and hardeners. Contact Dermatitis 1979;5(1):11–23.

143. Lim J, Balzer JL, Wolf CR, et al. Fiber glass reinforced plastics. Associated occupational health problems. Arch Environ Health 1970; 20(4):540–4.

144. Anavekar NS, Nixon R. Occupational allergic contact dermatitis to cobalt octoate included as an accelerator in a polyester resin. Australas J Dermatol 2006;47(2):143–4.

145. Bhushan M, Craven NM, Beck MH. Contact allergy to methyl ethyl ketone peroxide and cobalt in the manufacture of fibreglass-reinforced plastics. Contact Dermatitis 1998;39(4):203.

146. Minamoto K, Nagano M, Inaoka T, et al. Allergic contact dermatitis due to methyl ethyl ketone peroxide, cobalt naphthenate and acrylates in the manufacture of fibreglass-reinforced plastics. Contact Dermatitis 2002;46(1):58–9.

147. Hatch KL, Maibach HI. Textile dermatitis: an update (I). Resins, additives and fibers. Contact Dermatitis 1995;32(6):319–26.

148. Fowler JF, Skinner SM, Belsito DV. Allergic contact dermatitis from formaldehyde resins in permanent press clothing: an underdiagnosed cause of generalized dermatitis. J Am Acad Dermatol 1992;27(6 Pt 1):962–8.

149. Aalto-Korte K, Jolanki R, Estlander T. Formaldehyde-negative allergic contact dermatitis from melamine-formaldehyde resin. Contact Dermatitis 2003;49(4):194–6.

150. Lazarov A. Textile dermatitis in patients with contact sensitization in Israel: a 4-year prospective study. J Eur Acad Dermatol Venereol 2004;18(5):531–7.

151. Sommers S, Wilkinson SM, Dodman B. Contact dermatitis due to urea-formaldehyde resin in shin-pads. Contact Dermatitis 1999;40(3):159–60.

152. Peck SM, Palitz LL. Sensitization to facial tissues with urea-formaldehyde resin (wet-strength). J Am Med Assoc 1956;160(14):1226–7.

153. Finch M, Prais L, Foulds I. Allergic contact dermatitis from medium-density fibreboard containing melamine formaldehyde resin. Contact Dermatitis 1999;41(5):291.

154. Bell HK, King CM. Allergic contact dermatitis from urea-formaldehyde resin in medium-density fibreboard (MDF). Contact Dermatitis 2002;46(4):247.

155. L'Abbe KA, Hoey JR. Review of the health effects of urea-formaldehyde foam insulation. Environ Res 1984;35(1):246–63.

156. Isaksson M, Zimerson E, Bruze M. Occupational dermatoses in composite production. J Occup Environ Med 1999;41(4):261–6.

157. Ross JS, Rycroft JG, Bronin E. Melamine-formaldehyde contact dermatitis in orthopaedic practice. Contact Dermatitis 1992;26(3):203–4.

158. Fregert S. Formaldehyde dermatitis from a gypsum-melamine resin mixture. Contact Dermatitis 1981; 7(1):56.

159. Vale PT, Rycroft RJ. Occupational irritant contact dermatitis from fibreboard containing urea-formaldehyde resin. Contact Dermatitis 1988;19(1):62.

160. Dooms-Goossens AE, Debusschere KM, Gevers DM, et al. Contact dermatitis caused by airborne agents. A review and case reports. J Am Acad Dermatol 1986;15(1):1–10.

161. Berrens L, Young E, Jansen LH. Free formaldehyde in textiles in relation to formalin contact sensitivity. Br J Dermatol 1964;76:110–5.

162. Scheman AJ, Carroll PA, Brown KH, et al. Formaldehyde-related textile allergy: an update. Contact Dermatitis 1998;38(6):332–6.

163. Cockayne SE, McDonagh AJ, Gaskrodger DJ. Occupational allergic contact dermatitis from formaldehyde resin in clothing. Contact Dermatitis 2001;44(2):109–10.

164. Park SG, Lee EC, Hong WK, et al. A case of occupational allergic contact dermatitis due to PVC hose. J Occup Health 2008;50(2):197–200.

165. Vidovic R, Kansky A. Contact dermatitis in workers processing polyvinyl chloride plastics. Derm Beruf Umwelt 1985;33(3):104–5.

166. Schulsinger C, Mollgaard K. Polyvinyl chloride dermatitis not caused by phthalates. Contact Dermatitis 1980;6(7):477–80.

167. Tung RC, Taylor JS. Contact dermatitis from polyvinyl chloride identification bands. Am J Contact Dermat 1998;9(4):234–6.

168. Fregert S, Rorsman H. Hypersensitivity to epoxy resins used as plasticizers and stabilizers in polyvinyl chloride (PVC) resins. Acta Derm Venereol 1963;43:10–3.

169. Aalto-Korte K, Alanko K, Henriks-Eckerman ML, et al. Allergic contact dermatitis from bisphenol A in PVC gloves. Contact Dermatitis 2003;49(4):202–5.

170. Kanerva L, Jolanki R, Estlander T. Organic pigment as a cause of plastic glove dermatitis. Contact Dermatitis 1985;13(1):41–3.

171. Fregert S, Trulson L, Zimerson E. Contact allergic reactions to diphenylthiourea and phenylisothiocyanate in PVC adhesive tape. Contact Dermatitis 1982;8(1):38–42.

172. Huh WK, Masuji Y, Tada J, et al. Allergic contact dermatitis from a pyridine derivative in polyvinyl chloride leather. Am J Contact Dermat 2001; 12(1):35–7.

173. Aalto-Korte K, Alanko K, Henriks-Eckerman ML, et al. Antimicrobial allergy from polyvinyl chloride gloves. Arch Dermatol 2006;142(10):1326–30.

174. Estlander T, Jolanki R, Kanerva L. Dermatitis and urticaria from rubber and plastic gloves. Contact Dermatitis 1986;14(1):20–5.

175. Di Lernia V, Cameli N, Patrizi A. Irritant contact dermatitis in a child caused by the plastic tube of an infusion system. Contact Dermatitis 1989; 21(5):339–40.

176. Goh CL, Ho SF. An outbreak of acneiform eruption in a polyvinyl chloride manufacturing factory. Derm Beruf Umwelt 1988;36(2):53–7.

177. Sugiura K, Sugiura M, Hayakawa R, et al. A case of contact urticaria syndrome due to di(2-ethylhexyl) phthalate (DOP) in work clothes. Contact Dermatitis 2002;46(1):13–6.

178. Conde-Salazar L, Gonzalez MA, Guimaraens D, et al. Occupational allergic contact dermatitis from styrene. Contact Dermatitis 1989;21(2): 112.

179. Edwards EK Jr, Edwards EK Sr. Unusual cutaneous reaction to polystyrene in an otherwise healthy population. Contact Dermatitis 1998;38(1):50.

180. Sjoborg S, Fregert S, Trulsson L. Contact allergy to styrene and related chemicals. Contact Dermatitis 1984;10(2):94–6.

181. Uter W, Ruhl R, Pfahlberg A, et al. Contact allergy in construction workers: results of a multifactorial analysis. Ann Occup Hyg 2004;48(1):21–7.

182. Pegum JS. Penetration of protective gloves by epoxy resin. Contact Dermatitis 1979;5(5): 281–3.

183. Blanken R, Nater JP, Veenhoff E. Protection against epoxy resins with glove materials. Contact Dermatitis 1987;16(1):46–7.

184. Lachapelle JM. Preventive measures in allergic contact dermatitis. In: Dyall-Smith D, Marks R, editors. Dermatology at the millennium: the proceedings of the 19th World Congress of Dermatology. London: Informa Health Care; 1999. p. 234–8.

Hand Dermatitis: A Focus on Allergic Contact Dermatitis to Biocides

Lisa E. Maier, MD[a,b,*], Heather P. Lampel, MD, MPH[c],
Tina Bhutani, MD[d], Sharon E. Jacob, MD[e,f]

KEYWORDS

- Hand dermatitis • Contact dermatitis • Contact allergy
- Biocide • Preservative • Diagnosis

Hand dermatitis is a common affliction, affecting 2% to 10% of the general population.[1] It has multiple exogenous and endogenous causes, including allergic contact dermatitis (ACD), irritant dermatitis, atopic dermatitis, and dyshidrotic eczema.[1] Several studies have shown that irritant contact dermatitis (ICD) is the most common cause; however, ACD is not far behind.[2,3] Veien and colleagues[2] noted that 33% of 522 hand dermatitis patients had ICD, whereas 13% of male and 20% of female patients had ACD. Often, these 2 types of exogenous dermatitis can occur simultaneously in the same patient.[3]

Sufferers of chronic hand dermatitis experience a significantly decreased quality of life. They may feel shame, emotional upset, pain, pruritus, and decreased ability to perform activities of daily life.[4] Occupational hand dermatitis, 1 of the most common occupational diseases in many areas of the world,[5] may be devastating for workers and employers alike, because it is associated with job loss, lost work days, and decreased productivity.[6] Exposure to "wet work," which is defined as prolonged exposure to liquids, occlusive gloves, hand washing, and water-soluble irritants, increases the risk for developing hand dermatitis.[5,7] Those at risk include health care workers, janitors/cleaners, hairdressers, dental assistants, veterinarians, food preparation/service workers, and metalworkers.[1,6,8] Each of these careers have higher risks of developing contact dermatitis of the hands because of compromised skin barrier.[9,10]

Many of these "wet-work" jobs expose the worker to a variety of biocides, such as antimicrobials in scrubs, handwashes, cleaning fluids, and disinfectants,[11] and thus may result in allergic sensitization to these biocides. Identification of offending biocides in the workplace may be difficult because they may not be listed on material saftey data sheets (MSDSs). Biocides are important agents of ACD not only in occupational settings but also in nonoccupational settings.[12] These biocides are broadly used as preservatives in household products, including cosmetics, shampoos, moisturizers, topical medications, and home cleaning agents, allowing for exposure of a large portion of the population.[13] Despite their ability to cause sensitization, biocides are important in preventing decomposition and contamination of many household and occupational products by microorganisms, ultimately making

[a] Department of Dermatology, University of Michigan, 1910 A. Taubman Center 0314, 1500 East Medical Center Drive, Ann Arbor, MI 48109-0314, USA
[b] VA Ann Arbor Healthcare System, 2215 Fuller Road, Ann Arbor, MI 48105, USA
[c] Department of Dermatology, University of California, Irvine, 101 The City Drive South, Building 53 Room 302A, Ann Arbor, Orange, CA 92868, USA
[d] Department of Internal Medicine, University of California, San Diego, 200 West Arbor Drive, San Diego, CA 92103, USA
[e] Rady Children's Hospital, University of California, San Diego, 8010 Frost Street Suite 602, San Diego, CA, USA
[f] VA San Diego Healthcare System, 3350 La Jolla Village Drive, 111B San Diego, CA 92161, USA
* Corresponding author. Department of Dermatology, University of Michigan, 1910 A. Taubman Center 0314, 1500 E. Medical Center Drive, Ann Arbor, MI 48109-0314.
E-mail address: maierl@umich.edu (L.E. Maier).

Dermatol Clin 27 (2009) 251–264
doi:10.1016/j.det.2009.05.007
0733-8635/09/$ – see front matter. Published by Elsevier Inc.

products safer (from a microbial standpoint) and more efficacious.[14] Biocides also increase the longevity of many products.[14] These low–molecular weight chemicals are able to penetrate microbial cell surfaces and act intracellularly by different mechanisms.[11] It is this property of permeability that allows the same chemicals to potentially penetrate through the stratum corneum and cause allergenicity by conjugating with autologous proteins in the skin, forming tertiary structures that can be recognized by Langerhan cells.[15] As a consequence, preservatives and biocides are considered skin-sensitizing allergens that commonly cause contact dermatitis.[16]

In 2007, Warshaw and colleagues[12] published patch test data from the North American Contact Dermatitis Group (between 1994 and 2004) regarding ACD of the hands. They concluded that the most relevant allergens associated with hand-only ACD were preservatives, metals, rubber accelerators, fragrances, and topical antibiotics. Quaternium 15, a formaldehyde-releasing preservative was found to be the most common allergen accounting for 16.5% of clinically relevant positive patch test results in patients with hand-only ACD. Quaternium 15 was found to be responsible for more hand-only ACD than even nickel, a known strong sensitizer. This article attempts to provide more information and detail about some of the common biocides and preservatives known to cause ACD of the hands and briefly discusses the potential for these chemicals to cause other patterns of contact dermatitis. Some of the most common biocides causing ACD and potential sources of exposure are listed in **Table 1**.

FORMALDEHYDE

Formaldehyde is a widely used chemical substance found in a multitude of products and used for a variety of applications. It has been manufactured and marketed as a biologic preservative since the late 1800s.[17] It is often found in skin and hair care products, cosmetics, permanent press textiles, certain cleaning products, disinfectants, paper, and topical medications.[17] Metal working fluids,[18] paints and lacquers, construction material, and printing ink[19] may also contain formaldehyde or a formaldehyde releaser. Occupations that are associated with formaldehyde allergy include machinists, health care workers, painters, janitorial staff, and cosmetologists.[20] Because formaldehyde is present in many products encountered on a daily basis, allergy to this substance is quite common. The data from the North American Contact Dermatitis Group (NACDG), year 2003 to 2004, showed that

formaldehyde was positive in 8.7% of patients patch tested.[21] This prevalence of allergy has been stable during the previous decade.[21] Formaldehyde is also an important allergen inducing hand dermatitis. In analyzed data from 1994 to 2004 NACDG results on allergic contact *hand* dermatitis, formaldehyde ranked as the second most common allergen (trumped only by the formaldehyde releaser Quaternium 15) and accounted for 13% of positive patch test results.[12] It is an important cause of occupational hand dermatitis,[20] particularly affecting workers exposed to metalworking fluids and creams.[20]

Formaldehyde is patch tested as 1% in water or in the thin-layer rapid use epicutaneous (TRUE) test as 0.18 mg/cm^2 N-hydroxymethyl succinimide in polyvidone, which releases formaldehyde when in contact with the skin.[17] Formaldehyde patch tests must be interpreted carefully for several reasons. First, Formaldehyde is a notable irritant, so false-positive results may occur.[22] Clinical relevance determination may be difficult, because formaldehyde is nearly ubiquitous in everyday products. It may not be listed on ingredient labels, may be present as an impurity or may even be contained in the materials used to coat containers of various products.[23] Furthermore, many labeled products contain such small amounts that they may not cause dermatitis.[24] Lack of complete dose-response data makes predicting the allergic potential of these products difficult. Reported threshold responses are varied and range from 30 to 300 ppm.[24]

Patients with formaldehyde allergy commonly present with chronic hand and/or generalized dermatitis.[25,26] For these formaldehyde-allergic patients, slow recovery is to be expected, even with the strictest plan to avoid the allergen because patients may be unaware of, or unable to discontinue all potential sources of this chemical.[26]

FORMALDEHYDE-RELEASING PRESERVATIVES

Formaldehyde releasers are a group of chemicals that contain a small, detachable formaldehyde moiety.[23] The 5 most commonly used chemicals in this category are Quaternium 15, dimethyloldimethyl (DMDM) hydantoin, imidazolidinyl urea (IMID), diazolidinyl urea, and 2-bromo-2-nitropropane-1,3-diol (bronopol).[14] There are multiple formaldehyde releasers used specifically in industry, especially in cutting fluids that may cause allergic contact dermatitis of the hands.[27] These are not discussed in detail in this article, but the reader is directed to Schnuch and colleagues[27] for more information. Patients who are allergic to

Table 1
Common sensitizing biocides affecting the hands (in alphabetical order)

Biocide	Possible Sources of Exposure
Bronopol[a]	Shampoos Soaps Cosmetics Moisturizers Moist towelettes Topical medications Fabric dye Paint Cutting fluids Slimicides
DIAZ[a]	Cosmetics Hair care products Liquid soaps Baby wipes/moist towelettes Cleaning agents Detergents Topical medications
DMDM hydantoin[a]	Shampoos Liquid soaps Cosmetics Adhesives Paper Cutting oils Soaps Paints Ink Herbicides
Formaldehyde	Metalworking fluids Cosmetics Cleaning fluid Paints Ink Liquid soaps Topical medications Plastics Wood composites Nail polish Shampoos Tissue fixatives
Glutaraldehyde	Cold sterilizing solutions Disinfectants Embalming fluids Radiograph developers Waterless hand soaps Fabric softeners Paper slurry
IMID[a]	Cosmetics Topical medications
MCI/MI	Shampoos Slimicides Cosmetics Metalworking fluids Moist toilet paper Adhesives Topical medications Paints
MDBN/PE	Cosmetics Topical medications Cleansers Moist toilet paper Fuels Paints Solvents Sunscreen Lubricants
Quaternium 15[a]	Shampoos Conditioners Creams/lotions Metal working fluids Paper Cosmetics Shaving products Liquid soaps Paints Food packaging

[a] Formaldehyde releaser.
Data from Refs. [12,17–19,28,30,31,38,40,41,46,75–77,82,83,85,87,88]

formaldehyde alone may also need to avoid these formaldehyde releasers,[25] particularly Quaternium 15.[25,28] Cosensitivity among formaldehyde releasers does occur, possibly because of a primary formaldehyde allergy or from use of products containing more than 1 releaser. Some experts recommend that the patient with sensitivity to only 1 formaldehyde releaser avoid only that particular antigen.[24] However, when a patient is allergic to 2 or more formaldehyde releasers, the patient should avoid all of them because allergy may be due to the formaldehyde moiety.[25] Patch testing with these chemicals can be performed using petrolatum or aqueous vehicles; however, the petrolatum formulation was shown to be statistically more sensitive than aqueous solution for detecting allergy to these chemicals.[28,29]

QUATERNIUM 15

Quaternium 15 (1-[3-chloroallyl]-3,5,7-triaza-1-azoniaadamantane chloride) is a broad-spectrum preservative found in many cosmetics and personal care products because of its stability, water solubility, and relative pH insensitivity.[14]

Even at low concentrations, it is active against bacteria, fungi, and molds and is particularly effective against *Pseudomonas aeruginosa* and *P. cepacia*.[17] It is a ubiquitous preservative found in a variety of topical products, including shampoos, conditioners, lotions and creams, shaving products, bath gels, and liquid soaps—all with the potential of hand exposure and subsequent dermatitis.[17,28,30] Being water soluble, Quaternium 15 is most effective in the aqueous phase of formulations where it is intended, but as mentioned earlier, when testing for allergy to this preservative, petrolatum is the preferred testing vehicle.[28] Occupationally, Quaternium 15 may be found in metal working fluids, adhesives, paints,[28] cleansers/disinfectants, laundry soaps, gloves,[12] pigmented paper, paper and paperboard for packaging of foods, and polyurethane resins for food packaging.[31]

Quaternium 15 was the fifth most common allergen in the NACDG patch test results of 2003 to 2004;[21] however, for hand ACD specifically, it was the most common sensitizing agent tested.[12] Between 1983 and 1987, Parker and Taylor[28] found that moisturizers were by far the leading source of exposure to Quaternium 15, occurring in 79% of patients. Noncoloring hair care products accounted for exposure in one-third of patients, whereas cosmetics accounted for about one-eighth of exposures.[28] Data confirm that these exposure sources are still major perpetrators, but now soaps, detergents, cleansers, and disinfectants are also frequently responsible, particularly for ACD of the hands.[12] Thus, it is not surprising that occupations most affected included workers in food preparation, beauty salons, health care, and housekeeping/janitorial services. Quaternium 15 also seems to be an important sensitizer in the pediatric population. A study by Hogeling and Pratt[32] noted that 4% of their pediatric patch testing population (age 4–18 years) in Ottawa, Canada between 1996 and 2006 had a positive patch test to Quaternium 15. Similar rates (3.6%) were subsequently reported by the North American Contact Dermatitis Group.[33] This is not surprising, given the large number of pediatric personal hygiene formulations that contain this allergen.

Quaternium 15 is 1 of the strongest formaldehyde releasers. At 0.1% concentration, an estimated 100 ppm of free formaldehyde is released.[14] This formaldehyde release may play an important role in Quaternium15's allergic potential, as many Quaternium 15-sensitive patients are also allergic to formaldehyde.[25,28] However, the presence of patients with isolated Quaternium 15 sensitivity demonstrates its ability to act as a sensitizer independently of formaldehyde release.[25] Other "quaternium compounds" do not release formaldehyde and do not cross-react with Quaternium 15.[23]

IMIDAZOLIDINYL UREA

IMID, also known as Germall 115, is a formaldehyde-releasing biocide frequently used in cosmetics and topical medications.[14] This water-soluble preservative is active primarily against bacteria, including *Pseudomonas aeruginosa*.[34] It provides only weak antifungal activity, therefore it is often combined with other biocides to broaden the antimicrobial spectrum.[34] IMID is considered to be a safe cosmetic biocide, and allergic sensitization is low, given its widespread use.[14] In 1991, Fransway[25] demonstrated a low prevalence (2.2%) of positive patch tests to IMID in a group of 3700 patients. This rate has remained fairly stable in North America, as the NACDG 2003 to 2004 data demonstrated a 2.9% positive patch test result when tested as 2% IMID in petrolatum. IMID is also responsible for a low, but significant, number of hand dermatitis cases. The hand dermatitis data from the NACDG from 1994 to 2004 revealed that 3.8% of patients had clinically relevant allergy to IMID. As a low-level formaldehyde releaser, the entire molecule is more likely to cause allergy than the formaldehyde released.[25,35] Thus, IMID may be less likely to induce dermatitis in patients with formaldehyde sensitivity. Although overall rates of sensitivity are low, in the United Kingdom, the incidence of sensitivity is rising.[36] This increase has not been noted in the North American data.

DIAZOLIDINYL UREA

Diazolidinyl urea, a formaldehyde releaser, was first introduced in 1982 as Germall II.[14] It has a wider antimicrobial spectrum than IMID with excellent coverage against gram-positive and gram-negative bacteria and yeasts.[37] However, it must also be combined with other preservatives to obtain optimal antifungal activity. Most often, it is used in cosmetic products, creams, hair care products, liquid soaps, baby wipes, cleaning agents, detergents, and topical medications.[30,38] Diazolidinyl urea (DIAZ) has a greater sensitizing potential than IMID.[27] This is reflected in the higher rate of overall DIAZ allergy (3.5%) as reported by NACDG patch test results 2003 to 2004,[21] despite IMID's more widespread use.[27] Moreover, DIAZ tested positive in 1% petrolatum for 5.9% of hand-only dermatitis in NACDG hand dermatitis study.[12] As with other formaldehyde releasers, contact allergy to DIAZ may be caused by the released formaldehyde or to the compound it-self.[27] There does appear to be significant cosen-sitization with formaldehyde. In 1994, Hectorne and Fransway[37] demonstrated that among the DIAZ-sensitive patients tested, 81% had cross-reactivity to 2% aqueous formaldehyde. In contrast, there was very low coreactivity of 7% with the low-level formaldehyde releaser IMID, tested as 2% petrolatum. Thus one may want to advise formaldehyde-allergic patients to avoid DIAZ.

2-BROMO-2-NITROPROPANE-1,3-DIOL

2-Bromo-2-nitropropane-1,3-diol is also known most often as Bronopol for cosmetic use and as Myacide BT and Myacide AS in industrial uses; however, other trade names exist.[14,39] Bronopol has a broad range of strong antibacterial coverage, including many gram-positive and gram-negative bacteria. It also has some activity against yeasts and fungi.[14] Sources of exposure include personal hygiene products, such as sham-poos, soaps and baby wipes, cosmetics (blushes and eyebrow pencils), moisturizers,[40] and topical medications.[27,41] Occupations with possible Bro-nopol exposure include hairdressers, maids/cleaning service, farmers, painters, printers, and textile workers involved in dyeing fabrics.[42] Addi-tionally, occupations with industrial exposure to cutting fluids,[19] spin oil,[43] and papermill slimicides (products to prevent microbial overgrowth in the pulp paper precursor)[39] may be at risk.

Allergic contact dermatitis from Bronopol can arise from sensitivity to the molecule itself or from formaldehyde release. Formaldehyde release from this chemical increases with time, potentially increasing its ability to cause dermatitis in the formaldehyde-sensitive patient.[14] Increasing pH also promotes release of formaldehyde. Thus Bronopol may be more likely to induce allergy in formaldehyde-sensitive patients exposed to Bro-nopol-containing industrial cutting fluids, where the pH is elevated.[27] In a study by Peters and colleagues,[40] 33% of patients with positive patch reactions to Bronopol had cross-reactivity to form-aldehyde. Frosch and colleagues[44] found similar cross-sensitivity rates.

In cosmetics, Bronopol is found in concentra-tions of 0.01% to 1%. It is believed that prepara-tions containing less than 0.1% have minimal ability to cause ACD or ICD.[14,38,40] If used in concentrations greater than 1%, irritant dermatitis is common. Patch testing is generally accom-plished with concentrations of 0.5% in petro-latum.[38] The latest NACDG data showed a frequency of 2.3% positive reactions, which

was equal to that of DMDM hydantoin.[21] Evaluation of hand ACD only showed a frequency of 2.6% relevant positive reactions in North America.[12] It is also reported to be a clinically relevant antigen in pediatric contact dermatitis patients.[45]

DIMETHYLOLDIMETHYL HYDANTOIN

DMDM hydantoin, commercially known as Glydant, is a broad-spectrum biocide that was introduced in 1978.[38] After its introduction, DMDM hydantoin has become widely used and is found in a variety of cosmetics, moisturizers, sunscreens, topical medications[46] and other personal care products.[30,38] It is often used in rinse-off products, such as shampoos, body washes, and liquid hand soaps, because of its water solubility. These products may contain DMDM hydantoin in concentrations up to 1%.[47] DMDM hydantoin is also used in herbicides, cutting oils, paints, adhesives, copying paper, and inks.[38]

DMDM hydantoin is a formaldehyde releaser, and accordingly, can cause ACD in formalde-hyde-sensitive patients. De Groot and colleagues demonstrated that DM hydantoin, the formalde-hyde-releasing moiety, could cause patch test positivity in patients with formaldehyde allergy. Despite this, Uter and Frosch[46] evaluated patch test results from 67,915 European patients from 1994 to 2000 and found very few cross-sensitiv-ities between DMDM hydantoin and formalde-hyde, suggesting allergy that is independent of formaldehyde release.

Reported rates of sensitivity to DMDM hydan-toin are varied, likely based on geography and use patterns. Schnuch and colleagues[27] reported on patch test data from 11,485 European patients tested with preservative series. In this study, there was a very low rate of sensitization of 0.3% to DMDM hydantoin, tested in a concentration of 2% in petrolatum. Uter and Frosch[46] similarly demonstrated low levels of sensitivity in Europe. However, a study from the United States (NACDG Patch Test results, 2003–2004), showed a higher sensitivity rate of 2.3% when tested as 1% in petrolatum. For hand-only dermatitis, the NACDG reported a 4.7% rate of clinically relevant positive patch test to this chemical.[12] Very little information about occupational predilection has been pub-lished; however, Shaffer and Belsito[48] showed that health care workers were at slightly increased risk for allergy to DMDM hydantoin than non–health care workers (5.1% vs 3.6%). Patch testing for DMDM hydantoin is generally performed using concentrations of 1% in petrolatum in North America.[29]

METHYLDIBROMOGLUTARONITRILE/ PHENOXYETHANOL (MDGN/PE)

This preservative combination known as Euxyl K400 is a 1:4 mix of 1,2-dibromo-2,4-dicyanobutane and 2-phenoxyethanol. It is biostatic against bacteria, fungi, and yeasts at even low concentrations.[49] Euxyl K was first used in cosmetics and personal hygiene products, such as moist toilet paper and soaps, in the mid-1980s. It is also now used in a variety of other products including paper, latex paints, adhesives, and metalworking fluids.[17,23] For years, MDGN/PE has proven to be a significant contact sensitizer.[50] Warshaw and colleagues[12] found that MDGN/PE was related to hand dermatitis in approximately 6.3% of patients in North America, therefore making it 1 of the top 3 preservatives causing ACD of the hands. This is not surprising, given the wide variety of MDGN/PE-containing household products that contact the hands, such as liquid soaps and shampoos.[30] Of the MDGN/PE-sensitive patients in the aforementioned hand dermatitis study, 11.8% had hand dermatitis from occupational exposures, most commonly due to contact with solvents, oils, lubricants, fuels, and cosmetics.[12] MDGN-induced hand dermatitis may be quite robust and vesicular.[51] In addition to hand-only dermatitis, many MDGN-sensitive patients present with face and hand dermatitis, reflecting a pattern of cosmetic use.[27,51]

The most sensitizing component of Euxyl K400 appears to be MDGN, which also provides the main preservative activity.[38,52] MDGN is used in personal hygiene and cosmetic leave-on and rinse-off products in concentrations of up to 1000 ppm.[53] However, Pedersen and colleagues[53] demonstrated that the sensitivity threshold of some patients with MDGN allergy could be as low as 50 ppm in leave-on products. De Groot and Weyland[49] also reported that even concentrations as low as 0.001% could sensitize some patients. Therefore, even the lowest concentrations of Euxyl K400 may be allergenic in susceptible patients. Even rinse-off products containing MDGN may induce dermatitis. Jensen and colleagues[54] reported that 7 of 19 MDGN-sensitive patients developed positive reactions during repeated open application test of rinse-off MDGN-containing soaps (MDGN, 0.0999% and 0.0974%). A further complicating factor in rinse-off products is the fact that low concentrations used multiple times a day can be more sensitizing. Zachariae and colleagues[55] demonstrated that a daily exposure of 400 ppm is the same as 100 ppm applied 4 times a day. In Europe, because of sensitization concerns, MDGN has been banned from leave-on products, and in 2005, the European Scientific Committee for Cosmetic Products recommended eliminating it from rinse-off products.[56] These restrictions appear to already have resulted in decreasing incidence of clinically relevant allergy in the European Union.[57]

2-Phenoxyethanol (PE) alone is an uncommon sensitizer. It has rarely been implicated in hand dermatitis and contact urticaria.[12,58] Optimal concentration of MDGN/PE for patch testing is still debatable.[59] Tosti and colleagues[52] suggested that optimal patch test results for MDGN/PE are obtained at concentrations between 2% and 2.5% in petrolatum (at 2.5% the concentration of MDGN is 0.5%). In North America MDGN/PE is often tested at a concentration 2.5%.[21] Multiple investigators also recommended testing MDGN alone as 0.5 mg/cm^2 in petrolatum,[52,59,60] which is the current concentration provided on the European standard tray.[61]

METHYLCHLOROISOTHIAZOLINONE/ METHYLISOTHIAZOLINONE

Methylchloroisothiazolinone/methylisothiazolinone (MCI/MI) is an isothiazolinone mixture, namely 0.35% MI and 1.15% MCI in water with stabilizers. It is marketed under several names, including Kathon CG, Euxyl K100, and Amerstat 250. It has broad-spectrum activity at low concentrations against gram-positive and gram-negative bacteria as well as yeasts and fungi. MCI/MI is used both in industry (including paper mills, metalworking, jet fuels, and latex paint) and in consumer products (including shampoos, cosmetics, and moist wipes).[17,23]

After the introduction and use of MCI/MI in Europe in the 1980s, reports of allergy were of concern. Although some European studies found an initial prevalence of contact allergy to MCI/MI near 8%,[62,63] later studies in Europe and in the United States have found a prevalence of near 2% (1.8%, Marks and colleagues;[64] 2.3%, Pratt and colleagues (NACDG);[65] 2.0%–2.5%, Wilkinson and colleagues[66]). The NACDG reported decreasing prevalence of allergy, from 3.0% in study period from 1994 to 1996[65] to 2.2% in study period from 2003 to 2004.[21] Some speculate that the previously reported high rates of sensitization in Europe were because of exposure to higher concentrations of MCI/MI in products themselves and/or patch testing with 200 to 300 ppm MCI/MI. This is well above the accepted 100 ppm concentration for patch testing, and these elevated tested concentrations could have elicited false positives[17,23] or even sensitization.[67] With regard to hand-only ACD, NACDG data demonstrated a relevant positive patch test frequency of 4.1% when tested in a concentration of 100 ppm in aqueous solution.[12]

Because of elevated sensitization in Europe and widespread use of MCI/MI, restriction of its use as a preservative has been implemented. Japan allows its use only in rinse-off products, such as shampoos, and concentrations must remain at 15 ppm or less.[17] It is considered "safe with qualifications" by the Cosmetic Ingredient Review, with maximum standards of 15 ppm MCI/MI or less in rinse-off products and 7.5 ppm or less in leave-on products.[68] MCI/MI use has also been restricted to 15 ppm in cosmetics by the European Economic Community countries.[17] This is within the preservative's range of action, as MCI/MI continues to provide coverage in the concentration range of 3 to 15 ppm.[69] Occupational exposure remains of interest, as reports of sensitization and burns after exposure to MCI/MI have been reported.[70–74]

GLUTARALDEHYDE

Glutaraldehyde is a powerful biocide that may be found in sterilizing solutions, disinfectants, waterless hand soaps, fabric softeners, embalming fluids, cosmetics, paper slurry and radiograph developers.[39,75–77] It is active against a variety of bacteria, viruses, and fungi, including human immunodeficiency virus and *Mycobacterium tuberculosis*.[76] Glutaraldehyde is a known irritant and contact sensitizer, and it is a significant cause of allergic hand dermatitis.[12,48] In the NACDG hand dermatitis study, rates of clinically relevant positive patch tests of glutaraldehyde were similar to that of MCI/MI.[12] Studies suggest that glutaraldehyde is the most common occupational biocide causing ACD in health care workers,[75] and that these employees are at a significantly higher risk for glutaraldehyde sensitivity than those who are not health care workers.[48] Those working in dentistry are most often affected.[75,78] Of non–health care workers, janitorial staff are more likely to have glutaraldehyde sensitivity.[48] Because it is difficult to avoid in many health care jobs, occupational ACD secondary to glutaraldehyde tends to be chronic and unremitting.[48] Glutaraldehyde is also implicated in irritant and allergic occupational asthma.[79,80] Because of the occupational exposure risk, the National Institute for Occupational Safety and Health has released guidelines for safe working practices with glutaraldehyde.[81] They recommend the use of gloves and aprons made of nitrile or butyl rubber, as latex gloves are more easily penetrated by glutaraldehyde.[35,81] Goggles, face shields, local exhaust ventilation,

and fume hoods are also recommended.[81] These regulations have been placed to minimize exposure; however, it appears that even levels lower than recommended limits may result in allergic and irritant reactions.[80] Glutaraldehyde is often tested in concentrations of 0.5% aqueous or 1.0% in petrolatum.[9,21]

CHLOROXYLENOL (P-CHLORO-M-XYLENOL)

Chloroxylenol, also known as parachlorometaxylenol, is a biocide that is effective against bacteria, algae, and fungi. It is found in cleaning fluids used in medical facilities and institutions, and it is used as a preservative for paints, adhesives, and metal working fluids.[23,82] Additionally, hand washes, bar and liquid soaps/cleansers, skin disinfectants, and various topical medications may contain this biocide.[30,75,83] The NACDG reported that chloroxylenol was 1 of the top 4 preservatives causing ACD in health care workers.[75] Chloroxylenol is implicated also in ACD of the hands.[83] In the NACDG study of hand-only ACD, it was reported to have a relevant positive patch test frequency of 2.6%. Testing is often done as 1% in petrolatum, and it is found in the North American Contact Dermatitis Series.[61] Positive reactions often have high clinical relevance.[84]

PARABENS

"Paraben" is an abbreviation of para-hydroxybenzoic acid; "parabens" refers to a group of alkyl esters with substitutions at the para site of the hydroxybenzoic acid benzene ring.[13,85] Although 5 paraben esters are commonly used as preservatives in cosmetics and other topicals, the most prevalent are the methylparaben and propylparaben esters. Also used widely are the benzylparaben, ethylparaben, and butylparaben esters.[23] The antimicrobial properties of parabens are greater against fungi than bacteria, and are more effective against gram-positive than gram-negative bacteria, particularly *P. aeruginosa*.[23] Therefore, they are often combined with other preservatives, namely formaldehyde releasers, to increase the spectrum of coverage.[86] Because of parabens' low toxicity profile, low cost, antimicrobial activity, colorless and odorless properties, and stability in the range of pH of cosmetics,[23,85,87] they are used widely in makeup, medicaments, and various skin products.[88]

In a review of cosmetic ingredients, 87% to 93% cosmetic products contained at least 1 parabens preservative.[87,89] Despite the high prevalence of parabens in cosmetics and consumer products, allergy is relatively low. In the 2003 to 2004

NACDG patch-test results, 1.1% of 5142 subjects tested positive to paraben mix of 12% in petroleum.[21] Additionally, Schnuch and colleagues[27] reported that only 1.6% of subjects patch tested in their multicenter screening of over 28,000 individuals were reported to test positive to parabens. For hand ACD, the frequency of paraben allergy was reported as 1.3% in North America.[12]

Patients with paraben allergy may only react if the biocide in used on inflamed skin. Thus, clinically, paraben allergy may present as a dermatitis that fails to respond or that worsens in response to creams and topical medications. Fisher[90] first described this "paraben paradox" in 1973. He proposed that the parabens concentration in the products was too low to cause sensitization on normal skin. Further explanation has been provided by Cashman and Warshaw,[85] who suggest an "esterase hypothesis" and a "microbial metabolite hypothesis." In the former, disruption of the epidermis in dermatitic skin allows decreased short-chain ester processing by keratinocyte esterase and deeper penetration of all esters. This would support increased penetration of parabens, thus increased allergen exposure. In the microbial metabolite hypothesis, repeated application of parabens-containing products to compromised skin may encourage development of parabens-resistant microorganisms. These organisms may metabolize the parabens to hydroxybenzoic acid and subsequent remaining side chains, thus potentiating or even causing sensitization.[85]

Patch testing of parabens can be accomplished with different concentrations and formulations of the individual esters.[87] In the United States, a mixture of 4% each of methylparaben, ethylparaben, propylparaben, and butylparaben for a total concentration of 16% is routinely used in patch testing.[13] If parabens patch testing is positive, then each of the esters may be patch tested individually.[85]

IODOPROPYNYL BUTYLCARBAMATE

Iodopropynyl butylcarbamate (IPBC) is a preservative that has been used for years in the wood industry, and it has broad-spectrum activity against bacteria, fungi, and mites.[91] In 1996, formulations of up to 0.1% IPBC in topical products and cosmetics were approved by the Cosmetic Ingredient Review Expert Panel in the United States[92] with similar legislation passed in Europe.[93] Although IPBC is often found in cosmetics at a concentration of 0.0125% or less, it is not used in aerosolized products because of pulmonary toxicity in animal models.[94]

ACD to IPBC is rare. The data from the NACDG reported 24 positive results from patch testing 5137 patients.[21] A report from Bryld and colleagues[95] in 1997 reported 3 of 311 Danish patients patch tested positive to IPBC, with other data reporting 7 of 3168 patients testing positive. The Information Network of Departments of Dermatology (IVDK) in Germany reported 16 positive patch tests to IPBC in a group of 4883.[96] Although each of these groups patch tested IPBC in a 0.1% formulation in petroleum, some groups have recommended higher test concentrations. In the series from the IVDK, 43 doubtful reactions were reported, with concern that some of these may have been false negatives. Thus, the authors recommended consideration of a higher test concentration of IPBC.[96] Patch testing was subsequently performed using concentrations 0.1%, 0.2%, 0.3%, and 0.5% IPBC, and Brasch and colleagues[97] concluded that testing with 0.2% IPBC is superior to testing with a concentration of 0.1%, and testing with 0.2% rather than higher concentrations limits false-positive results. Therefore, 0.2% IPBC was recommended as the standard patch testing concentration. The NACDG has increased its IPBC patch testing concentration to 0.2% in petroleum.[23] Use of a higher concentration of IPBC in patch testing may capture false negatives previously missed.

IPBC remains a potential allergen in the workplace also. It functions as a biocide in wood products, paints and wallpaper,[23] as well as adhesives and textiles.[38] It is frequently found in metalworking fluids and cutting oils. Henriks-Eckerman and colleagues[98] found IPBC in 9 of 17 analyzed metalworking fluids. However, only 1 of 9 MSDSs reported IPBC as an ingredient. Although the highest concentration of IPBC detected in this analysis of metalworking fluids was 0.09%, IPBC is commonly used in industry in concentrations of 0.1% to 0.2%.[38] IPBC remains a potential consumer and occupational sensitizer and should be considered in the differential of hand dermatitis.

DISCUSSION

Hand dermatitis is a common problem encountered by physicians. For the patient it can cause emotional and physical discomfort and can interfere significantly with normal daily activities.[5,99] It also contributes to increased health care costs[4] and lost productivity.[6] Warshaw and colleagues[12] used data from the North American Contact Dermatitis Group to identify the common allergens inciting hand dermatitis. They found that preservatives/biocides accounted for the highest frequency of ACD, with Quaternium 15 being the most common sensitizer.[12]

Identifying the etiology of hand dermatitis can be difficult because it can arise as a result of multiple exogenous and endogenous causes, including irritant dermatitis, atopic dermatitis, and ACD.[2] The diagnosis of ACD can be straightforward if the area of inflammation corresponds exactly to the area contacted by the allergen and the patient makes a temporal association. However, when considering contact dermatitis to biocides and preservatives, this may not be the case. These products are routinely applied to the hands, primarily and as a means of applying the allergen-containing product diffusely to another area (eg, shampoo, body lotion). Therefore, the diagnosis and work-up may be more complicated. The clinician may be aided by noting patterns of dermatitis, which may suggest a biocide-containing product as a cause. For example, combined facial and hand dermatitis may suggest a cosmetic as the etiologic agent,[100] and hand dermatitis with concomitant perianal/genital dermatitis may implicate moist toilet paper containing a biocide, such as MCI/MI[101,102] and MDGN.[102]

Erythema, pruritic papules, and vesicles may characterize acute ACD. However, constant unknowing reexposure to the allergen can produce chronic ACD that most often manifests as lichenified pruritic plaques.[5] On the hands, this can often lead to chronically fissured and painful skin. This pattern is not specific, because it may also result from ICD and atopic dermatitis.[3] Some suggest that ACD hand dermatitis may favor the fingertips, dorsum of the hands and wrists, and less commonly involves the palms.[12] These patterns may be helpful, yet they are not diagnostic.[3] Identifying the cause of hand-predominant dermatitis may be further complicated by the existence of multiple diagnoses. For example, ICD often predisposes to and precedes ACD, and thus patients may experience both conditions concomitantly.[9,103] A new change in pattern of a stable dermatitis may be a clue that more than one condition is present and allergic contact dermatitis may be superimposed.[45,103] Because chronic ICD and ACD appear identical clinically and histologically, patch testing is important to help diagnose ACD and to begin to differentiate it from ICD.[10] A positive patch test must be carefully interpreted, because it should have clinical relevance to the patient's exposures.

Biocide sensitivity may result in other patterns of ACD. Many products containing biocides are designed to be applied to a widespread body area, thus it is not surprising that biocides can instigate dermatitis in a scattered generalized distribution (SGD). SGD is defined by the North American Contact Dermatitis Group as dermatitis affecting "more than 3 body sites" or "3 sites if the sites were trunk, arms, and legs."[104] The 3 most important biocides for SGD were Quaternium 15, formaldehyde, and MDGN/PE. Again, in widespread dermatitis cases, multiple etiologies may be present. Worsening (spreading to new areas) of noncontact dermatitis, such as localized atopic dermatitis and stasis dermatitis, may suggest a contact etiology.[45] In such a case, preservatives may be involved, because they are found in many of the topical medications and creams used to treat the original dermatitis.[105] In the uncommon case of intense sensitization, ACD may affect the entire integument (ie, erythroderma, exfoliative dermatitis, etc).[106] In these cases, the initial site of dermatitis often provides the best clue regarding the potential cause of ACD.[88]

Systemic contact allergic dermatitis may also result from ingestion, inhalation, or transdermal introduction of an allergen.[107] Clinically, systemic contact dermatitis can present as a flare of dermatitis at previously affected sites, widespread dermatitis, pompholyx, vasculitis, or intertriginous/flexural dermatitis.[108,109] The preservative methylparaben has been implicated in systemic contact dermatitis affecting a patient who ingested an oral mucolytic that contained methylparaben. Initial sensitization to parabens likely occurred from a topical paraben-containing cream in this patient.[110] Several other reports also identify parabens as a cause of systemic contact dermatitis.[111,112] Other preservatives reported to cause systemic contact dermatitis include sorbic acid,[113] thimerosol,[114,115] and phenoxyethanol.[23]

The mainstay of treatment for ACD is avoidance of the allergen.[116] By finding the suspect allergen, patch testing can improve a patient's quality of life by helping patients avoid these substances.[117] In addition, because careful avoidance of the allergen often results in clinical improvement, patch testing can also greatly reduce the cost of therapy for patients.[118] Many dermatologists perform patch testing using the commercially available TRUE test, which, in selected patients, can identify relevant allergies in as many as one-half of affected patients.[119] In many cases, however, more extensive patch testing is required with referral to a tertiary care, comprehensive patch testing center.[120] Patch testing to the patient's own suspected allergen source is often helpful in identifying and confirming the allergen that is responsible for hand eczema.[121] Patient education regarding avoidance of specific chemicals to which they are allergic, and education addressing compounds to which cross-reactions can occur is vital to the success of patch testing.

An important tool in avoidance is the Contact Allergen Replacement Database (CARD) of the American Contact Dermatitis Society, which allows physicians to tailor lists of products free of their allergens (and cross-reactors) for the patient.[122] The CARD is particularly useful in helping patients with ACD to preservatives to avoid their allergens, because these chemicals may not be listed on ingredient labels or may be referred to by alternate names. Another useful resource is the US Health and Human Services Household Product Database.[30]

Even if a clinically relevant allergen is found in a patient suffering from hand dermatitis, because coexisting ICD and ACD are common, one must not discount possible irritants as contributing factors. Patients should be educated on use of protective devices, such as gloves, because these can be important preventive and treatment measures.[123] Frequent emollient use also helps to repair irritant damaged skin barrier function.[124]

Topical corticosteroids are often used as an initial therapy for ACD of the hands.[103] It is important to use the CARD for its medicament index because some patients have been reported to be allergic to the active ingredients in topical corticosteroids whereas others have been reported to be allergic to vehicle chemicals, such as emulsifiers (sorbitan)[125] and preservatives (ie, formaldehyde releasers and parabens).[105] Prolonged topical steroid use should be avoided to decrease risk for skin atrophy and barrier dysfunction.[126] For recalcitrant cases, however, newer treatment modalities exist. Topical immunomodulators (TIMs), such as Tacrolimus (Protopic)[127,128] and Pimecrolimus (Elidel),[129] have been shown to be effective. ACD to the aforementioned TIMs has been reported both to the active and vehicle ingredients.[130–132] A wide range of systemic treatments, including phototherapy, systemic glucocorticoids, cyclosporine, and mycophenolate mofetil have been used for the treatment of chronic ACD recalcitrant to avoidance and first-line therapies. For more information, the reader is directed to the following resources.[103,121,133]

SUMMARY

Preservatives are low–molecular weight chemicals selected for their ability to prevent the overgrowth of bacteria and fungi in a wide range of products from cosmetics to cutting fluids. A large number of people have become sensitized by contact with these biocides and therefore are at risk for developing delayed-type hypersensitivity reactions on repeat exposure. This includes distressing and debilitating dermatitis of the hands. The prevalence of patients affected and the cost to society indicate a need for industry to follow published guidelines of safe use and continue further research to find the ideal preservative, which has high antimicrobial efficacy and low sensitizing potential. In addition, compulsory product ingredient labeling, accurate MSDS labeling, and disclosure of potential sensitizers would improve public education and potentially reduce exposure risk.

REFERENCES

1. Elston DM, Ahmed DDF, Watsky KL, et al. Hand dermatitis. J Am Acad Dermatol 2002;47(2): 291–9.
2. Veien NK, Hattel T, Laurberg G. Hand eczema: causes, course, and prognosis I. Contact Dermatitis 2008;58(6):330–4.
3. Diepgen TL, Andersen KE, Brandao FM, et al. Hand eczema classification: a cross-sectional, multicentre study of the aetiology and morphology of hand eczema. Br J Dermatol 2009;160(2):353–8.
4. Fowler JF, Ghosh A, Sung J, et al. Impact of chronic hand dermatitis on quality of life, work productivity, activity impairment, and medical costs. J Am Acad Dermatol 2006;54(3):448–57.
5. Diepgen TL, Coenraads PJ. The epidemiology of occupational contact dermatitis. Int Arch Occup Environ Health 1999;72(8):496–506.
6. Cvetkovski RS, Zachariae R, Jensen H, et al. Prognosis of occupational hand eczema: a follow-up study. Arch Dermatol 2006;142(3):305–11.
7. Flyvholm M-A, Lindberg M. OEESC-2005–summing up on the theme irritants and wet work. Contact Dermatitis 2006;55(6):317–21.
8. Skoet R, Olsen J, Mathiesen B, et al. A survey of occupational hand eczema in Denmark. Contact Dermatitis 2004;51(4):159–66.
9. Nettis E, Colanardi MC, Soccio AL, et al. Occupational irritant and allergic contact dermatitis among healthcare workers. Contact Dermatitis 2002;46(2): 101–7.
10. Rietschel R, Fowler J. Hand dermatitis due to contactants. In: Reitschel RL, Fowler JF, editors. Fisher's contact dermatitis. 6th edition. Hamilton (ON): BC Decker Inc; 2008. p. 319–37.
11. McDonnell G, Russell AD. Antiseptics and disinfectants: activity, action, and resistance. Clin Microbiol Rev 1999;12(1):147–79.
12. Warshaw EM, Ahmed RL, Belsito DV, et al. Contact dermatitis of the hands: cross-sectional analyses of North American Contact Dermatitis Group Data,

1994–2004. J Am Acad Dermatol 2007;57(2): 301–14.

13. Sasseville D. Hypersensitivity to preservatives. Dermatol Ther 2004;17(3):251–63.

14. Fransway AF. The problem of preservation in the 1990s. I. Statement of the problem, solution(s) of the industry, and the current use of formaldehyde and formaldehyde-releasing biocides. Am J Contact Dermat 1991;2(1):6–23.

15. Rietschel R, Fowler JF Jr. Pathogenesis of allergic contact hypersensitivity. In: Reitschel RL, Fowler JF, editors. Fisher's contact dermatitis. 6th edition. Hamilton (ON): BC Decker Inc.; 2008. p. 1–10.

16. Basketter DA, Clapp CJ, Safford BJ, et al. Preservatives and skin sensitization quantitative risk assessment. Dermatitis 2008;19(1):20–7.

17. Marks J, Elsner P, DeLeo V. Standard allergens. In: Elsner P, Marks JG, DeLeo VA, editors. Contact and occupational dermatology. St. Louis (MO): Mosby, Inc.; 2002. p. 65–139.

18. Geier J, Lessmann H, Hellriegel S, et al. Positive patch test reactions to formaldehyde releasers indicating contact allergy to formaldehyde. Contact Dermatitis 2008;58(3):175–7.

19. Flyvholm MA. Preservatives in registered chemical products. Contact Dermatitis 2005;53(1):27–32.

20. Aalto-Korte K, Kuuliala O, Suuronen K, et al. Occupational contact allergy to formaldehyde and formaldehyde releasers. Contact Dermatitis 2008;59(5): 280–9.

21. Warshaw EM, Belsito DV, DeLeo VA, et al. North American Contact Dermatitis Group patch-test results, 2003–2004 study period. Dermatitis 2008; 19(3):129–36.

22. Trattner A, Johansen JD, Menne T. Formaldehyde concentration in diagnostic patch testing: comparison of 1% with 2%. Contact Dermatitis 1998;38(1):9–13.

23. Rietschel RL, Fowler JL. Preservatives and vehicles in cosmetics and toiletries. In: Rietschel RL, Fowler JL, editors. Fisher's contact dermatitis. Hamilton (ON): BC Decker, Inc.; 2008. p. 266–318.

24. Herbert C, Rietschel RL. Formaldehyde and formaldehyde releasers: how much avoidance of cross-reacting agents is required? Contact Dermatitis 2004;50(6):371–3.

25. Fransway AF, Schmitz NA. The problem of preservation in the 1990s. II. Formaldehyde and formaldehyde releasing biocides: incidences of cross-reactivity and the significance of the positive response to formaldehyde. Am J Contact Dermat 1991;1991(2):78–88.

26. Agner T, Flyvholm MA, Menne T. Formaldehyde allergy: a follow-up study. Am J Contact Dermat 1999;10(1):12–7.

27. Schnuch A, Geier J, Uter W, et al. Patch testing with preservatives, antimicrobials and industrial biocides. Results from a multicentre study. Br J Dermatol 1998;138(3):467–76.

28. Parker LU, Taylor JT. A 5-year study of contact allergy to quaternium-15. Am J Contact Dermat 1991;2(4):231–4.

29. Rietschel RL, Warshaw EM, Sasseville D, et al. Sensitivity of petrolatum and aqueous vehicles for detecting allergy to imid azolidinylurea, diazolidinylurea, and DMDM hydantoin: a retrospective analysis from the North American Contact Dermatitis Group. Dermatitis 2007;18(3):155–62.

30. United States Department of Health and Human Services. Household products database. Available at: http://householdproducts.nlm.nih.gov/. Accessed November 8, 2008.

31. Dow Chemical Company. Dow biocides. Available at: http://www.dow.com/biocides/prod/dowicil.htm. Accessed December 4, 2008.

32. Hogeling M, Pratt M. Allergic contact dermatitis in children: the Ottawa hospital patch-testing clinic experience, 1996 to 2006. Dermatitis 2008;19(2):86–9.

33. Zug KA, McGinley-Smith D, Warshaw EM, et al. Contact allergy in children referred for patch testing: North American Contact Dermatitis Group data, 2001–2004. Arch Dermatol 2008;144(10): 1329–36.

34. Berke PA, Rosen W. Germall, a new family of antimicrobial preservatives for cosmetics. American Perfumer and Cosmetics 1970;85:55–9.

35. Jordan SL, Stowers MF, Trawick EG, et al. Glutaraldehyde permeation: choosing the proper glove. Am J Infect Control 1996;24(2):67–9.

36. Jong CT, Statham BN, Green CM, et al. Contact sensitivity to preservatives in the UK, 2004–2005: results of multicentre study. Contact Dermatitis 2007;57(3):165–8.

37. Hectorne KJ, Fransway AF. Diazolidinyl urea: incidence of sensitivity, patterns of cross-reactivity and clinical relevance. Contact Dermatitis 1994; 30(1):16–9.

38. Marks JG, EP, DeLeo VA. Preservatives and vehicles. In: Marks JG Jr, Elsner P, DeLeo VA, editors. Contact and occupational dermatology. St. Louis (MO): Mosby, Inc.; 2002. p. 140–71.

39. BASF Chemical. Paper industry biocides. Available at: http://www2.basf.us/biocides/pdfs/PIB_Brochure. pdf. Accessed January 20, 2009.

40. Peters MS, Connolly SM, Schroeter AL. Bronopol allergic contact dermatitis. Contact Dermatitis 1983;9(5):397–401.

41. Choudry K, Beck MH, Muston HL. Allergic contact dermatitis from 2-bromo-2-nitropropane-1,3-diol in metrogel. Contact Dermatitis 2002;46(1):60–1.

42. Specialized Information Services, National Library of Medicine, National Institutes of Health, U.S. Department of Health and Human Services. Hazmap occupational health database. Available at:

http://www.hazmap.nlm.nih.gov. Accessed December 10, 2008.

43. Podmore P. Occupational allergic contact dermatitis from both 2-bromo-2-nitropropane-1,3-diol and methylchloroisothiazolinone plus methylisothiazolinone in spin finish. Contact Dermatitis 2000;43(1):45.

44. Frosch PJ, White IR, Rycroft RJ, et al. Contact allergy to bronopol. Contact Dermatitis 1990; 22(1):24–6.

45. Jacob SE, Burk CJ, Connelly EA. Patch testing: another steroid-sparing agent to consider in children. Pediatr Dermatol 2008;25(1):81–7.

46. Uter W, Frosch PJ. Contact allergy from DMDM hydantoin, 1994–2000. Contact Dermatitis 2002; 47(1):57–8.

47. de Groot AC, van Joost T, Bos JD, et al. Patch test reactivity to DMDM hydantoin. Relationship to formaldehyde allergy. Contact Dermatitis 1988;18(4): 197–201.

48. Shaffer MP, Belsito DV. Allergic contact dermatitis from glutaraldehyde in health-care workers. Contact Dermatitis 2000;43(3):150–6.

49. de Groot A, Weyland JW. Contact allergy to methyldibromoglutaronitrile in the cosmetics preservative Euxyl K 400. Am J Contact Dermat 1991;2(1): 31–2.

50. Gruvberger B, Andersen KE, Brando FM, et al. Patch testing with methyldibromo glutaronitrile, a multicentre study within the EECDRG. Contact Dermatitis 2005;52(1):14–8.

51. Zachariae C, Rastogi S, Devantier C, et al. Methyldibromo glutaronitrile: clinical experience and exposure-based risk assessment. Contact Dermatitis 2003;48(3):150–4.

52. Tosti A, Vincenzi C, Trevisi P, et al. Euxyl K 400: incidence of sensitization, patch test concentration and vehicle. Contact Dermatitis 1995;33(3):193–5.

53. Kynemund Pedersen L, Agner T, Held E, et al. Methyldibromoglutaronitrile in leave-on products elicits contact allergy at low concentration. Br J Dermatol 2004;151(4):817–22.

54. Jensen CD, Johansen JD, Menna T, et al. Methyldibromoglutaronitrile in rinse-off products causes allergic contact dermatitis: an experimental study. Br J Dermatol 2004;150(1):90–5.

55. Zachariae C, Johansen JD, Rastogi SC, et al. Allergic contact dermatitis from methyldibromo glutaronitrile–clinical cases from 2003. Contact Dermatitis 2005;52(1):6–8.

56. Jong CT, Statham BN. Methyldibromoglutaronitrile contact allergy–the beginning of the end? Contact Dermatitis 2006;54(4):229.

57. Johansen JD, Veien N, Laurberg G, et al. Decreasing trends in methyldibromo glutaronitrile contact allergy–following regulatory intervention. Contact Dermatitis 2008;59(1):48–51.

58. Birnie AJ, English JS. 2-phenoxyethanol-induced contact urticaria. Contact Dermatitis 2006;54(6): 349.

59. Schnuch A, Kelterer D, Bauer A, et al. Quantitative patch and repeated open application testing in methyldibromo glutaronitrile-sensitive patients. Contact Dermatitis 2005;52(4):197–206.

60. Bruze M, Gruvberger B, Goossens A, et al. Allergic contact dermatitis from methyldibromoglutaronitrile. Dermatitis 2005;16(2):80–6, quiz: 55–6.

61. Dormer Laboratories. Available at: http://www. dormer.com. Accessed June 17, 2009.

62. de Groot AC. Methylisothiazolinone/methylchloroisothiazolinone (Kathon CG) allergy: an update review. Am J Contact Dermat 1990;1:151–6.

63. Tosti A. Prevalence and sources of Kathon CG sensitization in Italy. Contact Dermatitis 1988; 18(3):173–4.

64. Marks JG Jr, Moss JN, Parno JR, et al. Methylchloro-isothiazolinone/methylisothiazolinone (Kathon CG) biocide: second United States multicenter study of human skin sensitization. Am J Contact Dermat 1993;4:87–9.

65. Pratt MD, Belsito DV, DeLeo VA, et al. North American Contact Dermatitis Group patch-test results, 2001–2002 study period. Dermatitis 2004;15(4): 176–83.

66. Wilkinson JD, Shaw S, Andersen KE, et al. Monitoring levels of preservative sensitivity in Europe. A 10-year overview (1991–2000). Contact Dermatitis 2002;46(4):207–10.

67. Bjorkner B, Bruze M, Dahlquist I, et al. Contact allergy to the preservative Kathon CG. Contact Dermatitis 1986;14(2):85–90.

68. Cosmetic Ingredient Review (CIR). J Am Coll Toxicol 1992;11(1):75–128.

69. Cohen DE, Brancaccio RR. What is new in clinical research in contact dermatitis. Dermatol Clin 1997;15(1):137–48.

70. Isaksson M, Gruvberger B, Bruze M. Occupational contact allergy and dermatitis from methylisothiazolinone after contact with wallcovering glue and after a chemical burn from a biocide. Dermatitis 2004;15(4):201–5.

71. Nethercott JR, Rothman N, Holness DL, et al. Health problems in metalworkers exposed to a coolant oil containing Kathon 886 MW. Am J Contact Dermat 1990;1:94–9.

72. Madden SD, Thiboutot DM, Marks JG Jr. Occupationally induced allergic contact dermatitis to methylchloroisothiazolinone/methylisothiazolinone among machinists. J Am Acad Dermatol 1994; 30(2 Pt 1):272–4.

73. Kanerva L, Tarvainen K, Pinola A, et al. A single accidental exposure may result in a chemical burn, primary sensitization and allergic contact dermatitis. Contact Dermatitis 1994;31(4):229–35.

74. Primka EJ 3rd, Taylor JS. Three cases of contact allergy after chemical burns from methylchloroisothiazolinone/methylisothiazolinone: one with concomitant allergy to methyldibromoglutaronitrile/phenoxyethanol. Am J Contact Dermat 1997; 8(1):43–6.

75. Warshaw EM, Schram SE, Maibach HI, et al. Occupation-related contact dermatitis in North American health care workers referred for patch testing: cross-sectional data, 1998 to 2004. Dermatitis 2008;19(5):261–74.

76. Abbott L. The use and effects of glutaraldehyde: a review. Occup Health (Lond) 1995;47(7):238–9.

77. Weaver JE, Maibach HI. Dose response relationships in allergic contact dermatitis: glutaraldehyde-containing liquid fabric softener. Contact Dermatitis 1977;3(2):65–8.

78. Suneja T, Belsito DV. Occupational dermatoses in health care workers evaluated for suspected allergic contact dermatitis. Contact Dermatitis 2008;58(5):285–90.

79. Rideout K, Teschke K, Dimich-Ward H, et al. Considering risks to healthcare workers from glutaraldehyde alternatives in high-level disinfection. J Hosp Infect 2005;59(1):4–11.

80. Burge PS. Occupational risks of glutaraldehyde [letter]. BMJ 1989;299(6695):342.

81. National Institute for Occupational Safety and Health. Department of Health and Human Services. Centers for Disease Control and Prevention, Glutaraldehyde. Occupational hazards in hospitals. Available at: http://www.cdc.gov/niosh/docs/2001-115/. Accessed June 16, 2009.

82. United States Environmental Protection Agency. Prevention pesticides and toxic substances. R.E.D. Facts: chloroxylenolol. EPA-738-94-028. Available at: http://epa.gov/oppsrrd1/REDs/factsheets/3045fact.pdf. Accessed December 11, 2008.

83. Wilson M, Mowad C. Chloroxylenol. Dermatitis 2007;18(2):120–1.

84. Mowad C. Chloroxylenol causing hand dermatitis in a plumber. Am J Contact Dermat 1998;9(2):128–9.

85. Cashman AL, Warshaw EM. Parabens: a review of epidemiology, structure, allergenicity, and hormonal properties. Dermatitis 2005;16(2):57–66, quiz: 55–6.

86. Fisher AA. Cosmetic dermatitis. Part II. Reactions to some commonly used preservatives. Cutis 1980;26(2):136–7, 141–2, 147–8.

87. Rastogi SC, Schouten A, de Kruijf N, et al. Contents of methyl-, ethyl-, propyl-, butyl- and benzylparaben in cosmetic products. Contact Dermatitis 1995;32(1):28–30.

88. Biebl KA, Warshaw EM. Allergic contact dermatitis to cosmetics. Dermatol Clin 2006;24(2):215–32, vii.

89. Rastogi SC. Analytical control of preservative labelling on skin creams. Contact Dermatitis 2000;43(6):339–43.

90. Fisher AA. The paraben paradoxes. Cutis 1973;12:830–2.

91. Rossmore H. Handbook of biocide and preservative use. Glasgow (UK): Blackie Academic and Professional; 1995.

92. Bergfield W, Belsito DV, Carlton WW, et al. A final report approved by the expert panel of the cosmetic ingredient review: iodopropynyl butycarbamate (IPBC) 1996; Washington, DC.

93. EU Commission, Cosmetics Directive 95/34/EF and 96/41/EF. Milieu og Energiministeries 1996: 805(1). Available at: http://ec.europa.eu/enterprise/cosmetics/html/cosm_judgements.htm. Accessed June 16, 2009.

94. Final report on the safety assessment of iodopropynyl butylcarbamate (IPBC). Int J Toxicol 1998; 6(S5):1–37.

95. Bryld LE, Agner T, Menne T. Allergic contact dermatitis from 3-iodo-2-propynyl-butylcarbamate (IPBC)—an update. Contact Dermatitis 2001; 44(5):276–8.

96. Schnuch A, Geier J, Brasch J, et al. The preservative iodopropynyl butylcarbamate: frequency of allergic reactions and diagnostic considerations. Contact Dermatitis 2002;46(3):153–6.

97. Brasch J, Schnuch A, Geier J, et al. Iodopropynyl-butyl carbamate 0.2% is suggested for patch testing of patients with eczema possibly related to preservatives. Br J Dermatol 2004;151(3):608–15.

98. Henriks-Eckerman ML, Suuronen K, Jolanki R. Analysis of allergens in metalworking fluids. Contact Dermatitis 2008;59(5):261–7.

99. Agner T, Andersen KE, Brandao FM, et al. Hand eczema severity and quality of life: a cross-sectional, multicentre study of hand eczema patients. Contact Dermatitis 2008;59(1):43–7.

100. Jacobs MC, White IR, Rycroft RJ, et al. Patch testing with preservatives at St John's from 1982 to 1993. Contact Dermatitis 1995;33(4):247–54.

101. Timmermans A, De Hertog S, Gladys K, et al. 'Dermatologically tested' baby toilet tissues: a cause of allergic contact dermatitis in adults. Contact Dermatitis 2007;57(2):97–9.

102. de Groot AC. Vesicular dermatitis of the hands secondary to perianal allergic contact dermatitis caused by preservatives in moistened toilet tissues. Contact Dermatitis 1997;36(3):173–4.

103. Warshaw E, Lee G, Storrs FJ. Hand dermatitis: a review of clinical features, therapeutic options, and long-term outcomes. Am J Contact Dermat 2003;14(3):119–37.

104. Zug KA, Rietschel RL, Warshaw EM, et al. The value of patch testing patients with a scattered generalized distribution of dermatitis: retrospective cross-sectional analyses of North American Contact Dermatitis Group data, 2001 to 2004. J Am Acad Dermatol 2008;59(3):426–31.

105. Coloe J, Zirwas MJ. Allergens in corticosteroid vehicles. Dermatitis 2008;19(1):38–42.

106. Encarnacion LA, Celis-Versoza M. Contact allergy presenting as erythroderma. Dermatitis 2006; 17(1):45–7.

107. Jacob SE, Zapolanski T. Systemic contact dermatitis. Dermatitis 2008;19(1):9–15.

108. Thyssen JP, Maibach HI. Drug-elicited systemic allergic (contact) dermatitis—update and possible pathomechanisms. Contact Dermatitis 2008;59(4): 195–202.

109. Veien N, Menne T. Systemic contact dermatitis. In: Frosch P, Menne T, Lepoittevin J-P, editors. Contact dermatitis. Washington, DC: Birkhauser; 2006. p. 295–307.

110. Sánchez-Pérez J, Ballesteros Diez M, Alonso Pérez A, et al. Allergic and systemic contact dermatitis to methylparaben. Contact Dermatitis 2006;54(2):117–8.

111. Carradori S, Peluso AM, Faccioli M. Systemic contact dermatitis due to parabens. Contact Dermatitis 1990;22(4):238–9.

112. Aeling JL, Nuss DD. Letter: systemic eczematous "contact-type" dermatitis medicamentosa caused by parabens. Arch Dermatol 1974;110(4):640.

113. Raison-Peyron N, Meynadier JM, Meynadier J. Sorbic acid: an unusual cause of systemic contact dermatitis in an infant. Contact Dermatitis 2000;43(4):247–8.

114. Tosti A, Melino M, Bardazzi F. Systemic reactions due to thiomersal. Contact Dermatitis 1986;15(3):187–8.

115. Zenarola P, Gimma A, Lomuto M. Systemic contact dermatitis from thimerosal. Contact Dermatitis 1995;32(2):107–8.

116. Hogan DJ. The prognosis of occupational contact dermatitis. Occup Med 1994;9(1):53–8.

117. Woo PN, Hay IC, Ormerod AD. An audit of the value of patch testing and its effect on quality of life. Contact Dermatitis 2003;48(5):244–7.

118. Rajagopalan R, Anderson RT, Sarma S, et al. An economic evaluation of patch testing in the diagnosis and management of allergic contact dermatitis. Am J Contact Dermat 1998;9(3):149–54.

119. Militello G, Woo DK, Kantor J, et al. The utility of the TRUE test in a private practice setting. Dermatitis 2006;17(2):77–84.

120. Jacob SE, Steele T. Contact dermatitis and workforce economics. Semin Cutan Med Surg 2006; 25(2):105–9.

121. Diepgen TL, Agner T, Aberer W, et al. Management of chronic hand eczema. Contact Dermatitis 2007; 57(4):203–10.

122. Caperton C, Jacob SE. Improving post-patch-test education with the contact allergen replacement database. Dermatitis 2007;18(2):101–2.

123. Kwon S, Campbell LS, Zirwas MJ. Role of protective gloves in the causation and treatment of occupational irritant contact dermatitis. J Am Acad Dermatol 2006;55(5):891–6.

124. Yokota M, Maibach HI. Moisturizer effect on irritant dermatitis: an overview. Contact Dermatitis 2006; 55(2):65–72.

125. Castanedo-Tardan MP, Jacob SE. Allergic contact dermatitis to sorbitan sesquioleate in children. Contact Dermatitis 2008;58(3):171–2.

126. Kao JS, Fluhr JW, Man MQ, et al. Short-term glucocorticoid treatment compromises both permeability barrier homeostasis and stratum corneum integrity: inhibition of epidermal lipid synthesis accounts for functional abnormalities. J Invest Dermatol 2003; 120(3):456–64.

127. Pacor ML, Di Lorenzo G, Martinelli N, et al. Tacrolimus ointment in nickel sulphate-induced steroid-resistant allergic contact dermatitis. Allergy Asthma Proc 2006;27(6):527–31.

128. Saripalli YV, Gadzia JE, Belsito DV. Tacrolimus ointment 0.1% in the treatment of nickel-induced allergic contact dermatitis. J Am Acad Dermatol 2003;49(3):477–82.

129. Queille-Roussel C, Graeber M, Thurston M, et al. SDZ ASM 981 is the first non-steroid that suppresses established nickel contact dermatitis elicited by allergen challenge. Contact Dermatitis 2000;42(6):349–50.

130. Andersen KE, Broesby-Olsen S. Allergic contact dermatitis from oleyl alcohol in Elidel cream. Contact Dermatitis 2006;55(6):354–6.

131. Saitta P, Brancaccio R. Allergic contact dermatitis to pimecrolimus. Contact Dermatitis 2007;56(1): 43–4.

132. Shaw DW, Maibach HI, Eichenfield LF. Allergic contact dermatitis from pimecrolimus in a patient with tacrolimus allergy. J Am Acad Dermatol 2007;56(2):342–5.

133. Jacob SE, Castanedo-Tardan MP. Pharmacotherapy for allergic contact dermatitis. Expert Opin Pharmacother 2007;8(16):2757–74.

Patterns of Cosmetic Contact Allergy

Mari Paz Castanedo-Tardan, MD, Kathryn A. Zug, MD*

KEYWORDS

- Contact dermatitis • Cosmetic • Toiletries
- Personal care product • Facial • Eyelid • Neck • Cheilitis

The use of toiletries is a long-standing practice that extends worldwide and reaches virtually one and all. Practically everyone uses some form of toiletry in daily life, from common items, such as soap, toothpaste, or deodorant, to elaborate facial cosmetics and glamorous fragrances. It has been estimated that approximately 800 raw materials, vehicles, and fragrance ingredients are used in making toiletries,[1] and although most ingredients are safe to use by the majority of consumers, a significant minority of people experience adverse reactions to personal care products.[2]

In the United States, toiletries regulation falls under the governance of the Food and Drug Administration (FDA), which defines the term "cosmetic" as "articles intended to be rubbed, poured, sprinkled, sprayed on, introduced into, or otherwise applied to the human body...for cleansing, beautifying, promoting attractiveness, or altering the appearance."[3] Among the products included in this definition are skin moisturizers, perfumes, lipsticks, fingernail polishes, eye and facial makeup, shampoos, permanent waves, hair colors, toothpastes, and deodorants, as well as any material intended for use as a component of a cosmetic product—with the interesting exception of soap, which is legislated as a separate category. (In this article, the terms cosmetic, toiletry, and personal care product will be used interchangeably).

ADVERSE REACTIONS TO COSMETICS

Cosmetics are widely used, and yet, given the massive volume of sales and the range of product availability, there is remarkably little information on the exact incidence and prevalence of their detrimental effects.[4] Potential adverse reactions to cosmetics comprise a broad spectrum of cutaneous reactions that include irritant reactions, delayed-type hypersensitivity, contact urticaria, photosensitization (phototoxic or photoallergic), pigmentary disorders, damage of hair and nails, paronychia, acneiform eruptions, folliculitis, and worsening of preexisting dermatoses.[5]

The exact frequency of adverse reactions to toiletries in the general population is difficult to estimate,[6] mainly because most people who experience such reactions seldom consult a physician and simply discontinue using the product suspected of triggering the reaction.[7] (In an Italian poll published in 2006, more than 50% of the people who experienced an adverse reaction to a cosmetic did not seek medical advice.)[8] A recent survey of a non-selected population in the United Kingdom revealed that 23% of women and 13.8% of men experience some sort of adverse reaction to a personal care product over the course of a year, with an increase in overall rates of 51.4% and 38.2% over a lifetime.[9] Although they are quite common, only a minority of adverse reactions to cosmetics in the general population have been shown to be allergic in origin[10–12] highlighting that despite the widespread use of personal care products, the rates of allergic reactions to their ingredients are relatively low. Several studies in Europe and the United States have found a prevalence rate of cosmetic allergy of less than 1% among the general population.[1,13–19]

When looking at selected patients seen by a dermatologist and referred for patch testing for suspected allergic contact dermatitis (ACD), the

Department of Medicine, Section of Dermatology, Dartmouth-Hitchcock Medical Center, 1 Medical Center Drive, Lebanon, NH 03756, USA
* Corresponding author.
E-mail address: Kzug@hitchcock.org (K.A. Zug).

Dermatol Clin 27 (2009) 265–280
doi:10.1016/j.det.2009.05.014

prevalence rates of cosmetic allergy vary significantly from those seen in the general population and range from 2.4% to 36.3%, with most studies reporting prevalence rates between 4% and 9%.[1,13–16,19,20] In a 2006 review of ACD to cosmetics, Biebl and Warshaw[28] identified a weighted prevalence rate of 0.4% for the general population and 9.8% for patients referred for patch testing.

In the latest and largest US-based study of selected patients with suspected ACD, the North American Contact Dermatitis Group (NACDG) patch tested a total of 10,061 patients (6621 females and 3440 males) over a period of 7 years.[21] From the total of patients studied, 1582 females (23.8%) and 611 males (17.8%) had at least 1 allergic patch test reaction associated with a cosmetic source. Although slightly higher than the figures found by Biebl and Warshaw, the numbers are consistent with most major reviews. This and other studies also identified, not surprisingly, that the population most affected with cosmetic sensitivity are females[14–16,22] between 20 to 55 years of age.[1,13–15]

Most adverse reactions to cosmetics are irritant in nature, which can be further subdivided into subjective and objective reactions. Subjective irritation consists of the sensation of burning or stinging without visual changes, associated with the application of cosmetics.[5,23] Although most often patients do not seek medical attention for such reactions, they are believed to be the most common source of dissatisfaction with cosmetics.[20] Objective irritation, on the other hand, is defined as nonimmunologically mediated skin inflammation with visible skin changes.[20] The development of delayed type sensitization and ACD to cosmetics is less common,[12,24] and depends on several factors that include the product composition and concentration of potentially allergenic ingredients, the inherent sensitizing potential of an allergen, the application site, the amount of product applied, the frequency and duration of the exposure, the presence of penetration-enhancing factors, and finally the integrity of the skin barrier function.[25–27] Sensitization often occurs after repeated applications or application to damaged skin.[28]

When considering ACD to cosmetics, reactions can be classified according to the body region affected (site of dermatitis) and the likely allergens encountered at such region; or by the type of cosmetics (ie, eye cosmetics, nail cosmetics, hair cosmetics) and the possible allergens contained within.[12] Most of the available literature approaches the topic by type of cosmetic; in an attempt to provide a broader perspective, this article overviews ACD to cosmetics with a combined approach, but with special focus on the patterns of dermatitis that cosmetics might incite, followed by a brief description of the potential culprit allergens.

PATTERNS OF ALLERGIC CONTACT DERMATITIS CAUSED BY PERSONAL CARE PRODUCTS

Cosmetic contact allergy manifests when an offending allergen is directly applied, airborne, or transferred (often from the hands). The sites most commonly involved in cosmetic contact allergy include the face, eyelids, lips, and neck.

FACIAL DERMATITIS

The face is a common site for ACD. Schnuch and colleagues analyzed the data of 18,572 patients patch tested in the Information Network of Departments of Dermatology (IVDK) between 1995 and 2007, and found that the face was the main anatomic site involved.[29] Among patients with facial dermatitis, females were more predominant than men, and were most commonly affected by cosmetic-associated allergens such as fragrance mix (10.8% vs 8.3%), paraphenylenediamine (PPD) (4.0% vs 2.8%), lanolin alcohols (3.0% vs 2.2%), and Lyral (3.1% vs 2.0%).[29]

Allergens can be transferred to the face not only by direct contact but also indirectly from airborne or hand-to-face exposure. Facial cosmetic dermatitis is bilateral; however, even when a product is directly applied to the whole face, eczematous manifestations are often patchy, and therefore contact dermatitis might not be suspected because the involvement is not of the whole face. In addition to allergens found as ingredients in cosmetics, products used to apply them, such as cosmetic sponges, are reported to produce facial dermatitis in patients sensitive to rubber.[30] A similar situation is seen with nickel-plated objects used on the hair, such as bobby pins and curlers that may produce scalp and facial dermatitis in patients sensitive to nickel.[31]

Allergens applied to the scalp most often produce "run-off" patterns of dermatitis on the forehead and lateral face, eyelids, ears, neck, and hands, whereas the scalp remains uninvolved, suggesting that the scalp is particularly resistant to contact dermatitis.[31] Nevertheless, patients exquisitely sensitive to hair preparations such as PPD or glyceryl thioglycolate may show a marked scalp reaction with edema and crusting. PPD is 1 of the most potent sensitizers known and is widely used as an ingredient in hair dyes. PPD sensitization manifests on the face and scalp of female adult patients who had contact with a hair dye.[32–35] In a small Brazilian study, Duarte and colleagues[32] identified that in patients with positive patch test reactions to PPD (mostly females between 41 and 60 years of age), 70% had face or scalp involvement, and 48% had hair dye as the agent responsible for the sensitization.

EYELID DERMATITIS

The eyelids are one of the most sensitive skin areas, and they are highly susceptible to irritants and allergens. This does not mean that every case of eyelid dermatitis is allergic or irritant in origin, and other diagnoses, such as seborrheic dermatitis, atopic dermatitis, psoriasis, and nonspecific xerosis, should also be considered.[36] The particular vulnerability of eyelids to contactants might be because of the thinness of the eyelid skin, 0.55 mm, as compared to the rest of the facial skin, measuring approximately 2.0 mm.[31] Transfer of small amounts of allergens used on the scalp, face, or hands might be enough to cause an eczematous reaction of the eyelids, whereas the primary sites of contact remain unaltered. Volatile agents may affect the eyelids first and exclusively, causing airborne eyelid contact dermatitis.

Cosmetic sources of contact dermatitis of the eyelids include mascara, eye liners and eye shadows, adhesive in fake eyelashes, and nickel and rubber in eyelash curlers. Furthermore, marked edema of the eyelids is often a feature of hair dye dermatitis. Eyelids are also characterized for being a typical site for "ectopic contact dermatitis." Alexander A. Fisher coined this concept to describe the dermatitis caused by nail lacquer, since the allergic reaction does not occur in the periungual area, but on "ectopic" areas where fingernails touch, particularly the eyelids but also the neck, lips, and face.[37]

In 2007, the NACDG published the results of 5145 patients routinely tested with a 65-allergen screening series over a 2-year study period (2003–2004).[38] In 5.2% (n = 268) of the patients studied, eyelid dermatitis was the sole site of involvement and ACD was the final diagnosis of the cause of the dermatitis. Sixty-five percent of the cases were caused by 1 of 26 clinically relevant contact allergens identified in the study. The NACDG suggested in conclusion that these top 26 allergens would constitute "a potential screening series for the evaluation of patients with eyelid dermatitis, without other areas of involvement" (**Box 1**). This list includes mostly allergens found as ingredients in cosmetics, but

---

Box 1
NACDG suggested screening series for the evaluation of patients with only eyelid dermatitis

Allergen

1. Gold sodium thiosulfate 0.5% pet
2. Fragrance mix I 8% pet
3. *Myroxylon pereirae* (balsam of Peru [BOP]) 25% pet
4. Nickel sulfate 2.5% pet
5. Neomycin 20% pet
6. Methyldibromo glutaronitrile 2% pet
7. Quaternium-15 2% pet
8. Methylchloroisothiazolinone/methylisothiazolinone (MCI/MI) 100 ppm aq
9. Cobalt chloride 1% pet
10. 3'-Demethoxy-3o-Demethylmatairesinol (DMDM) hydantoin 1% aq
11. Amidoamine 0.1% aq
12. Cocamidopropyl betaine (CABP) 1% aq
13. Thiuram mix 1% pet
14. Bacitracin 20% pet
15. Cinnamic aldehyde 1% pet
16. d-α-Tocopherol acetate 100%
17. Tosylamide formaldehyde resin (TSFR) 10% pet
18. Propylene glycol 30% aq
19. Tixocortol pivalate 1% pet
20. Formaldehyde 1% aq
21. Colophony 20% pet
22. Ylang ylang oil 2% pet
23. Lanolin 30% pet
24. Ethyl acrylate 0.1% pet
25. Methyl methacrylate 2% pet
26. Budesonide 0.1% pet

Abbreviations: aq, aqueous; pet, petrolatum; ppm, parts per million.

Data from Rietschel RL, Warshaw EM, Sasseville D, et al. Common contact allergens associated with eyelid dermatitis: Data from the North American Contact Dermatitis Group 2003–2004 study period. Dermatitis 2007;18(2):78–81.

---

also topical antibiotics and certain metals such as gold. An interesting feature of gold allergy is the propensity for facial and eyelid dermatitis to occur.[39] In the NACDG analysis, gold was the most common allergen that accounted for pure eyelid dermatitis. It has been observed that upon contact with hard particles such as titanium dioxide (which is used to opacify facial cosmetics and is used in sunscreens as a physical blocker of ultraviolet [UV] light), gold found in jewelry may abrade, encouraging the release of gold particles that can then make occasional contact with facial and eyelid skin, causing dermatitis.[40] Aside from gold, fragrances and preservatives have been found to be the main cosmetic allergens to cause pure eyelid dermatitis in NACDG and other series.[38,41]

NECK DERMATITIS

The neck is also a highly reactive site for ACD. Cosmetics applied to the face, scalp, or hair often initially affect the neck.[31] Nail polish is also a common culprit in this region. Lazzarini and colleagues recently studied ACD from nail varnish according to the site of dermatitis and found that the most affected sites were the face and neck. Toluenesulfonamide formaldehyde resin, presently tosylamide formaldehyde resin (TSFR), the chemical added to nail polish to facilitate adhesion to the nail, was the most common allergen in the group studied.[42] Furthermore, as a cultural practice, perfumes are sprayed on the neck. In fragrance-sensitized people, this practice of repeated application of fragrances to the anterior neck may result in the appearance of a dermatitic plaque in that particular region, which has been coined the "atomizer sign."[43] Such a sign can be a particularly useful clue to the diagnosis of fragrance-based ACD, and its recognition may allow for early initial therapeutic intervention, notably fragrance avoidance.

ALLERGIC CONTACT CHEILITIS

Cheilitis is an inflammatory condition of the lips that can manifest as itching, burning, dryness, erythema, fissuring, crusting, and edema.[44] The factors contributing to this condition may be endogenous to the individual, like an atopic diathesis; exogenous to the individual, like allergens and irritants; or a combination of both.[45]

Allergic contact cheilitis (ACC) has been reported to result from the use of a wide array of products, including foods, metals, and cosmetics (such as lip balms, lipsticks, lip glosses, moisturizers, sunscreens, nail products, and oral hygiene products [mouthwashes, toothpastes, and dental floss]).[46,47]

A notable feature among patients with cheilitis is the evident female predominance, with most studies reporting a range of 70.7% to 90% female patients.[48–50] In a recent Greek study, Katsarou and colleagues studied a group of 106 patients with eczematous cheilitis of whom 75.5% (n = 80) were females.[51] Similarly, of 10,061 patients patch tested from 2001 to 2004 by the NACDG, 196 (2%) patients had lips as the sole involvement site, and females accounted for 84.2% of the cheilitis population.[45] (This is likely explained by the assumption that women wear more cosmetics and lip products than men do).

Approximately one-third of the patients with cheilitis are typically found to have an allergen as a contributing factor.[48,49] In accordance with this trend, 38.3% (n =75) of the 196 patients studied for cheilitis by the NACDG, were diagnosed with ACC after patch testing. Most of the studies on cheilitis have reported fragrance mix as the most common cause of allergy in patients who were patch tested.[48,49,52] In the NACDG cheilitis study, fragrance mix was the most common allergen identified, followed by *Myroxylon Pereirae* (balsam of Peru [BOP]) and nickel (**Box 2**). Overall, the most common sources for the top allergens causing ACC are cosmetics (including lip products).[45,48,49,52] Sources for nickel might include jewelry (causing ectopic dermatitis), metal lipsticks casings, or habitual sucking of metallic objects.[51]

An interesting contrast to the general patch test population is that patients with only lip involvement have few patch test reactions to preservatives. This might be as a result of the innate formulation of lip products, which are mostly waxy, water-free

---

Box 2
Top 18 clinically relevant allergens identified in patients with ACC patch tested to the NACDG standard series

Allergen

1. Fragrance mix I 8% pet
2. *Myroxylon pereirae* (BOP) 25% pet
3. Nickel sulfate 2.5% pet
4. Gold sodium thiosulfate 0.5% pet
5. Neomycin sulfate 20% pet
6. Cobalt chloride 1% pet
7. Propylene glycol 30% aq
8. Lanolin 30% pet
9. Cinnamic aldehyde 1% pet
10. Bacitracin 20% pet
11. Benzophenone-3 3% pet
12. Methyldibromo glutaronitrile/phenoxy ethanol 2% pet
13. Tea tree oil, oxidized 5% pet
14. Budesonide 0.1% pet
15. Mercaptobenzothiazole 1% pet
16. Formaldehyde 1% aq
17. Potassium dichromate 0.25% pet
18. TSFR 10% pet

Abbreviations: aq, aqueous; pet, petrolatum.
  Data from Zug KA, Kornik R, Belsito DV. Patch testing North American lip dermatitis patients: Data from the North American Contact Dermatitis Group 2001–2004. Dermatitis 2008;19(4):202–8.

mixtures, consequently requiring fewer and lower concentrations of preservatives.[45] Another particularity is the presence of some uncommonly reported allergens relevant to the lip location, namely benzophenone-3 and gallates. Benzophenone-3, a major constituent in many sunscreens, is also a common ingredient in many lip products and is increasingly reported as a culprit for ACC. Schram and colleagues recently reported a patient with severe cheilitis who had a strong patch test reaction to both benzophenone-3 and his own lip balm.[53] Similarly, Nedorost[54] and Aguirre and colleagues[55] reported 1 patient each with cheilitis who reacted to irradiated and nonirradiated benzophenone-3 patches. Notably, benzophenone-3 was an ingredient in the lip products used by both patients. Gallates, on the other hand, are antioxidants used in waxy or oily products, such as lip balms, lipsticks, and lip glosses, and have also shown to play a potential role in ACC.[56]

PERIORAL DERMATITIS AS A MANIFESTATION OF ALLERGIC CONTACT DERMATITIS

Perioral dermatitis (POD) is a distinct condition that usually presents as a persistent acneiform eruption composed of tiny (2–3 mm) erythematous papules or papulopustules distributed primarily around the mouth and sparing the vermillion border of the lips.[57] POD predominantly affects women between 16 and 45 years of age, with constitutionally dry skin or a history of mild atopic dermatitis. Without treatment, POD tends to run a fluctuating course. Its pathogenesis remains unclear; however, a number of factors have been implicated, including atopy, infective agents, contact allergens and irritants, occlusive topical cosmetic products, hormonal factors (premenstrual period, pregnancy, oral contraceptives),[58] glucocorticosteroids, and ultraviolet (UV) light. POD might represent a localized form of rosacea.[59] If rosacea-type POD and atopic dermatitis are ruled out by history or examination, or if appropriate treatment fails, ACC should be suspected and patch testing should be pursued.[59] In a medical pearl for the evaluation of POD, Nedorost recommended patch testing with a standard and bakery series in addition to photo patch testing to a sunscreen series, when ACD is the suspected cause of POD.[59] Such series would allow the identification of potential relevant allergens such as topical antibiotics (neomycin and bacitracin), cinnamic aldehyde (the flavorant used in most commercially available toothpastes), benzophenone-3,

and propolis (both frequently found as ingredients of lip products).

CONNUBIAL/CONSORT DERMATITIS

ACD may not be caused by direct exposure of a patient to an allergen, but by passive exposure via social contacts (partners, family members, friends, or coworkers). This phenomenon has been termed "consort" or "connubial" dermatitis, to describe the skin reaction as a result of a substance used by someone other than the person affected. Connubial dermatitis is most commonly a result of fragrances;[60] however, various case reports have proven that many other cosmetic-related allergens could be potentially involved. These include a case of compositae-mix contact allergy from exposure to a consort's "natural" cosmetics;[61] a case of facial dermatitis in a mother following face-to-face contact with her benzoyl peroxide-treated son;[62] and a case of severe hand dermatitis as a result of PDD in a man that regularly helped his wife color her hair with a PPD-containing hair dye,[63] among many others.

OCCUPATIONAL CONTACT ALLERGY TO COSMETIC-RELATED ALLERGENS

In cross-sectional data of 2193 patients with at least 1 allergic patch test reaction associated with a cosmetic source, the NACDG identified 125 patients with occupationally related allergic reactions associated with a cosmetic.[21] Cosmetics "not otherwise specified," hair care products, and moisturizers were the most common product categories which were occupationally related. For both men and women, the most common occupation which relates an allergic reaction to a cosmetic source is hairdressing (including barbers and cosmetologists). Up to 50% of hairdressers develop dermatitis of the hands (either irritant or allergic in origin) within 3 years of starting work.[64] Common culprits include allergens found in hair care products such as dyes (mainly PPD), permanent wave solution (glyceryl monothioglycolate), hair bleaches (ammonium persulfate), preservatives, surfactants, and fragrances.

In a 2008 Finnish study, Aalto-Korte and colleagues reported on occupational contact allergy to formaldehyde and formaldehyde releasing preservatives in people that come in contact with cosmetics in their working environment; these include masseurs, hairdressers, and workers in various fields that are required to use barrier creams or liquid soaps at work.[65]

POTENTIAL CULPRITS OF COSMETIC CONTACT ALLERGY

There are many allergens in cosmetics, and although this article concentrates on giving a brief description of the most common allergens[4] (**Box 3**), it is important to keep in mind that virtually any ingredient found in a cosmetic can have the potential to cause a contact allergy. As a group, the preservatives are the most common allergens, closely followed by fragrances.[66]

Preservatives

Formaldehyde

Formaldehyde is a colorless gas with preservative and disinfectant properties. The first mass commercial use of formaldehyde was in medical embalming, and soon after, it started to be used as a preservative for laboratory specimens. Currently there is a wide range of uses for formaldehyde (cleansing products, plywood, bonded leather, waterproof glues, fertilizers, biocides, and photographic developers), yet it is rarely used in cosmetics because it is a frequent sensitizer.[28] Formaldehyde is an irritant and an allergen,

and patch testing with it is important as it can serve as a marker to identify individuals allergic to formaldehyde related preservatives.

Formaldehyde releasing preservatives

Many manufacturers have replaced the use of formaldehyde with formaldehyde-releasing preservatives (FRPs) in an attempt to decrease contact sensitization to personal care products.[67] FRPs include: quaternium-15, imidazolidinyl urea (Germall), diazolidinyl urea (Germall II), 3′-demethoxy-3o-demethylmatairesinol (DMDM) hydantoin (Glydant), 2-bromo-2-nitropropane-1, 3-diol (Bronopol), and tris nitromethane (Tris Nitro).[68] (Tris Nitro is an industrial biocide and is not usually found in cosmetic products.) FRPs are added to many skin, hair, and makeup products; mouthwashes; baby wipes; and topical medications. Allergic reactions to FRPs may be caused by the preservative per se, by formaldehyde, or by both.[69] The rate of cross-reactivity between FRPs and formaldehyde varies, and allergy to 1 FRP may not necessitate a restriction of the entire class. Herbert and Rietschel have suggested that it is only necessary to avoid the specific preservatives to which an individual tests positive.[70]

Quaternium-15 deserves special mention since it is the most common cosmetic preservative allergen.[1,14] It was the fourth most frequently positive allergen (10.3%) in the most recent NACDG patch test results study (2005–2006 period), after nickel sulfate, *Myroxylon pereirae*, and fragrance mix I.[71] Quaternium-15 had a statistically significant higher prevalence rate of allergic reactions in the 2005–2006 cycle compared with the prior 10 years (1994–2004) ($P<.05$), showing that the frequency of positive patch tests to this preservative in the population tested by the NACDG continues to increase over time.

Parabens

With the exception of water, parabens are the most commonly used ingredient in cosmetic preparations; and are also the most widely used preservative in cosmetic products.[68,72] There are 5 types of paraben esters of which methylparaben and ethylparaben are the most frequently used. Despite their widespread use, allergic reactions to parabens are rare, with most studies showing a prevalence that ranges from 0% to 4.2%.[73–75] ACD to parabens has been most commonly reported when products containing parabens are used on damaged skin, for example in patients with long-standing dermatitis or leg ulcers.[76] Although frequently found in cosmetics, parabens are considered weak sensitizers in

---

Box 3
Most frequent sensitizers in cosmetics

- Preservatives:
  - Formaldehyde
  - Formaldehyde releasing preservatives:
    - Quaternium-15
    - Imidazolidinyl urea
    - Diazolidinyl urea
    - DMDM hydantoin
    - Bronopol
  - Parabens
  - Methyldibromo glutaronitrile/phenoxy ethanol (MDGN/PE)
  - MCI/MI
  - Iodopropynyl butylcarbamate
- Fragrances
- Lanolin
- Cocamidopropyl betaine
- Antioxidants
- UV absorbers
- PPD
- Glyceryl monothioglycolate
- TSFR
- Propylene glycol

Not in order of frequency.

Data from White IR, de Groot AC. Cosmetics and skin care products. In: Frosch PJ, Menné T, Lepoittevin J-P, editors. Contact dermatitis. 4th edition. Berlin: Springer Verlag; 2006. p. 493–503.

these formulations; and patients sensitive to parabens are often able to tolerate paraben-containing cosmetics when applied to normal intact skin. Sites of resolved dermatitis occasionally flare when paraben-containing products are applied to healthy skin that does not react.[77] This unique aspect of paraben sensitivity was termed the "parabens paradox" by Alexander Fisher more than 35 years ago.[78]

Methyldibromo glutaronitrile/phenoxyethanol
Methyldibromo glutaronitrile/phenoxyethanol (MDGN/PE) is a preservative commonly referred to in the literature as Euxyl K400. It is a combination of 2 active ingredients, 2-phenoxyethanol and 1,2-dibromo-2,4-dicyanobutane in a ratio of 4:1.[20] Shortly after being introduced to the market in the mid 1980s, MDBGN/PE was labeled as an emerging and increasingly important sensitizing agent[79] and unleashed what has been considered an "epidemic of allergic contact dermatitis."[80] This was followed by a ban in the European Union (EU) countries, first from stay-on cosmetics in 2005, and later from rinse-off cosmetics in 2007, in an attempt to decrease the rates of contact allergy. Following the regulatory intervention, a significant decreasing trend in the frequency of positive patch tests to MDGN/PE was found, from 4.6% in 2003 to 2.6% in 2007 ($P<.001$).[80]

Earlier, the vast majority of allergic reactions to MDGN/PE came from cosmetics, especially creams, lotions, and liquid soaps. MDGN/PE is not banned in cosmetics produced outside the EU, and therefore cosmetics bought outside of the EU may still contain MDGN/PE. Of 4437 patients patch tested to MDGN/PE (2.5% pet) by NACDG in the 2005–2006 study period, 5.8% had a positive patch test reaction to this allergen, of which 3.9% were considered of definitive and 44% of probable clinical relevance.[71]

Methylchloroisothiazolinone/ methylisothiazolinone
Methylchloroisothiazolinone/methylisothiazolinone (MCI/MI) is a broad-spectrum antimicrobial that consists of a mixture of 2 isothiazolinones. It is commonly referred to in the literature as Kathon CG. It can be found in many cosmetic products including rinse-off and leave-on products. The first reports of ACD to this preservative appeared in Europe in the mid 1980s, and many cases of ACD to this preservative resulted from the use of moisturizing creams. Sensitivity patterns to MCI/MI have followed a somehow similar pattern in the United States and in Europe, with an increase from the 1980s to the 1990s, followed by a decrease in the first part of this decade. MCI/MI is patch tested at 100 ppm aqueous, but the amount actually used in products is much lower.[28] Studies have suggested that concentrations of 15 ppm MCI/MI in rinse-off products and 7.5 ppm in leave-on products are unlikely to produce sensitization to this agent.[81]

Iodopropynyl butylcarbamate
Iodopropynyl butylcarbamate (IPBC) is a relatively new preservative and biocide used in many personal care products. It is currently used in shampoos, lotions, powders, makeup, creams, and baby products including cleansing wipes.[82] Structurally, it is a small, lipophilic molecule that potentially leads to sensitization after extensive and prolonged exposure.[83,84] However, there are only a few reported cases of ACD from IPBC in cosmetics, despite its increasingly widespread use.

Thimerosal
Thimerosal is a mercury derived preservative. Exposure sources vary widely between different populations (eg, Europe vs America) and include contact lens solutions, otic and ophthalmic solutions, solutions for intradermal testing, antiseptics (eg, merthiolate), and certain cosmetics; however, it is believed that most sensitization cases originate from its presence in vaccines.[85–87] While patch testing with thimerosal may indicate a positive test, relevance these days to the presenting dermatitis is uncommon. Because of this regular lack of identified relevant sources, the majority of US-based patch test experts have removed thimerosal from their standard screening trays.[88,89]

Fragrances
Fragrances are aromatic compounds that impart a smell or odor. They can be natural (from botanic or animal products) or synthetic in origin. In 2007, fragrances were named "Allergen of the Year" by the American Contact Dermatitis Society (ACDS) to recognize the importance of these allergens.[90] It has been estimated that between 1% and 4% of the general population is allergic to fragrances.[91,92] Fragrance allergy is 1 of the 2 top causes of contact allergy to cosmetics, and the typical sites of involvement include the face and hands, as well as behind the ears, neck, and axillae in addition to generalized contact dermatitis.[93,94]

Three main substances are currently used by most patch test groups for screening of subjects with suspected fragrance sensitivity. The first substance, fragrance mix I (8.0% in petrolatum), is a mixture of 8 fragrance allergens (cinnamic alcohol 1.0%, cinnamic aldehyde 1.0%, eugenol 1.0%, hydroxycitronellal 1.0%, isoeugenol 1.0%, geraniol 1.0%, oak moss absolute, and alpha-amyl cinnamic aldehyde 1.0%.)

The second material, *Myroxylon pereirae* (MP), also known as balsam of Peru (BOP), is a substance derived from *Myroxolon balsamum*, a tree that is native to El Salvador. Given that many of MP components are fragrance ingredients,[95] it is considered to be a good marker for fragrance allergy, and able to identify approximately 50% of fragrance allergic individuals.[96] MP smells of vanilla and cinnamon because it contains 60% to 70% cinnamein, a combination of cinnamic acid, benzoyl cinnamate, benzoyl benzoate, benzoic acid, vanillin, and nerodilol.[97] These are all potential allergens, making MP one of the 5 most prevalent allergens detected by the Thin-layer Rapid Use Epicutaneous (TRUE) test.[75] In addition to pharmaceutical preparations and cosmetic products such as perfumes, lotions, and lip products, MP-related substances can also be found in toothpastes and mouthwashes, as well as in scents and flavorings for foods and drinks. This explains the frequent association between MP and ACC.[52,98] Cross-reactions may occur between MP and other chemicals such as colophony (rosin), wood and coal tars, resorcinol monobenzoate, coniferyl benzoate, Tolu balsam, storax, propolis, turpentine, and benzoin.[31] Certain foods, such as tomatoes and tomato-containing products, citrus fruit peel/zest, chocolate, ice cream, wine, beer, vermouth, dark colored sodas, and spices such as cinnamon, cloves, curry, and vanilla, have chemical ingredients related to BOP.[99] In 2001, Salam and Fowler[99] drew attention to the ability of orally ingested balsam-related substances to induce systemic contact dermatitis; and they reported that almost half of the subjects with positive patch tests to MP who followed a BOP reduction diet in their study had a significant to complete improvement of their dermatitis.

It was originally estimated that over 90% of individuals allergic to fragrance would be detected by patch testing to fragrance mix I and MP;[100] however, fragrances used by the industry are evolving constantly, and more recent studies have suggested that these 2 testing substances now pick-up only 60% to 70% of individuals allergic to fragrances.[101] In answer to this, an additional mixture called fragrance mix II has been added to many screening series. Fragrance mix II (14% in petrolatum) is a mixture of 6 fragrance allergens (citronellol 0.5%, Lyral (hydroxyisohexyl 3-cyclohexene carboxaldehyde) 2.5%, hexyl cinnamal 5.0%, citral 1.0%, coumarin 2.5%, and farnesol 2.5%).

Regulation of fragrance ingredients in cosmetics is a complicated topic and differs widely between countries. The Fair Packaging and Labeling Act, for example, requires that every cosmetic product in the United States list all of its ingredients following the International Nomenclature of Cosmetic Ingredients (INCI). Fragrance formulas; however, are exempted from this rule, because they often constitute "trade secrets" or proprietary formulas.[102] Therefore, most products found in the United States simply list either "fragrance" or "perfume" on their ingredient list, whereas there is the possibility that hundreds of different fragrance ingredients were mixed together to form that final fragrance in any given product.

A recent seventh amendment to the European Cosmetic Directive regulates cosmetic products in the EU. This amendment establishes that 26 distinct fragrance allergens are now required to be disclosed on the labels of cosmetic products that contain them. (A list of the 26 fragrance ingredients can be found in **Box 4**.)[103]

Although some manufacturers do not consider essential oils to be fragrances, these plant extracts are natural sources of various fragrance ingredients, and therefore possible sources of fragrance contact allergy.[104] *Melaleuca alternifolia* oil (tea tree oil), *Cananga odorata* oil (ylang-ylang oil), *Jasminum officinale* oil (jasmine flower oil), *Mentha piperita* oil (peppermint oil), *Lavandula angustifolia* oil (lavender oil), and limonene (citrus oil) are all examples of essential oils known to cause contact allergy.

Another tricky aspect of fragrance allergy is the existence of so-called "covert fragrances." Covert fragrances are aromatic chemicals which can be used for purposes other than imparting an aroma, for example, they can be used as preservatives, and therefore they can be added to a "fragrance-free" product. Examples of covert fragrances include benzaldehyde, benzyl alcohol, bisabolol, citrus oil, and unspecified essential oils.

Vehicles, Emulsifiers, and Surfactants

Lanolin

Lanolin (or wool wax alcohols) is the sebaceous excretion from sheep; it is extracted from wool and used as an emollient for skin barrier protection and repair. It is often added to a variety of cosmetics including lip products (lipsticks, lip balms), moisturizers, powders, shaving creams, shampoos, and soaps, and it may be a source of allergy from cosmetic products.[105,106] Ointment bases for topical medicaments are another common source of lanolin exposure.

Patients with chronic dermatitis, especially lower-extremity venous stasis dermatitis, have been identified as a high-risk population for the development of contact dermatitis from lanolin.[107] Based on this, Wolf concluded that lanolin is a weak sensitizer in normal skin, whereas damaged skin is easily sensitized, and Wolf named this phenomenon the "lanolin paradox."[108]

Box 4
List of the 26 fragrance ingredients requiring labeling on cosmetic products in Europe

INCI name

Amyl cinnamal

Benzyl alcohol

Cinnamyl alcohol

Citral

Eugenol

Hydroxycitronellal

Isoeugenol

Amylcinnamyl alcohol

Benzyl salycilate

Cinnamal

Coumarin

Geraniol

Lyral

Anise alcohol

Benzyl cinnamate

Farnesol

Butylphenyl methylpropional

Linalool

Benzyl benzoate

Citronellol

Hexyl cinnamal

Limonene

Methyl 2-octynoate

Alpha isomethyl ionone

Evernia prunastri (Oak moss) extract

Evernia furfuracea (Tree moss) extract

Data from IFRA. Skin reactions to fragrances. Procedures for promptly supplying fragrance information to dermatologist. Available at: http://www.ifraorg.org/binarydata.aspx?type=doc/FinalProcedure_Dermatologists-Requests.pdf. Accessed January 30, 2009.

Sorbitans

Sorbitol-based emulsifiers are commonly used in personal care products and topical medicaments (corticosteroids, antibiotics, antifungals, and retinoids).[109] Sorbitan sesquioleate (SSO) is a water-in-oil emulsifier that allows oil and water to blend together into a homogeneous mixture that does not separate.[110] It is widely used in cosmetics such as moisturizers, cleansers, conditioners, eye makeup removers, exfoliating products, sunscreens, makeup, and baby products. ACD from sorbitol derivatives is uncommon. Cosmetics and topical medicaments have been reported as the most common sources for ACD in patients allergic to SSO. Closely related emulsifiers such as Span 20 (sorbitan monolaurate), Span 40 (sorbitan monopalmitate), span 60 (sorbitan monostearate), span 65 (sorbitan tristearate), span 80 (sorbitan monooleate), and Span 85 (sorbitan trioleate) can cross-react with SSO and therefore should be avoided in patients sensitive to SSO.[110]

Cocamidopropyl betaine

Cocamidopropyl betaine (CAPB) is derived from coconut oil and is a commonly used surfactant in foaming cleansers that appears in many shampoos, bath foams, and soaps.[111] Recently, there is evidence that impurities from the CAPB preparation, such as amidoamine[112,113] and 3-dimethylaminopropylamine,[114,115] may be the true sensitizers. With improved (less contaminated) manufacturing, sensitization to products containing CAPB may be reduced in the near future.[116] Currently, contact sensitization prevalence rates are between 3.0% and 7.2%.[117]

Antioxidants

Gallates

Gallates (propyl gallate, octyl gallate, and dodecyl gallate) are chemical compounds used as antioxidant preservatives. They are added to food or cosmetic products to prevent spoilage as a result of the oxidation of fats and oils.[118] In cosmetics, gallates are primarily found in waxy or oily products such as lip balms or lip sticks, but can also be found in creams. Because of its more frequent inclusion in cosmetic products since 1947, propyl gallate should be kept in mind when evaluating patients, especially women, presenting with cheilitis, and in consumers of creams and topical medicaments that contain these chemicals. Hausen and Beyer determined that the gallate with the most sensitizing potential is dodecyl gallate.[119] The exact prevalence of gallate allergy in the United States is not known because screening for gallate sensitivity is not done routinely. These chemicals are not included in the NACDG screening tray or in the TRUE test.

Because of the similarity of the base compounds, cross-reactions between gallates can occur. In general, if a patient is tested with only 1 gallate and has a positive reaction, he or she should avoid all gallates. However, if the patient is tested with all 3 gallates and reacts to only 1 of them, the patient needs to avoid only the specific gallate to which he or she reacted.[118]

Ultraviolet Absorbers

Benzophenone-3 (oxybenzone)

Benzophenone-3 (2-hydroxy-4-methoxy-5 acid benzophenone) is the most common sunscreen allergen.[120] Synonyms for benzophenone-3 include oxybenzone, Eusolex 4360, Uvinul M 40, and diphenylketone. In addition to its use in sunscreens, benzophenone-3 may be added to toiletries, cosmetics, perfumes, and other products to prevent color degradation.[121] It is also an ingredient in many lip products, and patients may be unaware of any sunscreen exposure when using a product such as a shampoo or a lip balm. Occupational hand dermatitis to benzophenone in hair products has been reported in a hairdresser,[122] and multiple cases of cheilitis as a result of benzophenone-3 are reported in the literature.

Compared with other contact allergens, the prevalence of oxybenzone allergy is relatively low. Between 2005 and 2006, only 0.7% of more than 4000 patients with suspected ACD patch tested by members of the NACDG reacted to benzophenone-3.[71] Oxybenzone can cause both immediate and delayed-type hypersensitivity reactions that can be photoallergic and non-photoallergic, and therefore regular patch testing and photo patch testing may be necessary to evaluate patients with a suspected sunscreen allergy.

Allergenic Ingredients Found in Hair Products

Paraphenylendiamine

PPD is an oxidizing agent commonly used as a permanent hair dye. More recently it has gained notoriety for its use in adulterating natural henna to make "black henna," a substance increasingly used to make temporary tattoos.[123,124] Hair dye, however, remains the main source of exposure to PPD.

Contact allergy to PPD often presents as facial dermatitis near the hairline, but it may also involve the eyelids and the neck, whereas the scalp may or may not be spared.[125] Both consumers and hairdressers who are exposed to PPD are at risk for sensitization. PPD has the potential to cross-react with other para-amino group chemicals such as para-aminobenzoic acid, sulfonylureas, hydrochlorothiazide, benzocaine, procainamide, and certain azo and aniline dyes.[126–128]

Glyceryl monothioglycolate

Glyceryl monothioglycolate (GMT) is a chemical substance used in permanent wave (perming) solutions. Known as an acid perm, GMT works by altering the disulfide bonds of hair keratin so that the hair may be curled or waved. The scalp is generally resistant to ACD, and reactions to hair care products often involve the forehead, eyelids, ears, and neck, sparing the scalp. GMT reactions, however, frequently manifest as intense scalp reactions with scaling, edema, and crusting.[129] As an occupational cosmetic allergen, reaction to GMT can be seen on the hands, forearms, face, and neck of hairdressers. GMT persists on the permed hair for months, and therefore a sensitized hairdresser may react while cutting or styling permed hair.[129]

Allergenic Ingredients Found in Nail Products

Tosylamide formaldehyde resin

TSFR is a chemical added to nail varnish to facilitate adhesion of the varnish to the nail. Despite the name, there is only a small amount of free formaldehyde in TSFR, and it is the actual resin that constitutes the allergen.[130] Allergic reactions to TSFR generally develop at sites that are remote from the fingernails, such as the eyelids, face, and neck. The prevalence of ACD to TSFR has been on a decrease for the past 20 years,[131] and although this allergen is still traditionally considered in the evaluation of eyelid dermatitis, it has been found to be a minor factor.[38] In the NACDG study of common contact allergens associated with eyelid dermatitis, TSFR represented only 1% of the cases (n = 4 of 268 patients),[38] whereas other studies done outside the United States, like the one from Duarte and colleagues, have reported a rate as high as 12%.[132]

Artificial nail products

Artificial nails are often used when natural nails are not of the desired length or shape. Preformed plastic nails may be glued over the natural nail using ethyl cyanoacrylate (the ingredient found in Super Glue), which has been reported as a potential sensitizer.[133] On the other hand, sculptured nails are usually made of acrylic created from a liquid monomer and a powder polymer that is cured with an accelerator, often benzoyl peroxide.[12] Sensitization to artificial nail products has been reported in both beauticians and their clients, and includes nail fold, fingertip, facial, and neck dermatitis, as well as paresthesia.[12] Some authors advocate screening for suspected contact allergy to artificial nail products, with an acrylate series containing methyl methacrylate 2%, bisphenol A 1%, tetraethylene glycol dimethacrylate 2%, ethylene glycol dimethacrylate 2%, dimethyl-p-toluidine 2%, and benzoyl peroxide 1%.[134]

Other Cosmetic Allergens

Propolis

Propolis, also known as "bee glue," is a wax-like resinous substance made by honeybees. Resins collected by the bee from a variety of tree buds and barks (particularly conifers and poplars) are partially digested by the bee and then combined with beeswax to form a complex mixture of approximately 180 to 300 constituents, primarily resins (45% to 55%) consisting of free aromatic acids (ie, benzoic and cinnamic); waxes (30%); essential oils (10%); vitamins A, B, C, and E; flavonoids; and various minerals.[135,136] Human uses of propolis are extensive and include cough syrups, lozenges, ointments, vitamins, and cosmetics, such as shampoos, conditioners, lip balms, lotions, and toothpastes.[136]

Cases of ACD[137] and ACC[138,139] have been reported in association with propolis, and most cases result from use of propolis-containing products either applied topically (cosmetics) or ingested orally.[135] The main allergen found in propolis is LB-1, which consists of 2 distinct allergens: 3-methyl-2- butenyl caffeate and phenylethyl caffeate.[140] 1.2% to 6.6% of patients who are patch tested for dermatitis are sensitive to propolis.[136]

Colophony

Colophony, also known as rosin, is a natural resin obtained from the pine tree. In cosmetics, it is used in lip products as well as eye makeup (mascara, eye shadows, and eye liners).[5] Cases of eyelid dermatitis, cheilitis, and perioral dermatitis have been reported, albeit uncommonly, in association with colophony. Abietic acid and dihydroabietyl alcohol have been determined as the allergens present in colophony.[5,141]

Propylene glycol

Propylene glycol is a solvent and humectant with antibacterial properties, widely used in cosmetics. It is a frequent cause of both irritant contact dermatitis and ACD, yet it is predominantly an irritant. In view of its propensity to cause irritation, the high prevalence rates of sensitization have been questioned.[142] The NACDG found that sensitization to propylene glycol 30% aqueous was 2.9% in 4439 patients patch tested from 2005 to 2006.[71] Notably, in another study by the same group, Zug and colleagues identified propylene glycol as 1 of the most frequently relevant positive contact allergens in patients with a scattered generalized distribution of dermatitis.[143]

Diagnosis

The first step in the diagnosis of ACD to cosmetics is a careful medical history, including a meticulous investigation of the products used by the patient (both in the household and working environments). This should be followed by a thorough physical examination, with special attention to the pattern of the dermatitis, because clinical signs can provide vital information regarding the precipitating factors.[144] Patch testing is considered the "cornerstone" procedure in the diagnosis of ACD and should be performed when there is a substantial clinical suspicion and a suggestive history. In patients presenting with dermatitis in sun exposed areas it may also be necessary to consider performing photo patch testing—even more now that UV filters are increasingly being introduced as ingredients in cosmetics. It is fundamental that all likely allergens are included in the patch test, and dermatologists should be aware of national differences in the formulations of products for particular populations. It is also necessary to continually update the patch test series according to changes in product formulation.

When considering cosmetic allergy, it is of foremost importance to include the patient's own products in the testing. Most types of leave-on products (products that are meant to stay on the skin for a prolonged period of time, such as lotions, creams, sunscreens, makeup, and deodorants) can be patch tested "as-is," but rinse-off products and products that contain obvious irritants (eg, shampoos, cleansers, bubble baths, toothpastes) need to be diluted. The appropriate dilution and the dilutional vehicle for each product should be estimated based on the product's composition, solubility, and pH.[145] Other types of cosmetic products with volatile solvents (eg, hairsprays, mascara), can be patch tested "as-is," but only after the product has been allowed to dry.[12]

The diagnosis of cosmetic allergy is usually based on a positive patch test; yet sometimes it can be based on a positive use test and/or repeated open application test (ROAT test).[15] In a ROAT test, potentially allergenic leave-on products are applied twice daily to the upper arm on a marked 1 cm × 1 cm area for 7 days and evaluated for an eczematous skin reaction.[146] In a use test, a patient uses the suspected substance in the same way as when the dermatitis developed,[147] for example, by applying a suspected facial cream to a small marked area (1 cm × 1 cm) on the face for 1 week. As with the ROAT test, if an eczematous skin reaction occurs during the test period, the test is considered positive. Both the ROAT test and the use test can also be helpful in determining clinical relevance of a particular patch test positive reaction. (Diagnostic pearls for cosmetic contact allergy are summarized in **Box 5**.)

General therapeutic strategy

Because allergen identification can be achieved through proper patch testing, there is a good potential for a sustained remission. Therefore identification and removal of the inciting agent (allergen avoidance) should always be the mainstay of treatment.[148]

Waiting for patch testing, patients are helpfully provided with what Dr. K.A. Zug has coined the "Lo.C.A.L. (Low Contact Allergen) Skin Diet." The Lo.C.A.L. Skin Diet consists of a list of topical products devoid of the most commonly identified contact allergens in patients with ACD, including fragrances, formaldehyde releasing preservatives, MCI/MI, MDGN/PE, lanolin, CAPB, and benzophenone-3. The list is short and does not eliminate all contact allergens; however, based on experience from interviewing and testing many allergic patients, the list does a good job eliminating the most common allergens.

Once patch testing has isolated the causal allergen(s), avoidance compliance generally requires the substitution of safe alternatives. A good tool to provide the patient with such safe alternatives is the Contact Allergen Replacement Database (CARD).[149] The CARD was developed by James A. Yiannias, MD, at the Mayo Clinic in Scottsdale, Arizona, and consists of a regularly updated database with over 2000 over-the-counter and prescription personal care products available in the United States, which enables the creation of an individualized list of allergen-free products that the allergic patient can use. It has been shown that patients' compliance rates of avoidance increase when the CARD is used.[150] Access to CARD is a benefit of membership in the ACDS.

Box 5
Diagnostic pearls for cosmetic contact allergy

Persistent itching and swelling may be indicative of allergy versus solely cosmetic irritation.

Facial, eyelids, lips, and neck patterns of dermatitis should raise the suspicion of a cosmetic-related contact allergy.

Facial, eyelid, lip, and neck dermatitis can be caused by ectopic allergens.

Keep in mind the possibility of airborne and occupationally-related ACD to cosmetics.

In addition to screening series (including a routine and cosmetic tray), patients should be patch tested to their own cosmetics.

Both ROAT test and use test can be helpful when patch tests give negative results, or when the relevance of a positive reaction is in question.

REFERENCES

1. Eiermann HJ, Larsen W, Maibach HI, et al. Prospective study of cosmetic reactions: 1977–1980. J Am Acad Dermatol 1982;6:909–17.
2. Scheman A. Adverse reactions to cosmetic ingredients. Dermatol Clin 2000;18:685–98.
3. US FDA/CFSAN/Office of Cosmetics and Colors. Is it a cosmetic, a drug, or both? (Or is it soap?). July 8, 2002. Available at: http://www.cfsan.fda.gov/~dms/cos-218.html. Accessed January 14, 2009.
4. White IR, De Groot AC. Cosmetics and skin care products. In: Frosch PJ, Menné T, Lepoittevin J-P, editors. Contact dermatitis. 4th edition. Berlin: Springer Verlag; 2006. p. 493–506.
5. Engasser PG. Cosmetics and contact dermatitis. Dermatol Clin 1991;9:69–80.
6. De Groot AC. Labeling cosmetics with their ingredients. BMJ 1990;300:1636–8.
7. Mehta SS, Reddy BS. Cosmetic dermatitis—current perspectives. Int J Dermatol 2003;42:533–42.
8. Di Giovanni C, Arcoraci V, Gambardella L, et al. Cosmetovigilance survey: are cosmetics considered safe by consumers? Pharmacol Res 2006;53(1):16–21.
9. Willis CM, Shaw S, De Lacharriere O, et al. Sensitive skin: an epidemiological study. Br J Dermatol 2001;145:258–63.
10. De Groot AC, Beverdam E, Ayong C, et al. The role of contact allergy in the spectrum of adverse effects caused by cosmetics and toiletries. Contact Dermatitis 1988;19:195–201.
11. De Groot AC, Nater J, Van der Lende T, et al. Adverse effects of cosmetics and toiletries: a retrospective study in the general population. Int J Cosmet Sci 1987;9:255–9.
12. Orton DI, Wilkinson JD. Cosmetic allergy: incidence, diagnosis, and management. Am J Clin Dermatol 2004;5(5):327–37.
13. Romaguera C, Camarasa JMG, Alomar A, et al. Patch tests with allergens related to cosmetics. Contact Dermatitis 1983;6:167–8.

14. Adams RM, Maibach HI. A five-year study of cosmetic reactions. J Am Acad Dermatol 1985; 13:1062–9.

15. De Groot AC. Contact allergy to cosmetics: causative ingredients. Contact Dermatitis 1987;17:26–34.

16. Kohl L, Blondeel A, Song M. Allergic contact dermatitis from cosmetics: Retrospective analysis of 819 patch tested patients. Dermatology 2002; 204:334–7.

17. Skog E. Incidence of cosmetic dermatitis. Contact Dermatitis 1980;6:449–51.

18. Nielsen NH, Menné T. Allergic contact sensitization in an unselected Danish population. The Glostrup Allergy Study, Denmark. Acta Derm Venereol 1992;72:456–60.

19. Nielsen NH, Linneberg A, Menné T, et al. Allergic contact sensitization in an adult Danish population: two cross-sectional surveys eight years apart (The Copenhagen Allergy Study). Acta Derm Venereol 2001;81:31–4.

20. Wolf R, Wolf D, Tuzun B, et al. Contact dermatitis to cosmetics. Clin Dermatol 2001;19:502–15.

21. Warshaw EM, Buchholz HJ, Belsito DV, et al. Allergic patch test reactions associated with cosmetics: retrospective analysis of cross-sectional data from the North American Contact Dermatitis Group, 2001–2004. J Am Acad Dermatol 2009;60(1):23–38.

22. Penchalaiah K, Handa S, Lakshmi SB, et al. Sensitizers commonly causing allergic contact dermatitis from cosmetics. Contact Dermatitis 2000;43:311–3.

23. Zeller S, Warshaw E. Allergic contact dermatitis. Minn Med 2004;87:38–42.

24. De Groot AC, Bruynzeel DP, Bos JD, et al. The allergens in cosmetics. Arch Dermatol 1988;124(10):1525–9.

25. Dooms-Goossens A. Cosmetics and causes of allergic contact dermatitis. Cutis 1993;52:316–20.

26. De Groot AC, Weyland JW, Nater JP. Contact allergy to cosmetics. In: De Groot AC, Weyland JW, Nater JP, editors. Unwanted effects of cosmetics and drugs in dermatology. 3rd edition. New York: Elsevier; 1994. p. 452–68.

27. Robinson MK, Gerberick GF, Ryan CA, et al. The importance of exposure estimation in the assessment of skin sensitization risk. Contact Dermatitis 2000;42:251–9.

28. Biebl KA, Warshaw EM. Allergic contact dermatitis to cosmetics. Dermatol Clin 2006;24:215–32.

29. Schnuch A, Szliska C, Uter W, IVDK. Facial allergic contact dermatitis. Data from the IVDK and review of literature [abstract]. Hautarzt 2009;60(1):13–21. [in German].

30. Furman D, Fisher AA, Leider M. Allergic eczematous contact-type dermatitis caused by rubber sponges used for the application of cosmetics. J Invest Dermatol 1950;15:223–31.

31. Rietschel RL, Fowler JF. Regional contact dermatitis. In: Rietschel RL, Fowler JF, editors. Fisher's contact dermatitis. 6th edition. Hamilton (ON): BC Decker Inc.; 2008. p. 66–87.

32. Duarte I, Fusaro M, Lazzarini R. Etiology of paraphenylenediamine sensitization: hair dye and other products. Dermatitis 2008;19(6):342.

33. Chan YC, Ket S, Goh CL. Positive patch test reactions to paraphenylenediamine, their clinical relevance and the concept of clinical tolerance. Contact Dermatitis 2001;45:217–20.

34. Katugampola RP, Statham BN, English JS. A multicenter review of hairdressing allergens tested in UK. Contact Dermatitis 2005;53:130–2.

35. Patel S, Basketter DA, Jefferies D, et al. Patch test frequency to paraphenylenediamine: follow up over the last 6 years. Contact Dermatitis 2007;56:35–7.

36. Guin JD. Eyelid dermatitis: a report of 215 patients. Contact Dermatitis 2004;50:87–90.

37. Fisher AA. Allergic contact dermatitis and patch testing in childhood. Cutis 1994;54:230–2.

38. Rietschel RL, Warshaw EM, Sasseville D, et al. Common contact allergens associated with eyelid dermatitis: data from the North American Contact Dermatitis Group 2003–2004 study period. Dermatitis 2007;18(2):78–81.

39. Fowler J Jr, Taylor S, Storrs F, et al. Gold allergy in North America. Am J Contact Dermatol 2001;12:3–5.

40. Nedorost S, Wagman A. Positive patch test reactions to gold: Patients' perception of relevance and the role of titanium dioxide in cosmetics. Dermatitis 2005;16(2):67–70.

41. Guin JD. Eyelid dermatitis: experience in 203 cases. J Am Acad Dermatol 2002;47:755–65.

42. Lazzarini R, Duarte I, de Farias DC, et al. Frequency and main sites of allergic contact dermatitis caused by nail varnish. Dermatitis 2008;19(6):319–22.

43. Jacob SE, Castanedo-Tardan MP. A diagnostic pearl in allergic contact dermatitis to fragrances: the atomizer sign. Cutis 2008;82(5):317–8.

44. Fisher AA. Contact stomatitis, glositis, and cheilitis. Otolaryngol Clin North Am 1974;7:827–43.

45. Zug KA, Kornik R, Belsito DV. Patch testing North American lip dermatitis patients: data from the North American Contact Dermatitis Group 2001 to 2004. Dermatitis 2008;19(4):202–8.

46. Ophaswongse S, Maibach HI. Allergic contact cheilitis. Contact Dermatitis 1995;33:365–70.

47. Francalanci S, Sertoli A, Giorgini S, et al. Multicenter study of allergic contact cheilitis from toothpastes. Contact Dermatitis 2000;43:216–22.

48. Lim SW, Goh CL. Epidemiology of eczematous cheilitis at a tertiary dermatological referral center in Singapore. Contact Dermatitis 2000;43:322–6.

49. Zoli V, Silvani S, Vincenzi C, et al. Allergic contact cheilitis. Contact Dermatitis 2006;54:296–7.

50. Freeman S, Stephens R. Cheilitis: analysis of 75 cases referred to a contact dermatitis clinic. Am J Contact Dermatol 1999;10:198–200.

51. Katsarou A, Armenaka M, Vosynioto V, et al. Allergic contact cheilitis in Athens. Contact Dermatitis 2008;59:123–5.

52. Strauss RM, Orton DI. Allergic contact cheilitis in the United Kingdom: a retrospective study. Am J Contact Dermat 2003;14:75–7.

53. Schram SE, Glesne LA, Warshaw EM. Allergic contact cheilitis from benzophenone-3 in lip balm and fragrance/flavorings. Dermatitis 2007;18(4):221–4.

54. Nedorost ST. Facial erythema as a result of benzophenone allergy. J Am Acad Dermatol 2003;49(5): S259–61.

55. Aguirre A, Izu R, Gardeazabal J, et al. Allergic contact cheilitis from a lipstick containing oxybenzone. Contact Dermatitis 1992;27:267–8.

56. Serra-Baldrich E, Puig LL, Gimenez Arnau A, et al. Lipstick allergic contact dermatitis from gallates. Contact Dermatitis 1995;32:359–60.

57. Hafeez ZH. Perioral dermatitis: an update. Int J Dermatol 2003;42:514–7.

58. Macdonald A, Feiwel M. Perioral dermatitis: aetiology and treatment with tetracycline. Br J Dermatol 1972;87(4):315–9.

59. Nedorost ST. Medical pearl: the evaluation of perioral dermatitis: use of an extended patch test series. J Am Acad Dermatol 2007;56:S100–2.

60. Rycroft RJG, Menné T, Frosch PJ, et al, editors. Textbook of contact dermatitis. Berlin: Springer Verlag; 1992. p. 276–7.

61. Bernedo N, Audicana MT, Uriel O, et al. Allergic contact dermatitis from cosmetics applied by the patient's girlfriend. Contact Dermatitis 2004;50: 252–3.

62. Hernandez-Nunez A, Sanchez-Perez J, Pascual-Lopez M, et al. Allergic contact dermatitis from benzoyl peroxide transferred by a loving son. Contact Dermatitis 2002;46:302.

63. Gass JK, Todd PM. PPD: Is this a connubial dermatitis? Contact Dermatitis 2006;55:309.

64. Worth A, Arshad SH, Sheikh A. Occupational dermatitis in a hairdresser. BMJ 2007;335:399.

65. Aalto-Korte K, Kuuliala O, Suuronen K, et al. Occupational contact allergy to formaldehyde and formaldehyde releasing preservatives. Contact Dermatitis 2008;59:280–9.

66. Warshaw EM, Belsito DV, DeLeo VA, et al. North American Contact Dermatitis Group patch test results, 2003–2004 study period. Dermatitis 2008; 19(3):129–36.

67. Scheman A, Jacob S, Zirwas M, et al. Contact allergy: alternatives for the 2007 North American Contact Dermatitis Group (NACDG) standard screening tray. Dis Mon 2008;54(1-2):7–156.

68. Sasseville D. Hypersensitivity to preservatives. Dermatol Ther 2004;17(3):251–63.

69. Brancaccio RR. What's new in contact dermatitis. Am J Contact Dermatitis 1993;4:55–7.

70. Herbert C, Rietschel RL. Formaldehyde and formaldehyde releasers: how much avoidance of cross-reacting agents is required? Contact Dermatitis 2004;50:371–3.

71. Zug KA, Warshaw EM, Fowler JF Jr, et al. Patch-test results of the North American Contact Dermatitis Group 2005-2006. Dermatitis 2009;20(3): 149–60.

72. Richardson EL. Update frequency of preservative use in cosmetic formulas as disclosed to FDA. Cosmetic and Toiletries, FDA Report 1977;92:85.

73. Elder RL. Final report on the safety assessment of methylparaben, ethylparaben, propylparaben, and butylparaben. J Am Coll Toxicol 1984;3:147–209.

74. Menné T, Hjorth N. Routine patch testing with parabens esters. Contact Dermatitis 1988;19:189–91.

75. Krob HA, Fleischer AB, D'Agostino R, et al. Prevalence and relevance of contact dermatitis allergens: a meta-analysis of 15 years of published T.R.U.E. test data. J Am Acad Dermatol 2004; 51(3):349–53.

76. Fisher AA. Paraben dermatitis due to a new medicated bandage: the "parabens paradox". Contact Dermatitis 1979;5:273–4.

77. Cashman AL, Warshaw EM. Parabens: a review of epidemiology, structure, allergenicity, and hormonal properties. Dermatitis 2005;16(2):57–66.

78. Fisher AA. The parabens paradoxes. Cutis 1973; 12:830–1.

79. Van Ginkel C, Rundervoort G. Increasing incidence of contact allergy to the new preservative 1,2-dibromo-2,4-dicyanobutane (methyldibromo glutaronitrile). Br J Dermatol 1995;132:918–20.

80. Johansen JD, Veien N, Laurberg G, et al. Decreasing trends in methyldibromo glutaronitrile contact allergy – following regulatory intervention. Contact Dermatitis 2008;59:48–51.

81. Cardin CW, Weaver JE, Bailey PT. Dose response assessment of Kathon biocide. Contact Dermatitis 1986;15:10–6.

82. Bryld LE, Agner T, Rastogi SC, et al. Iodopropynyl butylcarbamate: a new contact allergen. Contact Dermatitis 1997;36:156–8.

83. Pazzaglia M, Tosti A. Allergic contact dermatitis from 3-iodo-2-propynyl-butylcarbamate in a cosmetic cream. Contact Dermatitis 1999;41:290.

84. Bryld LE, Agner T, Menné T. Allergic contact dermatitis 3-iodo-2-propynyl-butylcarbamate (IPBC) – an update. Contact Dermatitis 2001;44:276–8.

85. Audicana MT, Munoz D, del Pozo MD, et al. Allergic contact dermatitis from mercury antiseptics and derivatives: study protocol of tolerance to intramuscular injections of thimerosal. Am J Contact Dermat 2002;13:3–9.

86. Schafer T, Enders F, Przybilla B. Sensitization to thimerosal and previous vaccination. Contact Dermatitis 1995;32:114–6.

87. Osawa J, Kitamura K, Ikezawa Z, et al. A probable role for vaccines containing thimerosal in thimerosal hypersensitivity. Contact Dermatitis 1991;24:178–82.

88. Marks JG Jr, Belsito DV, DeLeo VA, et al. North American Contact Dermatitis Group patch test results, 1998 to 2000. Am J Contact Dermat 2003;14:59–62.

89. Freiman A, Al-Layali A, Sasseville D. Patch testing with thimerosal in a Canadian center: an 11-year experience. Am J Contact Dermat 2003;14:138–43.

90. Storrs FJ. Fragrance. Dermatitis 2007;18:3–7.

91. Larsen WG. How to test for fragrance allergy. Cutis 2000;65:39–41.

92. Schnuch A, Uter W, Geier J, et al. Contact allergy to farnesol in 2021 consecutively patch tested patients. Results of the IVDK. Contact Dermatitis 2004;50:117–21.

93. de Groot AC, Frosch PJ. Adverse reactions to fragrances: a clinical review. Contact Dermatitis 1997;36:57–86.

94. Tomar J, Jain VK, Aggarwal K, et al. Contact allergies to cosmetics: testing with 52 cosmetic ingredients and personal products. J Dermatol 2005;32:951–5.

95. Api AM. Only Peru Balsam extracts or distillates are used in perfumery. Contact Dermatitis 2006;54:179.

96. Larsen WG. Perfume dermatitis. J Am Acad Dermatol 1985;12:1–9.

97. Hjorth N. Eczematous allergy to balsams, allied perfumes and flavoring agents, with special reference to balsam of Peru. Acta Derm Venereol 1961;41(Suppl 46):1–216.

98. Magnusson B, Wilkinson DS. Cinnamic aldehyde in toothpaste. Contact Dermatitis 1975;1:70–6.

99. Salam TN, Fowler JF Jr. Balsam-related systemic contact dermatitis. J Am Acad Dermatol 2001;45:377–81.

100. Larsen W, Nakayama H, Lindberg M, et al. Fragrance contact dermatitis: a 144 DM, January/February 2008 worldwide multicenter investigation (part I). Am J Contact Dermatitis 1996;7:77–83.

101. Larsen W, Nakayama H, Fischer T, et al. Fragrance contact dermatitis: a worldwide multicenter investigation (part III). Contact Dermatitis 2002;46:141–4.

102. Jackson EM. AAD drafts position statement to label fragrance allergens in cosmetics. Cosmet Dermatol 1999;12:47–51.

103. IFRA. Skin reactions to fragrances. Procedures for promptly supplying fragrance information to dermatologist. Available at: http://www.ifraorg.org/binarydata.aspx?type=doc/Final Procedure_DermatologistsRequests.pdf. Accessed January 30, 2009.

104. Simpson EL, Law SV, Storrs FJ. Prevalence of botanical extract allergy in patients with contact dermatitis. Dermatitis 2004;15:67–72.

105. Hasan T, Rantanen T, Alanko K, et al. Patch test reactions to cosmetic allergens in 1995–1997 and 2000–2002 in Finland–a multicentre study. Contact Dermatitis 2005;53:40–5.

106. Wakelin SH, Smith H, White IR, et al. A retrospective analysis of contact allergy to lanolin. Br J Dermatol 2001;145:28–31.

107. Lee B, Warshaw E. Lanolin allergy: history, epidemiology, responsible allergens, and management. Dermatitis 2008;19(20):63–72.

108. Wolf R. The lanolin paradox. Dermatology 1996;192:198–202.

109. Asarch A, Scheinman PL. Sorbitan sesquioleate: an emerging contact allergen. Dermatitis 2008;19(6):339–41.

110. Castanedo-Tardan MP, Jacob SE. Sorbitan sesquioleate. Dermatitis 2008;19(4):E22–3.

111. de Groot AC, van der Walle HB, Weyland JW. Contact allergy to cocamidopropyl betaine. Contact Dermatitis 1995;33:419–22.

112. Fowler JF, Fowler LM, Hunter JE. Allergy to cocamidopropyl betaine may be due to amidoamine: a patch test and product use test study. Contact Dermatitis 1997;37:276–81.

113. Fowler JF Jr, Zug KM, Taylor JS, et al. Allergy to cocamidopropyl betaine and amidoamine in North America. Dermatitis 2004;15:5–6.

114. Foti C, Bonamonte D, Mascolo G, et al. The role of 3-dimethylaminopropylamine and amidoamine in contact allergy to cocamidopropyl betaine. Contact Dermatitis 2003;48:194–8.

115. Angelini G, Foti C, Rigano L, et al. 3-Dimethylaminopropylamine: a key substance in contact allergy to cocamidopropyl betaine? Contact Dermatitis 1995;32:96–9.

116. Hunter JE, Fowler JF. Safety to human skin of cocamidopropyl betaine: a mild surfactant for personal care products. J Surf Det 1998;1(2):235–9.

117. Jacob SE, Amini S. Cocamidopropyl betaine. Dermatitis 2008;19(3):157–60.

118. Jacob SE, Caperton CV. Allergen avoidance. Gallates. Dermatitis 2007;18(3): Last two pages of journal. No numbers given.

119. Hausen BM, Beyer W. The sensitizing capacity of the antioxidants propyl, octyl, and dodecyl gallate and some related gallic acid esters. Contact Dermatitis 1992;26(4):253–8.

120. Rietschel RL, Fowler JF Jr. Photocontact dermatitis. In: Rietschel RL, Fowler JF Jr, editors. Fisher's contact dermatitis. 5th edition. Philadelphia: Lippincott Williams & Wilkins; 2001. p. 397–411.

121. Fisher A. Sunscreen dermatitis: part III – the benzophenones. Cutis 1992;50:331–2.

122. Alanko K, Jolanki R, Estlander T, et al. Occupational allergic contact dermatitis from benzophenone-4 in hair care products. Contact Dermatitis 2001;44(3):188.

123. Neri I, Guareschi E, Savoia F, et al. Childhood allergic contact dermatitis from henna tattoo. Pediatr Dermatol 2002;19(6):503–5.

124. Chung WH, Chang YC, Yang LJ, et al. Clinicopathologic features of skin reactions to temporary tattoos and analysis of possible causes. Arch Dermatol 2002;138(1):88–92.

125. Zapolanski T, Jacob SE. para-Phenylenediamine. Dermatitis 2008;19(3):E20–1.

126. Leysat SD, Boone M, Blondeel A, et al. Two cases of cross-sensitivity in subjects allergic to paraphenylenediamine following ingestion of polaronil. Dermatology 2003;206:379–80.

127. Arroyo MP. Black henna tattoo reaction in a person with sulfonamide and benzocaine allergy. J Am Acad Dermatol 2003;48(2):301–2.

128. Paraphenylenediamine. Available at: http://www.aad.org/public/publications/pamphlets/skin_allergic.html. Accessed October 31, 2008.

129. Parsons LM. Glyceryl monothioglycolate. Dermatitis 2008;19(6):E51–2.

130. Fisher AA. Contact dermatitis. 3rd edition. Philadelphia: Lea & Febiger; 1986. p. 383–384.

131. Stechschulte SA, Avashia N, Jacob E. Tosylamide formaldehyde resin. Dermatitis 2008;19(3):E18–9.

132. Duarte I, Lazzarini R, Kobata CM. Contact dermatitis in adolescents. Am J Contact Dermat 2003; 14:200–2.

133. Guin JD, Baas K, Nelson-Adesokan P. Contact sensitization to cyanoacrylate adhesive as a cause of severe onychodystrophy. Int J Dermatol 1998;37: 21–6.

134. Freeman S, Lee MS, Gudmundsen K. Adverse contact reactions to sculptured acrylic nails: 4 case reports and a literature review. Contact Dermatitis 1995;33:381–5.

135. Giusti F, Miglietta R, Pepe P, et al. sensitization to propolis in 1225 children undergoing patch testing. Contact dermatitis 2004;51:255–8.

136. Walgrave SE, Warshaw EM, Glesne LA. Allergic contact dermatitis from propolis. Dermatitis 2005; 16:209–15.

137. Ting PT, Silver S. Allergic contact dermatitis to propolis. J Drugs Dermatol 2004;3:685–6.

138. Jacob SE, Chimento S, Castanedo-Tardan MP. Allergic contact dermatitis to propolis and carnauba wax from lip balm and chewable vitamins in a child. Contact Dermatitis 2008;58:242–3.

139. Pasolini G, Semenza D, Capezzera R, et al. Allergic contact cheilitis induced by repeated contact with propolis-enriched honey. Contact Dermatitis 2004; 50:322–3.

140. Hausen BM, Wollenweber E, Senff H, et al. Propolis allergy (I). Origin, properties, usage and literature review. Contact Dermatitis 1987;17:163–70.

141. Karlberg AT, Bergstedt E, Boman A, et al. Is abietic acid the allergenic component of colophony? Contact dermatitis 1985;13:209–15.

142. Wahlberg JE. Propylene glycol: search for a proper and non-irritant patch test preparation. Am J Contact Dermat 1994;5:156–9.

143. Zug KA, Rietschel RL, Warshaw EM, et al. The value of patch testing patients with a scattered generalized distribution of dermatitis: retrospective cross-sectional analyses of North American Contact Dermatitis Group data, 2001 to 2004. J Am Acad Dermatol 2008;59(3):426–31.

144. Belsito DV. A Sherlockian approach to contact dermatitis. Dermatol Clin 1999;17:705–13.

145. Jolanki R, Estlander T, Alanko K, et al. Patch testing with a patient's own materials handled at work. In: Kanerva L, editor. Handbook of occupational dermatology. New York: Springer; 2000. p. 375–83.

146. Gelpi CB, Jacob SE. Instructions for educating patients on ROAT testing in conjunction with patch testing. Dermatol Nurs 2008;20(2):139–43.

147. Bashir SJ, Maibach HI. Contact urticaria syndrome. In: Chew AL, Maibach HI, editors. Irritant dermatitis. Berlin: Springer; 2006. p. 63–70.

148. Jacob SE, Castanedo-Tardan MP. Pharmacotherapy for allergic contact dermatitis. Expert Opin Pharmacother 2007;8(16):2757–74.

149. Yiannias JA. Contact Allergen Replacement Database (CARD): a topical skin care product database sneak preview. Available at: http://www.contactderm.org/CARDPreview03.ppt. Accessed January 30, 2009.

150. Kist JM, El-azhary RA, Henz JG, et al. The Contact allergen replacement database and treatment of allergic contact dermatitis. Arch Dermatol 2004; 140:1448–50.

Clinical Patterns of Hand and Foot Dermatitis: Emphasis on Rubber and Chromate Allergens

Susan Nedorost, MD

KEYWORDS

- Rubber • Thiruam • Carbamates • Chromate
- Hand dermatitis

HAND AND FOOT DERMATITIS
Hand and Foot Versus Hand or Foot

Pattern of presentation can offer important diagnostic clues that guide the physician when obtaining history to evaluate dermatitis. Pattern of dermatitis also must correlate with history of exposure in order for a positive patch test to be considered relevant.

Hand dermatitis without foot dermatitis, especially if there is involvement of the face or neck, is more likely to be because of allergic contact, as opposed to hand dermatitis presenting with foot dermatitis. Hand dermatitis presenting with foot dermatitis is more likely to be a result of a systemic, "endogenous" cause.

Contactants for hands are many and include occupational exposures, personal care products, and hobby exposure, whereas contactants for feet are usually limited to footwear and medicaments; therefore there are few common exposures. Sometimes, hand and foot dermatitis occur together because of medicaments applied to both. Alternatively, when hand and foot dermatitis occur together, there may be a common allergen, such as mercaptobenzothiazole, with occupational hand exposure to corrosion inhibitors and/or nitrile gloves and feet exposure to mercaptobenzothiazole in rubber shoe components (Figs. 1–3).

More commonly, hand and foot dermatitis presenting together are because of an endogenous process such as dietary metal sensitivity (Fig. 4). The article on chronic vesicular hand dermatitis in this issue further discusses the endogenous dermatoses.

Hand and foot dermatitis resulting from contact allergy may not occur synchronously given the different routes of exposure (Figs. 5 and 6). Because hands are also subject to irritation from wet/dry cycles during handwashing and wet work and sometimes from patients picking or paring away scales, irritant dermatitis can also be superimposed upon another primary dermatosis, such as psoriasis or dermatomyositis. Irritant dermatitis can appear spongiotic histologically, such that skin biopsy from the hands and feet must be interpreted with caution.

Allergic contact dermatitis resulting from medicament may be limited to hands and feet (Fig. 7) in patients with disorders such as underlying tinea or palmar/plantar psoriasis. The presence of spongiosis prevents histological diagnosis of psoriasis in most of these cases. When hands and feet are the only affected areas, the clinician should maintain diagnostic suspicion for underlying psoriasis, dermatomyositis, chronic hyperkeratotic hand dermatitis, or chronic vesicular dermatitis.

Chronic hyperkeratotic hand dermatitis is symmetrically located on the middle portion of the palms and/or soles with painful fissures.[1] A 10-year follow-up study of 32 adults with hyperkeratotic dermatitis of the palms revealed that only 1 developed psoriasis during the decade of follow-up, and that the patient developed only a plaque on the elbow. There was no increased

University Hospitals Case Medical Center, 11100 Euclid Avenue, Cleveland, OH 44106, USA
E-mail address: stn@case.edu

Dermatol Clin 27 (2009) 281–287
doi:10.1016/j.det.2009.05.008

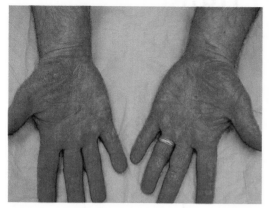

Fig. 1. Hand dermatitis due to mercaptobenzothiazole in corrosion inhibitors at work and subsequent use of nitrile gloves containing mercaptobenzothiazole.

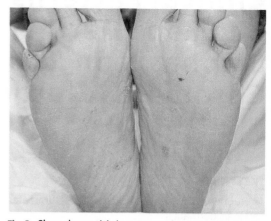

Fig. 3. Shoe dermatitis in same patient as in Fig. 1; relevant to thioureas and/or mercaptobenzothiazole in shoe insoles.

prevalence of family history of psoriasis, and all of the 9 patients who underwent skin biopsy of the palm showed spongiotic dermatitis.[2] This diagnosis does not respond well to treatment and tends to be stable and chronic.

Frictional hand dermatitis also often involves the palms, but it is directly a result of chronic rubbing, usually of an occupational contactant, and has a good prognosis when the friction is eliminated. Antiimpact gloves have been reported to be of benefit for this condition.[3] Grenz ray treatment was reportedly successful in a single case of a dermatological surgeon with frictional hyperkeratotic hand and foot dermatitis, who had failed topical and systemic corticosteroids, topical tacrolimus, calcipotriene, and bexarotene gel.[4]

Other Affected Areas in Addition to Hand or Foot

The pattern of hand dermatitis with forearm or with facial dermatitis can suggest the causative allergen. Allergic contact dermatitis resulting from sticky substances, such as acrylate nail products, or other resins, such as plant resin or colophony, often involves the fingertips and facial skin (**Fig. 8**). Allergy to preservatives in personal care products often involves the hands with a more generalized distribution of skin affected; if occupational biocides are the only exposure to these chemicals, dermatitis is usually limited to the hands and forearms. These allergens are discussed in other articles in this issue.

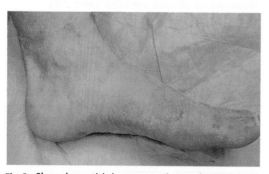

Fig. 2. Shoe dermatitis in same patient as in Fig. 1; positive patch tests to mercaptobenzothizole and potassium dichromate, both likely relevant; also positive patch test to mixed dialkyl thiourea.

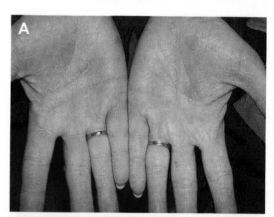

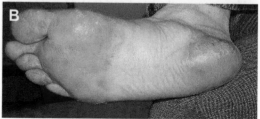

Fig. 4. (*A, B*) Hand and foot dyshidrotic eczema as a result of systemic nickel dermatitis in a candy maker.

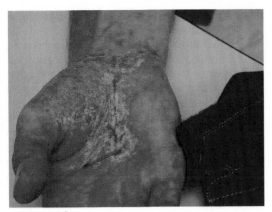

Fig. 5. Allergy due to foam rubber glove insert on palm.

This article focuses on allergic contact dermatitis of the hands and feet resulting from rubber and chromate; dermatitis from these allergens almost always involves the hands or feet. For patients with positive patch tests to rubber chemicals, 78% have hand dermatitis.[5] Rubber and chromate sensitization often coexist in construction workers, with 67% of rubber-allergic patients also sensitized to chromates in a 1991 study.[5]

RUBBER CHEMICALS

In addition to allergy to natural rubber latex discussed in the section on glove pattern dermatitis, allergy to chemicals used to accelerate the vulcanization of natural latex or synthetic rubber or to reduce degradation of rubber is common. There

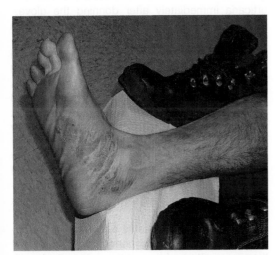

Fig. 6. Same patient as in Fig. 5, after 5 years, with dermatitis due to rubber in shoes during episode of increased perspiration. Cleared entirely with avoidance of rubber, despite psoriasiform appearance.

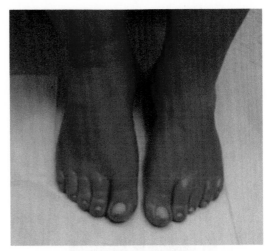

Fig. 7. Dermatitis caused by medicament: positive relevant patch tests to econazole nitrate, lanolin, and iodopropynyl butyl carbamate.

is an overlap between the products where these chemicals are used, but some patterns emerge and are described here for each of the common rubber allergens.

Hand/Foot Dermatitis Due to Black Rubber

Black rubber mix (N-isopropyl-N-phenyl-4-phenylenediamine and N-cyclohexyl-N-phenyl-4-phenylenediamine and N, N-diphenyl-4-phenylenediamine) is a patch test screen for paraphenylenediamine-related antioxidants used in making black or gray rubber. Black rubber is frequently used in occupational personal protective equipment (Fig. 9). Cross-reaction with 4-phenylenediamine base can occur, but most patients allergic to N-isopropyl-N-phenyl-4-phenylenediamine-type antioxidants do not react to paraphenylenediamine.

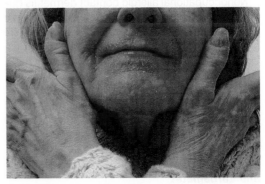

Fig. 8. Allergy to nail polish and ethylcyanoacrylate (Superglue) used to treat fissures on fingers, with ectopic dermatitis on face.

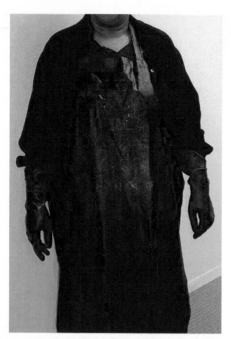

Fig. 9. Allergy to black rubber apron and gloves in a worker with hand, forearm, and neck dermatitis, who tested positive to black rubber mix.

Palmar/Grip Pattern

Black rubber is used to make solid objects that are often present in an industrial environment. Tire workers sensitized to N-isopropyl-N-phenyl-4-phenylenediamine and its related chemicals often have dermatitis on the palms and extensor wrists.[6] Related antioxidants are the most common causes of allergic contact dermatitis in tire workers.

Other devises made of black rubber can cause occupational dermatitis. Hyperkeratotic palmar dermatitis, worse on the right hand, was reported to occur from handling an egg stamper made of black rubber.[7]

Nonoccupational allergic contact dermatitis due to black rubber mix usually occurs as a palmar "grip pattern", as the most common sources are grips on exercise equipment or orthopedic assistive devices, such as canes and wheelchairs. Hard rubber that has a gray color is often manufactured with these antidegradant chemicals.

Black rubber on an escalator handrail caused palmar and perioral contact dermatitis in 1 case report.[8]

Hand/Foot Dermatitis Due to Thiurams and Carbamates

Thiuram is tested as a mix of tetramethylthiuram monosulfide, tetramethylthiuram disulfide, tetraethylthiuram disulfide, and dipentamethylene-thiuram disulfide because these components do not always cross-react. Carba mix contains N, N-diphenylguanidine (a cross-reacting noncarbamate), zinc diethyldithiocarbamate, and zinc dibutyldithiocarbamate. Thiurams are the most common causes of contact dermatitis to rubber gloves.[9] Many patients are patch test positive to thiuram and carba mixes; 92% of patients with a positive patch test to dithiocarbamates also react to thiurams.[9] Even if carba mix patch tests are negative, patients with positive patch tests to thiuram mix may be intolerant of gloves containing carbamates.[10]

Whenever allergens are tested as a mix, the concentration of the individual allergens may be too low and cause a false-negative reaction. Therefore, if there is a high degree of suspicion of rubber allergy, a rubber series containing the individual allergens and testing with thin pieces of the suspect rubber should be performed.[6]

Dorsal Hand and Finger Dermatitis with Cut-off at Wrist

Many patients with this pattern are allergic to rubber chemicals in gloves, especially thiuram and carbamates. Many patients have dermatitis of the thenar and hypothenar eminence also. Vinyl gloves are an acceptable substitute for most patients allergic to rubber gloves. The American Contact Dermatitis Web site offers members a database of gloves free of various rubber accelerators for sterile and nonsterile use.

Allergy to natural rubber latex can also cause glove dermatitis, but there is usually a history of urticaria immediately after donning the gloves. Immediate hypersensitivity to latex was a common problem in the late 1980s and 1990s, when adoption of universal precautions suddenly increased usage of gloves and possibly led to decreased quality of manufacturing. Work-up for patients with a history of urticaria from gloves should include a radioallergosorbent test to the latex protein, Hevea braziliensis (which is not entirely sensitive because of differences in the latex proteins from different sources), and testing of pieces of the glove. Prick or scratch testing should be performed only with the presence of appropriate emergency assistance because of the risk for anaphylaxis.[11]

Atopic dermatitis patients often react to occlusion with inflammatory response[12] and may exhibit the same pattern of dermatitis as do patients with glove allergy. This diagnosis must be considered in the atopic dermatitis patient with negative patch tests to an extended screening series. To improve the dermatitis, patients should wear thin cotton gloves under occlusive gloves to prevent perspiration from irritating the skin and to prevent maceration of the skin, which causes fissuring due to rapid drying upon removal of the gloves in low humidity conditions.

Eyelid Dermatitis

Eyelid dermatitis may result from use of rubber cosmetic applicators or removal pads and the edge of eyelash curlers. Airborne patterns of dermatitis occasionally result from nonrubber exposures to thiurams in insecticides and fungicides.[6]

Pattern of Shoe Dermatitis

Thiuram, carbamate, meracapto, and thiourea are chemicals that can all cause shoe dermatitis. **Figs. 10A, B** show the typical pattern of dermatitis due to rubber or rubber adhesives in the soles of shoes with sparing of the instep and the interdigital webs. The dorsum of the foot under the tongue of the shoe is often involved as well.

Hand/Foot Dermatitis Due to Mercaptobenzothiazole

Mercaptobenzothiazole is a common cause of shoe dermatitis. Mercaptobenzothiazole is tested on the standard series alone and as part of the mercapto mix along with N-cyclohexylbenzothiazyl sulfenamide, dibenzothiazyl disulfide, and morpholinylmercaptobenzothiazole.

Dorsal Hand/Foot Sparing Webspace Pattern

Mercaptobenzothiazole is frequently found in shoes, but it is sometimes detected in rubber gloves also.[13] Use of mercaptobenzothiazole-related chemicals in gloves increased in the late 1990s.[9] In this investigator's experience, mercaptobenzothiazole is the rubber allergen most likely responsible for allergic contact dermatitis affecting the hands and feet. A predisposing occupation may be mechanics and machinists, who are exposed to mercaptobenzothiazole in corrosion-inhibiting fluids. Nitrile gloves are often provided to protect the worker from these fluids, and the gloves themselves often contain mercaptobenzothiazole. Sensitized workers may then develop shoe dermatitis from mercpatobenzothiazole in work boots or athletic shoes (see **Figs. 1–3**).

Hand Dermatitis Involving Webspace

If the hand dermatitis is due to mercaptobenzothiazole in a corrosion inhibitor, there may be

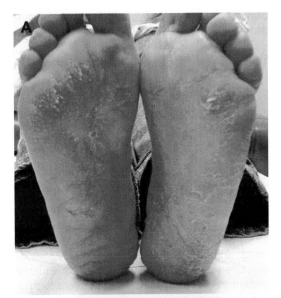

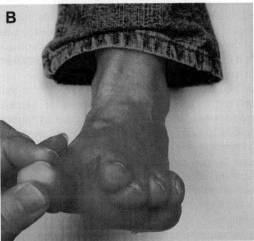

Fig. 10. (A, B) Shoe dermatitis usually spares the interdigital webs and plantar arch with involvement of the remainder of the plantar aspect and often the dorsal foot under the tongue of the shoe. This patient was allergic to thiuram mix.

patchy dermatitis with webspace involvement rather than the glove pattern.

Nonrubber dermatitis due to mercaptobenzothiazole is also rarely described from flea and tick powders for pets.

Hand/Foot Dermatitis Due to Thioureas

Thioureas are accelerators most often tested as a mix containing diethyl thiourea and dibutyl thiourea. Thioureas are often used in neoprene orthopedic braces and wetsuits. Similar to mercaptobenzothiazole, dibutyl thiourea can be used as an anticorrosive, or they may be used in paint and adhesive removers and may cause hand dermatitis.[6]

Sole of Foot/Glove Pattern Hand Dermatitis

Thioureas are often used in insoles that patients insert into shoes after purchase. This may lead to a chronic, scaly plantar dermatitis. Thioureas are also occasionally used in neoprene gloves.

CHROMATE ALLERGY

Chromate frequently causes chronic hand dermatitis in metal workers and construction workers.[14] Men are more likely to be sensitized than women.[15] Hexavalent and trivalent chromium can cause allergy. Hexavalent chromium is more irritating, and in the 1980s, Scandinavian countries mandated adding ferrous sulfate to construction cement to cause reduction of hexavalent to trivalent chromium. Incidence of chromate dermatitis decreased after this initiative, but there is debate regarding whether the use of ferrous sulfate was of benefit or whether reduced usage of chromate and industrial hygiene played a role.[16] Hexavalent chromium is more likely to be systemically absorbed than trivalent, and a study in Taiwan that compared urinary chromium levels in cement workers before and after introduction of ferrous sulfate to cement in 2004 showed that systemic absorption was significantly reduced in workers after ferrous sulfate was added, especially those workers with hand dermatitis.[17] However, there was no difference in prevalence of hand dermatitis 3 months after addition of ferrous sulfate was instituted.

Cobalt is a common cosensitizer in chromium-allergic patients, especially those sensitized from cement.[15] Thiuram is the next most common cosensitizer as discussed in a previous section.

Pattern of Hand/Foot Dermatitis Due to Chromates

Allergic contact dermatitis resulting from chromates in cement occurs on the hands and wrists, especially the back of the dominant hand.[16] Cement is a common irritant; irritant dermatitis due to cement is more likely to be limited to the hands, whereas allergic dermatitis to cement may also affect the forearms, feet, and face.[17] Because chromates are used to tan leather, use of leather gloves can cause hand dermatitis. Allergy to leather can also cause hand and foot pattern dermatitis because of exposure to leather gloves and shoes. Hand dermatitis alone is the most common pattern of presentation of chromate allergy, accounting for about 35% of cases,

followed by hand with foot dermatitis in 15%, generalized pattern in 20%, and feet only in about 6%.[15]

Hyperkeratotic lesions on the elbow are reported in patients with dyshidrotic hand eczema to nickel and chromate. These lesions demonstrate dermatitis rather than psoriasis on biopsy, and usually flare with dietary metal exposure.[18]

Dietary Exposure Patterns in Chromate Allergy

Chromate-allergic patients may develop vesicles with experimental immersion of a finger into a metal solution more consistently than cobalt- or nickel-allergic patients.[19] Dietary ingestion of metals is often implicated in chronic vesicular hand dermatitis and is discussed in another article in this issue. A few patients with nonvesicular hand dermatitis, with or without positive patch tests to chromate, may flare with oral chromate challenge.[20] Dietary metal restriction is a low-risk therapeutic option in patients with recalcitrant hand dermatitis, especially men who have risk factors for occupational chromate sensitization.

MANAGEMENT OF DERMATITIS DUE TO RUBBER AND CHROMATES

Glove manufacturers report the types of chemicals used in published sources.[21] Vinyl gloves are a safe alternative for rubber-allergic patients, but they are not appropriate for all occupational hazards.

Shoe dermatitis poses a more difficult problem, as there is usually no way to determine the rubber chemicals used in shoes. Some patients improve with control of pedal hyperhidrosis, as perspiration permits leaching of rubber and chromates from footwear. Application of aluminum chloride hexahydrate to the feet to decrease perspiration lessens shoe dermatitis in some patients. Purchase of new socks is recommended, as rubber chemicals from previous shoes[22] or from previously applied allergenic medicaments may be retained in socks even after laundering.

Vinyl work boots are available. Also, insoles free of rubber chemicals can be used to replace existing insoles. Finally, custom shoemakers can create shoes free of specified allergens. Scheman et al[21] provide specific sources for these alternatives.

SUMMARY

Rubber chemicals and chromates, along with medicaments and adhesives, are common causes of dermatitis of the hands and feet. Patch testing to an extended standard series, shoe series, including rubber chemicals and textile dyes, and an extended medicament series is the best way to diagnosis allergic contact dermatitis of the hands and feet. When hand and foot dermatitis occur together, investigation for a primary systemic cause, such as psoriasis or chronic vesicular hand dermatitis, is indicated.

REFERENCES

1. Warshaw EM. Therapeutic options for chronic hand dermatitis. Dermatol Ther 2004;17(3):240–50.
2. Hersle K, Mobacken H. Hyperkeratotic dermatitis of the palms. Br J Dermatol 1982;107(2):195–201.
3. Sandy M. Slotnicki-Grant. Presented at the American Contact Dermatitis Society Meeting. Montreal, Quebec, Canada, Saturday, August 30, 2008.
4. Walling HW, Swick BL, Storrs FJ, et al. Frictional hyperkeratotic hand dermatitis responding to Grenz ray therapy. Contact Dermatitis 2008;58(1):49–51.
5. von Hintzenstern J, Heese A, Koch HU, et al. Frequency, spectrum and occupational relevance of type IV allergies to rubber chemicals. Contact Dermatitis 1991;24(4):244–52.
6. Rietschel R, Fowler JF. Rubber. In: Fisher's contact dermatitis. 6th edition. Hamilton: BC Decker; 2008. p. 581–604.
7. Kroft EB, van der Valk PG. Occupational contact dermatitis of both hands because of sensitization of black rubber. Contact Dermatitis 2008;58(2):125–6.
8. Dooms-Goossens A, Degreef H, De Veylder H, et al. Unusual sensitization to black rubber. Contact Dermatitis 1987;17(1):47–8.
9. Geier J, Lessmann H, Uter W, et al. Information Network of Departments of Dermatology (IVDK). Occupational rubber glove allergy: results of the Information Network of Departments of Dermatology (IVDK), 1995–2001. Contact Dermatitis 2003;48(1):39–44.
10. van Ketel WG, van den Berg WH. The problem of the sensitization to dithiocarbamates in thiuram-allergic patients. Dermatologica 1984;169(2):70–5.
11. Heese A, van Hintzenstern J, Peters KP, et al. Allergic and irritant reactions to rubber gloves in medical health services. Spectrum, diagnostic approach, and therapy. J Am Acad Dermatol 1991;25(5 Pt 1):831–9.
12. Kobaly K, Somani AK, McCormick TS, et al. Effects of occlusion on the skin of atopic dermatitis patients. Manuscript in preparation.
13. Knudsen BB, Hametner C, Seycek O, et al. Allergologically relevant rubber accelerators in single-use medical gloves. Contact Dermatitis 2000;43(1):9–15.
14. Shah M, Palmer IR. An ultrastructural study of chronic chromate hand dermatitis. Acta Derm Venereol 2002;82(4):254–9.
15. Olsavszky R, Rycroft RJ, White IR, et al. Contact sensitivity to chromate: comparison at a London contact dermatitis clinic over a 10-year period. Contact Dermatitis 1998;38(6):329–31.
16. Fisher AA. Cement injuries: part I. Cement hand dermatitis resulting in "chrome cripples". Cutis 1998;61(2):64.
17. Chou TC, Chang HY, Chen CJ, et al. Effect of hand dermatitis on the total body burden of chromium after ferrous sulfate application in cement among cement workers. Contact Dermatitis 2008;59(3):151–6.
18. Kaaber K, Sjølin KE, Menné T. Elbow eruptions in nickel and chromate dermatitis. Contact Dermatitis 1983;9(3):213–6.
19. Nielsen NH, Kristiansen J, Borg L, et al. Repeated exposures to cobalt or chromate on the hands of patients with hand eczema and contact allergy to that metal. Contact Dermatitis 2000;43(4):212–5.
20. Veien NK, Hattel T, Justesen O, et al. Oral challenge with metal salts (I). Vesicular patch-test-negative hand eczema. Contact Dermatitis 1983;9(5):402–6.
21. Scheman A, Jacob S, Zirwas M, et al. Contact Allergy: alternatives for the 2007 North American contact dermatitis group (NACDG) Standard Screening Tray. Dis Mon 2008;54(1–2):7–156.
22. Rietschel RL. Role of socks in shoe dermatitis. Arch Dermatol 1984;120(3):398.

Unusual Patterns in Contact Dermatitis: Medicaments

Mark D.P. Davis, MD

KEYWORDS

- Contact dermatitis • Hypersensitivity • Patch tests
- Topical drug administration • Adverse effects

A medicament is defined as an agent that treats, prevents, or alleviates the symptoms of disease. However, when topically applied, medications may cause multiple direct adverse effects; irritant contact dermatitis, allergic contact dermatitis, and contact urticaria are common adverse effects. For particular medicaments, other adverse effects may be observed: atrophy, striae, hypertrichosis, hyperpigmentation or hypopigmentation, acne, rosacea or perioral dermatitis, lichenoid skin eruptions, purpura, necrosis, and erythema multiforme.

This article focuses on the adverse effects of allergic contact dermatitis. Epidemics of allergy to topically applied medications have occurred for decades, directly paralleling the use of the topical prepared medicaments. The most notorious sensitizer was topical penicillin; its use was abandoned because of this problem.[1] So common are reactions to the antibiotics neomycin and bacitracin that bacitracin was named Contact Allergen of the Year in 2003 by the American Contact Dermatitis Society, to draw attention to the fact that these topical antibiotics are frequently associated with allergic contact dermatitis. Sulfonamides, mercurial products, and topically applied antihistamines are also well-known sensitizers, and their use has been substantially curtailed also because of this adverse effect. Increasingly recognized for the capability of causing allergic contact dermatitis are other popular topical antibiotics, topical anesthetics, and corticosteroids, among others.

Contact dermatitis due to topically applied medicaments may be caused by allergy not only to the agent but also to the preservatives or vehicle of the medication. For example, the stabilizer ethylenediamine (used in an antifungal cream in the 1970s and 1980s) was a well-known sensitizer. Allergic reactions to 1,3-butylene glycol,[2] benzyl alcohol,[3] and plant extracts in "alternative" topical medications[4] have been described. Paraben preservatives in topical antibiotics have also been recognized to be common sensitizers.

Clinical presentation of allergy to a medicament may have bizarre patterns that reflect the direction and site of its application to the skin or how it was inadvertently transferred on the skin from 1 area to another. Round patches of dermatitis may be a result of allergic contact dermatitis caused by the application of a medicament, with the pattern corresponding to the circular motion used during the application (Fig. 1). Certain areas of the skin seem to be more prone to contact allergy to medications. For example, perianal or genital dermatoses may be exacerbated by allergic contact dermatitis because of the medicament used for the dermatosis.

INCIDENCE AND PREVALENCE OF ALLERGIC CONTACT DERMATITIS TO MEDICAMENTS

In a prospective study, Edman and Moller[5] calculated that contact allergy to topical medications accounted for a startling 40% of all contact allergies observed. This percentage was equivalent to an annual incidence of 43 cases per 100,000 persons. They further observed that incidence was greater in patients who were older (mean age, 57 years) and male and in dermatitis cases involving the lower leg and anogenital area. Goh[6–8] found a lesser incidence of medicament sensitivity (22.5%) at a contact dermatitis clinic in Singapore. He reported that the rate was approximately equal for men and women and among

Department of Dermatology, Mayo Clinic, 200 First Street SW, Rochester, MN 55905, USA
E-mail address: davis.mark2@mayo.edu

Dermatol Clin 27 (2009) 289–297
doi:10.1016/j.det.2009.05.003

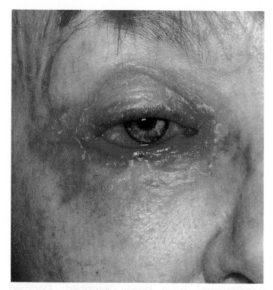

Fig. 1. Severe eyelid allergic contact dermatitis. A patient presented with a severe dermatitis involving her eyelids. Patch testing showed that the patient was allergic to the corticosteroid preparation she was using for her glaucoma. Discontinuation of the preparation and a switch to a different corticosteroid to which she was not allergic (with patch testing) led to resolution of the eyelid dermatitis.

races (Chinese, Malay, Indian, and others) and that most cases were on the limbs (upper and lower). Green and colleagues[9] noted that in the United Kingdom, contact allergy to topical medicaments was more common and numerous in patients older than 70 years.

RISK FACTORS FOR ALLERGIC CONTACT DERMATITIS TO MEDICAMENTS

Identified predisposing factors in this type of contact dermatitis include certain body sites (eg, lower extremities and body folds), use of occlusive dressings, use of transdermal medications, and preexisting dermatoses (eg, psoriasis, atopic dermatitis, otitis externa, vulvar and perianal dermatoses).

WHICH ALLERGENS IN TOPICAL MEDICATIONS CAUSE CONTACT DERMATITIS?

The culprit allergens in medicaments that cause contact dermatitis differ by geographic area and reflect local prescribing habits. Wilkinson and colleagues[10] found that in 2 adjacent areas of southeast England with the same climate, cultural backgrounds, and patch test methods, allergy to selected medications and their vehicles (lanolin, neomycin sulfate, parabens, iodochlorhydroxyquinoline, ethylenediamine, caine mix,

and chlorocresol) reflected the local prescribing habits.

The culprit allergens also change with time, reflecting changes in local prescribing habits. In 1985, Angelini and colleagues[11] described that penicillin, sulfonamide, promethazine, and neomycin were previously the most common culprits in contact dermatitis cases in Italy. The list is now headed by neomycin, benzocaine, and ethylenediamine, with antihistamines and parabens also frequently observed as sensitizers.

Also, the culprit allergens vary by report and, again, reflect the local prescribing habits. Edman and Moller[5] noted that the leading antigens were ethylenediamine, phenylbutazone, myristyl alcohol, chlorocresol, and cinchocaine. Green and colleagues[9] reported that the most frequent individual allergens were fragrance mix, *Myroxylon pereirae* (balsam of Peru), lanolins, local anesthetic agents, neomycin, gentamicin, and tixocortol pivalate; Goh[7] noted that common sensitizers included neomycin (7.8%), proflavine (7.1%), clioquinol (4.3%), colophony (3.3%), and wool alcohol (2.7%). In Singapore, Lim and colleagues[12] found that topical antibiotics (18.2%) and topical traditional Chinese medicaments (15.9%) were the most common causes of allergic contact dermatitis in a study of patients with leg ulcers.

Topical Antibiotics

Prevalence of allergy to topically applied antibiotics varies greatly by geographic location. In the United Kingdom, neomycin, clioquinol, and fusidic acid are widely used. A United Kingdom study that compared the frequency of patch test reactions positive to fusidic acid, clioquinol, and neomycin in 1119 patients found that medicament allergy to neomycin was 5 times more common than to clioquinol and 10 times more common than to fusidic acid.[13]

Neomycin, a widely used topical antibiotic, has become the most common allergen of all antibacterial preparations. In the latest North American Contact Dermatitis Group patch test reports, 11.6% of adults[14] and 8% of children[15] who received patch testing had an allergic patch test reaction to neomycin. Several drugs cross-react with neomycin, including streptomycin, kanamycin, gentamicin, tobramycin, and, commonly, bacitracin. Hence, bacitracin–polymixin B sulfate (Polysporin) ointment, which does not contain neomycin, may not be a safe option for neomycin-sensitive individuals. Notably, neomycin is often combined with corticosteroids in eye, ear, and skin preparations; in these preparations, the corticosteroids may mask the allergic contact dermatitis to neomycin. Patch test–induced "flare-up" reactions to neomycin at previous biopsy sites have been reported.[16]

Bacitracin coreacts frequently with neomycin, and 7.9% of patients have been reported to be sensitized.[14] It can also cause contact urticaria and contact anaphylaxis, and allergic contact dermatitis.

Penicillin was a frequent sensitizer in the past, but it has been taken off the market. Similarly, sulfonamides have been major sensitizers in the past, but they are less often found in topical preparations at present. They have been an integral part of many ophthalmic medications and vaginal medications and also of preparations used on leg ulcerations. Silver sulfadiazine used on burns is almost nonallergenic.

Chloramphenicol is a rare sensitizer, but sensitization has been reported in patients using eye drops containing this antibiotic. Sodium fusidate has been rarely reported to be associated with allergic contact dermatitis in patients with leg ulcerations, with the reports mainly from Europe. Tetracycline, clindamycin, and mupirocin are also rare sensitizers. Although the erythromycin base is a weak sensitizer, erythromycin salts (eg, erythromycin sulfate, erythromycin stearate, and erythromycin ethylsuccinate) can be sensitizing. Clioquinal and chlorquinaldol are weak sensitizers. Povidone iodine has rarely been reported to cause allergic contact dermatitis but has been reported to cause irritant contact dermatitis and contact urticaria. Quaternary ammonium compounds, such as benzalkonium chloride, contained in antiseptics, disinfectants, and eyedrops, have also been reported to cause irritant contact dermatitis.

Antifungal Agents

Antifungal agents, such as undecylenic acid and its derivatives (a natural fungicide that the US Food and Drug Administration approved in over-the-counter medications for skin disorders), allylamines (eg, naftifine and amorolfine), and polyene antimycotics (eg, nystatin) have all been reported to cause allergic contact dermatitis. Terbinafine has been associated with acute pustular exanthematous pustulosis. Imidazoles (eg, clotrimazole, tioconazole, and ketoconazole) are weak sensitizers; notably, ketoconazole has been reported in association with systemic contact dermatitis.

Antihistamines

Antihistamines are well-known sensitizers, and occasionally their sensitizing capacity exceeds their benefits. Topically applied diphenhydramine can cause allergic contact dermatitis and photoallergic contact dermatitis. Chlorpheniramine is a known sensitizer in eyedrops. Promethazine and chlorpromazine (an antipsychotic with antihistaminic properties) have been known to cause allergic contact dermatitis and photoallergic contact dermatitis. Doxepin (a tricyclic antidepressant with antihistaminic activity) can cause allergic and systemic contact dermatitis.

Nonsteroidal Antiinflammatory Drugs

Nonsteroidal antiinflammatory drugs are frequently used medications that are available by prescription and, often, over the counter. When topically applied, this class of drugs has a high incidence of adverse effects. Irritant contact dermatitis, allergic contact dermatitis, photoallergic contact dermatitis, phototoxicity, contact urticaria, erythema multiforme–like reactions, and systemic contact dermatitis have all been reported.

The arylpropionic acid derivatives, particularly ketoprofen, cause most allergic and photoallergic reactions. Photoallergic contact dermatitis to the nonsteroidal antiinflammatory drug ketoprofen[17] is increasingly recognized. Cross-reactivity of ketoprofen with ibuproxam, flurbiprofen, suprofen, oxybenzone, and fenofibrate have been documented; allergic and photoallergic contact dermatitis to these drugs has also been reported.

Bufexamac, diclofenac, and aceclofenac are all sensitizers; bufexamac use has also been reported in association with the development of erythema multiforme. Indomethacin and other pyrazolone derivatives have been described in association with allergic contact dermatitis and erythema multiforme–like reactions.

Topical Anesthetics

The term topical anesthetic drugs applies to numerous agents used to numb the skin. Topical anesthetics are used in an increasing number of skin care products, particularly for symptomatic relief of itch and pain. Although benzocaine was the chief offender in the past, other anesthetics are increasingly recognized as agents that may cause allergic contact dermatitis. Local anesthetics are used in burn remedies, external analgesics, athlete's foot remedies, lozenges, chewing gum, hemorrhoid products, pruritus vulvae treatment, and agents for toothache, canker sores, and denture irritation. Wherever these local anesthetics are used, they may cause allergic contact dermatitis.

The benzoic acid group is perhaps best known for causing allergic contact dermatitis. This group includes benzocaine, procaine (Novocain), and amethocaine (tetracaine). These agents are known to cross-react with *p*-aminobenzoic acid, *p*-phenylenediamine, sulfa drugs, thiazide diuretics, and azo and aniline dyes. Commonly used markers of allergy to this group in standard patch test series include benzocaine 5% in petrolatum.

The amide group is a less potent sensitizer and less commonly causes allergic contact dermatitis. This group includes lidocaine, dibucaine, mepivacaine, prilocaine, and bupivacaine. The commonly used marker of allergy to this group is lidocaine, used in various concentrations in the standard series (Mayo Clinic, 5%; North American Contact Dermatitis Group, 15%). Allergy to prilocaine (used in the eutectic mixture of lidocaine and prilocaine) has occasionally been reported.

It is important to patch test to multiple topical anesthetics. Of 10,061 patients who had patch testing performed by members of the North American Contact Dermatitis Group, 344 (3.4%) had an allergic reaction to at least 1 anesthetic.[18] Of the topical anesthetics tested, benzocaine was the most frequent allergen overall. More than 50% of allergic reactions to topical anesthetics in this study would have been missed had benzocaine been used as a single screening agent. Cross-reactivity patterns were not consistent with structural groups.

Simultaneous allergic contact dermatitis to classes (eg, amide, ester) of local anesthetic has been reported.[19]

Corticosteroids

Increasingly, topical corticosteroids have been recognized as a cause of allergic contact dermatitis. This finding has been the subject of numerous publications. For patients in whom corticosteroid allergy is suspected, patch test rates as high as 10.7% have been reported; allergy is often to multiple corticosteroids.[20] Allergic contact dermatitis to corticosteroids should be suspected when a patient with chronic dermatitis does not respond to topical corticosteroids.

Exposure to corticosteroids can occur through many routes, such as topical inhalation, oral exposure, and intravenous administration. Allergic reactions varying from eczema to purpura and urticaria have been reported. Type IV reactions are more common than type I reactions.

INVESTIGATIONS
Which Allergens are Recommended for a Standard Series?

In reports of various standard series, it is notable that numerous medicaments (predominantly antibiotics, corticosteroids, and topical anesthetics

and the vehicles and preservatives used in their preparation) are considered as sufficiently frequent sensitizers to be included in a standard series. For example, in the Mayo Clinic experience, medications accounted for approximately one-sixth of allergens in the standard tray. In order of decreasing frequency of positive allergic patch test result, the following allergens were included in the clinic's most recent report: neomycin, bacitracin, tixocortol pivalate, budesonide, benzocaine, hydrocortisone-17-butyrate, lidocaine, triamcinolone acetonide, clobetasol-17-proprionate, dibucaine, tetracaine hydrochloride, and prilocaine hydrochloride.[21]

Which Allergens Should Be Included in a Medicament Series?

Because contact allergies differ hugely depending on which agent is applied to the skin and according to the area of dermatitis, the best patch test to use is one with the products the patient uses and the components of a locally relevant patch test series.[22]

Interpretation of Patch Test Results

Some caveats to interpretation of patch test results must be born in mind. Patients may be able to tolerate a medication containing a preservative to which they are patch-test positive, because the concentration of the preservative in the commercial preparation is often below the threshold necessary to produce a clinical reaction.[23] Kellett and colleagues[24] reported 7 patients who reacted on patch testing to medicaments but who had negative reaction to the individual ingredients of the medicaments.

CLINICAL PRESENTATION AND SITES OF INVOLVEMENT

The areas of involvement in allergic contact dermatitis are generally related directly to where the topical medication is applied. On occasion, the medication may be transferred from 1 part of the skin to another and the consequent allergic contact dermatitis may be observed on 1 or both areas.

Unusual Patterns of Presentation

Unusual presentation patterns of contact dermatitis may be seen on the face, eyelids, forehead, scalp, lower face, lips, oral mucosa, neck, trunk, upper extremities, lower extremities (leg ulcer sensitization), or anogenital area (**Fig. 2**).

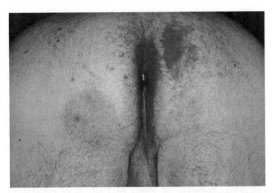

Fig. 2. Severe anogenital allergic contact dermatitis. This patient, a mail carrier, was on disability leave because of his severe anogenital dermatitis. On patch testing he was sensitive to the preservative methyl-chloroisothiazolinone and methylisothiazolinone that was in the moist toilet wipes he was using to clean this area after a bowel movement.

Transdermal Therapeutic Systems

Occlusion from transdermal therapeutic systems predispose to sensitization. There are numerous reports of reactions to active drugs contained in transdermal therapeutic systems, such as scopolamine, nitroglycerin, noresthisterone, clonidine, estradiol, nicotine, and testosterone. There are also reports of allergic contact dermatitis caused by the adhesive layer, including hydroxypropyl cellulose, methacrylate, ethanol, and polyisobutylene.

Scalp

Data from patch testing of 1320 patients with scalp dermatitis showed that medical products, hair tints and bleaches (predominantly those products that the patient used), and hair-cleansing products together caused nearly two-thirds of positive patch test reactions.[25]

Ear

Millard and Orton[26] found that a quarter of 179 patients with chronic inflammatory ear disease had medicament contact allergic dermatitis, evidence that supports the routine use of patch testing in these patients. The most common allergens in order of frequency of reaction were neomycin, framycetin sulfate, gentamicin, quinoline mix, and caine mix. Patch testing of 40 patients with chronic inflammatory ear disease showed medicament allergic contact dermatitis in 35%.[27] The most frequent sensitizers were neomycin, framycetin, clioquinol, and gentamicin. Wilkinson and Beck[28] reported that in their study of 9 patients with otitis externa, 4 had allergic

contact dermatitis, most commonly to corticosteroids and topical antibiotics used in the treatment of their dermatitis.

Lips

In a study of 75 patients with recalcitrant cheilitis who received patch testing, allergic contact dermatitis was diagnosed in 25%.[29] Medicaments applied to the lips were 1 of the culprits.

Eyes

Preservatives and active ingredients can cause allergic contact dermatitis. Allergic contact conjunctivitis to medicaments that are used in eyes can be confirmed with a provocative use test.

The best known of these agents in the past was the preservative thimerosal, a frequently used preservative in contact lens solution and eye medicaments. Substitute preservatives are now used in most eye solutions, and therefore its importance as an allergen in this context has waned.

Medications that have been reported to cause allergic contact conjunctivitis include β-adrenergic agents (levobutanol, thimalol, and befunolol), mydriatics (atropine, scopolamine, tropicamide, and phenylephrine), antibiotics (bacitracin, gentamicin, polymyxin B, neosporin, sulfathiazole, penicillin, and tetracycline), and antivirals (idoxuridine and trifluridine). In addition, antiinflammatory agents (chlorphenramine), antihistamines (ketolifen and amlexanox), corticosteroids (many agents), anesthetics (benzocaine, procaine, oxybuprocaine, proxymetacaine, proparacaine, and tetracaine), and other medications (eg, declofenac, penicillamine, pilocarpine) have been reported to be sensitizing.

Vulvar Dermatitis

The vulva is susceptible to irritant and allergic contact dermatitis to whatever medicaments are applied to the vulvar area.[30] Patients with lichen simplex chronicus, lichen sclerosus, pruritus vulvae, and pruritus ani apply many medicaments to the involved area. Occlusion in this area increases permeability of medications, increasing the chance of sensitization. High rates of sensitization have been reported in many studies, particularly to local anesthetics, antibiotics, corticosteroids, antiseptics, and preservatives.[30]

In a study of 61 women with vulvar lichen simplex chronicus, 47.5% had at least 1 positive patch test result.[31] Relevant positivities were observed in 26%, and the relevant allergens were usually medicaments and preservatives.

Marren and colleagues[32] similarly found that, of 135 patients with persistent vulval itch and discomfort who were evaluated, 63 (47%) had results positive for allergy. For 39 (29%) of these patients, the results were considered relevant to their clinical condition. Medicaments and their constituents were responsible for most of the reactions, and more than half of the patients had multiple allergies.

In a study of 121 women with pruritus vulvae, 57 (47%) had 1 or more relevant reactions positive for allergy.[33] Medicaments or their constituents were the most common allergens to cause the reactions. Out of the 16 patients with lichen sclerosus, 7 (44%) had positive reactions. In another study, Utaş and colleagues[34] reported that medications were frequent sensitizers in 50 women who received patch testing for pruritus vulvae.

Of 50 patients with vulvar symptoms, Brenan and colleagues[35] reported a similar incidence of allergic contact dermatitis: 42% of the patients had test results positive for allergy. Caine mix (6%) and ethylenediamine (8%) were among the identified culprits. Medicaments and fragrances were regarded as important allergens. Allergy to corticosteroids and imidazole was not a problem in this series of patients.

Peristomal Dermatitis

Peristomal allergic contact dermatitis caused by materials used for wound care has been well documented. Patch testing to a patient's own products should be performed, because avoidance of identified allergens may have a large impact on the patient's quality of life. Martin and colleagues[36] reported a case of a patient with stoma who had allergic contact dermatitis to Dansac soft paste (Dansac A/S, Hollister Inc, Chicago, Illinois), the wound care paste used on the patient's peristomal area.

Stasis Dermatitis and Chronic Leg Ulcerations

The risk for sensitization is high in patients with stasis dermatitis and leg ulcerations because patients apply multiple medicaments to remedy these conditions. The risk is heightened by the damaged skin barrier, the possibility of increased penetration of the applied medicament, and the use of occlusive dressings.

Patients may have allergic contact dermatitis caused by whatever medicine is applied to the skin. The most common example is allergic contact dermatitis to topical antibiotics, such as neosporin or bacitracin. Such dermatitis is a common and underrecognized phenomenon in patients with recalcitrant wounds. The many possible causes of this contact dermatitis include components of numerous treatments for wounds, such as topical antibiotics, adhesives in dressings, emollients, emulsifiers, and self-administered medicaments. When a wound is recalcitrant, allergic contact dermatitis is an important consideration for wound management.[37]

Reports of contact allergy in leg ulcerations reflect the pattern of use of wound care materials. In Singapore, Lim and colleagues[12] noted that the overall rate of contact sensitization in 44 patients with chronic leg ulcerations was 61.4%. Individually, colophony (11.3%), Saw Hong Choon skin ointment (Kam Bo Med, Hong Kong, Hong Kong) (11.3%), balsam of Peru (9.1%), and povidone iodine (9.1%) were among the most frequent allergens. The sensitization rate among users of topical traditional Chinese medicaments was notably high (41%).

Of 200 United Kingdom patients with venous leg ulcer, a similarly high rate of contact allergy (68%) was detected.[38] Multiple allergies occurred in 102 patients (51%). Among the most common sensitizers were antimicrobials (19.5%) and topical corticosteroids (8%); other most frequent allergen groups were fragrances (30.5%), topical excipients (19.5%), and rubber accelerators (13.5%). The investigators suggested that all patients with venous leg ulcer should receive patch testing with a locally relevant patch test series.

Other allergens identified include lanolin, bacitracin, clioquinol, corticosteroids, benzoyl peroxide, benzethonium chloride, neomycin, polymyxin B, sodium fusidate, parabens, and povidone iodine. Allergic contact dermatitis reactions to hydrocolloid dressings are often caused by the tackifying agent pentaerythritol ester of hydrogenated resin (Pentalyn),[39] carboxymethylcellulose,[40] or other chemicals.

Foot Dermatitis

In a study of patch testing to a shoe series for 230 patients with recalcitrant foot dermatitis, Holden and Gawkrodger[41] showed that medicament allergens were a prominent cause of allergic contact dermatitis, specifically, topical antibiotics (eg, neomycin) and topical corticosteroids (eg, tixocortol pivalate).

Systemic Contact Dermatitis

The term systemic allergic dermatitis is perhaps a better term to describe the rare development of a cutaneous allergic "hypersensitivity" reaction after systemic exposure to a hapten that reaches the skin through hematogenous transport.[42] Many drugs have been documented to induce this disorder (Box 1), but most drugs probably have the potential if the patient is sensitized and

Box 1
Drugs that have caused systemic allergic dermatitis

α-Blockers
Acetylsalicylic acid
Acyclovir
Alprenolol
Aminophylline
Amlexanox
5-Aminosalicylic acid
Amoxicillin
Barium sulfate
Captopril
Ceftriaxone
Cetirizine
Chloramphenicol
Cimetidine
Cinchocaine
Clindamycin
Clioquinol
Clobazam
Clonidine
Codeine
Corticosteroids
Cyclooxygenase-2 inhibitors
Dimethyl sulfoxide
Diphenhydramine
Doxepin
Ephedrine
Erythromycin
Estradiol
5-Fluorouracil
Fusidic acid
Gentamicin
Heparin
Hydromorphone
Hydroxyurea
Hydroxyzine
Intravenous human immunoglobulins
Iodinated radiocontrast media
Isoniazid
8-Methoxypsoralen
Miconazole
Mitomycin C
Neomycin
Nitroglycerin
Nonsteroidal antiinflammatory drugs
Norfloxacin
Nystatin
p-Amino compounds
Phenobarbital
Phenothiazines
Penicillins
Pristinamycin
Pseudoephedrine
Quinolones
Streptomycin
Sulfonamides
Suxamethonium
Terbinafine
Tetraethylthiuram disulfide

Valacyclovir
Virginiamycin

Includes symmetrical drug-related intertriginous and flexural exanthema and baboon syndrome. This box provides a partial list.

Data from Thyssen JP, Maibach HI. Drug-elicited systemic allergic (contact) dermatitis: update and possible pathomechanisms. Contact Dermatitis 2008;59(4):194–202.

the dose is high enough.[42] Many different routes of administration have been reported to cause systemic allergic contact dermatitis: topical, oral, rectal, vaginal, parenteral, and inhalational. With a latency period of a few hours or a few days after systemic exposure, a heterogeneous clinical picture occurs, many of which have received specific pattern designations or terms (**Box 2**). Described presentations include widespread, symmetrical maculopapular rash; pompholyx that consists of deeply seated vesicles and erythema in the palms and fingers; flexural dermatitis; baboon syndrome; and vasculitis-like lesions. Dermatitis may be seen as a flare-up reaction at sites of previously positive patch reactions or at sites of contact dermatitis, or both. Finally, the clinical picture may show erythroderma, erythema multiforme, or perhaps simply "intractable eczema." If systemic symptoms occur in systemic allergic dermatitis, they include headaches, fever, malaise, arthralgia, vomiting, and diarrhea. **Box 2** summarizes the described clinical presentations and previous designations. The medical literature on this topic continues to be sparse and confusing, but it has been neatly summarized by Thyssen and Maibach.[42]

Box 2
Terms used for systemic allergic dermatitis

Mercury exanthema
Internal-external contact-type
  hypersensitivity
Systemically induced allergic contact
  dermatitis—baboon syndrome
Systemic contact dermatitis
Paraptic eczema
Nonpigmented fixed drug eruption
Intertriginous drug eruption
Drug-induced intertrigo
Flexural (drug) eruption

Data from Thyssen JP, Maibach HI. Drug-elicited systemic allergic (contact) dermatitis: update and possible pathomechanisms. Contact Dermatitis 2008;59(4):194–202.

SUMMARY

Medicaments applied topically to the skin may cause many skin reactions, including allergic contact dermatitis. In cases of localized or generalized dermatitis, a list of the topical preparations applied to the affected areas or adjacent areas of the skin should be obtained. Patch testing, including use testing, should be used to ascertain the culprit allergen.

REFERENCES

1. Fisher AA. Topical medicaments which are common sensitizers. Ann Allergy 1982;49(2):97–100.
2. Oiso N, Fukai K, Ishii M. Allergic contact dermatitis due to 1,3-butylene glycol in medicaments. Contact Dermatitis 2004;51(1):40–1.
3. Sestini S, Mori M, Francalanci S. Allergic contact dermatitis from benzyl alcohol in multiple medicaments. Contact Dermatitis 2004;50(5):316–7.
4. Bruynzeel DP, van Ketel WG, Young E, et al. Contact sensitization by alternative topical medicaments containing plant extracts. The Dutch Contact Dermatoses Group. Contact Dermatitis 1992;27(4):278–9.
5. Edman B, Moller H. Medicament contact allergy. Derm Beruf Umwelt 1986;34(5):139–43.
6. Goh CL, Ling R. A retrospective epidemiology study of contact eczema among the elderly attending a tertiary dermatology referral centre in Singapore. Singapore Med J 1998;39(10):442–6.
7. Goh CL. Contact sensitivity to topical medicaments. Int J Dermatol 1989;28(1):25–8.
8. Goh CL. Epidemiology of contact allergy in Singapore. Int J Dermatol 1988;27(5):308–11.
9. Green CM, Holden CR, Gawkrodger DJ. Contact allergy to topical medicaments becomes more common with advancing age: an age-stratified study. Contact Dermatitis 2007;56(4):229–31.
10. Wilkinson JD, Hambly EM, Wilkinson DS. Comparison of patch test results in two adjacent areas of England, II: medicaments. Acta Derm Venereol 1980;60(3):245–9.
11. Angelini G, Vena GA, Meneghini CL. Allergic contact dermatitis to some medicaments. Contact Dermatitis 1985;12(5):263–9.
12. Lim KS, Tang MB, Goon AT, et al. Contact sensitization in patients with chronic venous leg ulcers in Singapore. Contact Dermatitis 2007;56(2):94–8.
13. Morris SD, Rycroft RJ, White IR, et al. Comparative frequency of patch test reactions to topical antibiotics. Br J Dermatol 2002;146(6):1047–51.
14. Pratt MD, Belsito DV, DeLeo VA, et al. North American Contact Dermatitis Group patch-test results, 2001–2002 study period. Dermatitis 2004;15(4):176–83 [Erratum in: Dermatitis 2005;16(2):106].
15. Zug KA, McGinley-Smith D, Warshaw EM, et al. Contact allergy in children referred for patch testing: North American Contact Dermatitis Group data, 2001–2004. Arch Dermatol 2008;144(10):1329–36.
16. Jacob SE, Barland C, ElSaie ML. Patch-test-induced "flare-up" reactions to neomycin at prior biopsy sites. Dermatitis 2008;19(6):E46–8.
17. Sugiyama M, Nakada T, Hosaka H, et al. Photocontact dermatitis to ketoprofen. Am J Contact Dermat 2001;12(3):180–1.
18. Warshaw EM, Schram SE, Belsito DV, et al. Patch-test reactions to topical anesthetics: retrospective analysis of cross-sectional data, 2001 to 2004. Dermatitis 2008;19(2):81–5.
19. Gunson TH, Greig DE. Allergic contact dermatitis to all three classes of local anaesthetic. Contact Dermatitis 2008;59(2):126–7.
20. Davis MD, el-Azhary RA, Farmer SA. Results of patch testing to a corticosteroid series: a retrospective review of 1188 patients during 6 years at Mayo Clinic. J Am Acad Dermatol 2007;56(6):921–7.
21. Davis MD, Scalf LA, Yiannias JA, et al. Changing trends and allergens in the patch test standard series: a Mayo Clinic 5-year retrospective review, January 1, 2001, through December 31, 2005. Arch Dermatol 2008;144(1):67–72.
22. Stewart LA. Patch testing to cosmetics and topical drugs. Am J Contact Dermat 1996;7(1):53–5.
23. Skinner SL, Marks JG. Allergic contact dermatitis to preservatives in topical medicaments. Am J Contact Dermat 1998;9(4):199–201.
24. Kellett JK, King CM, Beck MH. Compound allergy to medicaments. Contact Dermatitis 1986;14(1):45–8.
25. Hillen U, Grabbe S, Uter W. Patch test results in patients with scalp dermatitis: analysis of data of the information network of departments of dermatology. Contact Dermatitis 2007;56(2):87–93.
26. Millard TP, Orton DI. Changing patterns of contact allergy in chronic inflammatory ear disease. Contact Dermatitis 2004;50(2):83–6.
27. Holmes RC, Johns AN, Wilkinson JD, et al. Medicament contact dermatitis in patients with chronic inflammatory ear disease. J R Soc Med 1982; 75(1):27–30.
28. Wilkinson SM, Beck MH. Hypersensitivity to topical corticosteroids in otitis externa. J Laryngol Otol 1993;107(7):597–9.
29. Freeman S, Stephens R. Cheilitis: analysis of 75 cases referred to a contact dermatitis clinic. Am J Contact Dermat 1999;10(4):198–200.
30. Bauer A, Rodiger C, Greif C, et al. Vulvar dermatoses: irritant and allergic contact dermatitis of the vulva. Dermatology 2005;210(2):143–9.
31. Virgili A, Bacilieri S, Corazza M. Evaluation of contact sensitization in vulvar lichen simplex chronicus: a proposal for a battery of selected allergens. J Reprod Med 2003;48(1):33–6.

32. Marren P, Wojnarowska F, Powell S. Allergic contact dermatitis and vulvar dermatoses. Br J Dermatol 1992;126(1):52–6.

33. Lewis FM, Shah M, Gawkrodger DJ. Contact sensitivity in pruritus vulvae: patch test results and clinical outcome. Am J Contact Dermat 1997;8(3):137–40.

34. Utas S, Ferahbas A, Yildiz S. Patients with vulval pruritus: patch test results. Contact Dermatitis 2008;58(5):296–8.

35. Brenan JA, Dennerstein GJ, Sfameni SF, et al. Evaluation of patch testing in patients with chronic vulvar symptoms. Australas J Dermatol 1996;37(1):40–3.

36. Martin JA, Hughes TM, Stone NM. Peristomal allergic contact dermatitis: case report and review of the literature. Contact Dermatitis 2005;52(5):273–5.

37. Siegel DM. Contact sensitivity and recalcitrant wounds. Ostomy Wound Manage 2000;46(Suppl 1A):65S–74S.

38. Tavadia S, Bianchi J, Dawe RS, et al. Allergic contact dermatitis in venous leg ulcer patients. Contact Dermatitis 2003;48(5):261–5.

39. Timmer-de Mik L, Toonstra J. Allergy to hydrocolloid dressings. Contact Dermatitis 2008;58(2):124–5.

40. Koo FP, Piletta-Zanin P, Politta-Sanchez S, et al. Allergic contact dermatitis to carboxymethylcellulose in Comfeel hydrocolloid dressing. Contact Dermatitis 2008;58(6):375–6.

41. Holden CR, Gawkrodger DJ. 10 years' experience of patch testing with a shoe series in 230 patients: which allergens are important? Contact Dermatitis 2005;53(1):37–9.

42. Thyssen JP, Maibach HI. Drug-elicited systemic allergic (contact) dermatitis: update and possible pathomechanisms. Contact Dermatitis 2008;59(4):194–202.

Clinical Patterns of Phytodermatitis

Denis Sasseville, MD, FRCPC

KEYWORDS

- Allergic contact dermatitis • Irritant contact dermatitis
- Phytodermatitis • Phytophotodermatitis • Botanic extracts

Cutaneous exposure to plants occurs mostly through outdoor activity. Campers, hikers, forestry workers, farmers, and gardeners at times develop skin eruptions from close interaction with the vegetal kingdom. Plants are also present indoors and can adversely affect homemakers, housekeepers, florists, cooks, and grocery store workers. Botanic extracts and plant derivatives are ubiquitous and found in a wide range of products, from foods to building materials, and from fragrances to topical and oral medicaments.

Most published textbook reviews describe phytodermatitis from a pathophysiologic or botanic perspective.[1–3] The present article puts the emphasis on the clinical presentation of cutaneous reactions to plants, highlighting some classic and less common patterns of dermatitis.

POISON IVY DERMATITIS

Members of the family Anacardiaceae, 5 species of the genus *Toxicodendron* are widely distributed across the North American continent.[4] The 2 species of poison oak have different ranges, *T. diversilobum* being found along the Pacific coast, whereas *T. toxicarium* inhabits the southeastern United States. Poison ivy is represented by 2 species: *T. rydbergii*, which grows in the northern and midwestern United States and Canada as a low-lying shrub, and *T. radicans*, a climbing vine found all along the eastern coast of the United States. All 4 species have pinnate (compound) leaves divided in 3 leaflets. Those of poison oak are deeply notched, such as oak leaves, while poison ivy leaflets are spoon-shaped (**Fig. 1**). The habitat of *T. vernix*, or poison sumac, is restricted to the eastern United States and

Canada. A tree that grows in marshy areas, it bears 7 to 13 smooth-edged, lanceolate leaflets on a long central petiole.

When bruised, all parts of the plant exude a sticky, strongly allergenic oleoresin, called urushiol. It could theoretically sensitize 70% of individuals who come in contact with it, and up to 50% of North Americans are presumably already sensitized.[5,6] The allergens are penta- or heptadecylcatechols, benzene rings that bear hydroxyl groups at position 1 and 2, and aliphatic side chains at position 3. The length of the side chain and the number of its double bonds determine the allergenicity of the molecule.[7,8]

Once an individual is sensitized, repeated contact will elicit cutaneous lesions within 12 to 48 hours. The reaction is an acute eczema that begins with pruritic, edematous, erythematous papules and urticarial-looking plaques that rapidly become studded with vesicles and tense bullae. Lesions appear where the plant has brushed against the skin, typically on the legs, thighs, hands, and upper limbs. They classically display a linear morphology of crisscrossing streaks (**Fig. 2**). The sticky sap can be transferred from the fingers to more distant sites, such as the face, trunk, and genitals. It may at times produce a bizarre-shaped, severely edematous and vesicular perianal and genital eczema in the unfortunate hiker who used a handful of poison ivy leaves instead of toilet paper.

New lesions will continue to erupt for 1 to 2 weeks. It is not rare for insufficiently treated episodes to last 4 to 8 weeks, or to flare up after short courses of systemic corticosteroids. In subsequent episodes, lesions tend to become

No funding was available for this work.
Division of Dermatology, Department of Medicine, McGill University Health Centre, Royal Victoria Hospital, Room A 4.17, 687 Pine Avenue west, Montreal, QC H3A 1A1, Canada
E-mail address: denis.sasseville@mcgill.ca

Dermatol Clin 27 (2009) 299–308
doi:10.1016/j.det.2009.05.010

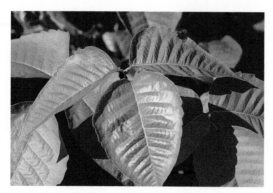

Fig. 1. *Toxicodendron rydbergii* (poison ivy) showing the three leaflets of its pinnate leaves.

more severe, and they tend to appear after a shorter interval following exposure.

Depending on the type of exposure, the classic, streaky pattern may be blurred or unrecognizable. This may occur with weed-wacker dermatitis.[9] The victim, often clad in shorts, trims weeds with a rotating strimmer that projects a puree of vegetal particles. The resulting dermatitis is a diffuse papulovesicular eruption that involves the exposed front half of the body and is more severe on the shins. Exposure to smoke from burning poison ivy plants results in an airborne pattern of dermatitis that spares covered areas. Lesions do not follow a specific pattern when the dermatitis is acquired by proxy, such as after handling contaminated garments or tools, or petting a dog that went cavorting in poison ivy.

SESQUITERPENE LACTONE DERMATITIS

The Asteraceae, or Compositae, family is the second largest of the vegetal kingdom. It comprises edible plants, such as lettuce, sunflower, tarragon, and artichoke; weeds like dandelion, ragweed, and thistle; and ornamental plants whose names cover the entire alphabet,

from aster to zinnia. Chrysanthemums, chamomile, coneflowers, dahlias, daisies, and black-eyed Susans, all belong to this family. Most of these plants bear small, tubular flowers densely packed on a flowering disk, or capitulum. The florets of the outer row are often ligulated, displaying rays of fused petals (**Fig. 3**).

Asteraceae produce chemicals known as sesquiterpene lactones (SLs), 15-carbon molecules made of a sesquiterpene linked to a lactone ring.[10] Approximately 750 of these molecules could theoretically sensitize, and allergenicity is increased by the presence of an α-methylene group attached to the lactone ring.[11] SLs are present in fresh plants, pollen, and in particles from dried plants.[12]

Classically, SL-induced dermatitis affects men more than women, and is rare in childhood. Outdoor workers, such as farmers and gardeners, have a higher risk for sensitization, but florists, nursery workers, and cooks have also been affected. Sensitization occurs through direct and airborne skin contact. Subacute eczematous lesions initially involve the face, the neck, and the exposed areas of the upper limbs. The dermatitis is seen in the growing season of the plants and abates during the winter. With repeated yearly exposure, however, the disease-free interval gets progressively shorter, and a chronic, severely pruritic, and extremely lichenified dermatitis becomes perennial. On the face, massive lichenification gives rise to a leonine facies reminiscent of cutaneous lymphoma or actinic reticuloid. This pattern of involvement simulates photodermatitis, but in many patients, true photosensitivity eventually supervenes and progresses to severe chronic actinic dermatosis or full-blown erythroderma. SLs are not phototoxic or photoallergic, and the cause

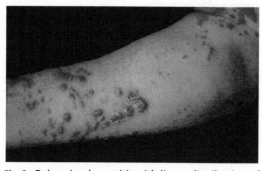

Fig. 2. Poison ivy dermatitis with linear distribution of papules and vesicles.

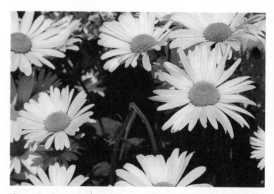

Fig. 3. *Leucanthemum vulgare* (oxeye daisy). Hundreds of tiny yellow florets are clustered on a flowering disk. The peripheral flowers bear white rays made of three fused petals.

of SL-associated photosensitivity therefore remains elusive.[13]

Asteraceae are not the only plants that produce SLs. They are also found in magnolias and laurels, and in liverworts, or bryophytes, moss-like organisms that grow on the bark of trees. *Frullania dilatata* and *F. tamarisci*, of the family Jubulaceae, have been identified as the cause of "cedar poisoning," an occupational dermatitis of forest workers.[14] It is clinically indistinguishable from Asteraceae dermatitis, except that it flares during the wet winter months of the Pacific northwest logging season.[15]

PRIMULA DERMATITIS

Among the 500 varieties of primroses, *Primula obconica* is a winter-flowering indoor plant that is still quite popular in Europe. It possesses broad and hairy leaves, and small goblet flowers that must be deadheaded to stimulate continuous blooming. Primin, or 2-methoxy-6-pentylbenzoquinone, is the main allergen, and its concentration in the plant is highest between the months of April and August.[16]

The dermatitis involves the fingertips, the dorsum of the fingers, and hands, sometimes the forearms. It presents as edematous papules and irregular or linear papulovesicular plaques. The eyelids, face, and neck may become secondarily affected by hand-borne transfer of the allergen.

Primin-free cultivars are now available and widely distributed. The beginning of the 2000s has seen a steady decline in the detection rate of primin allergy in Europe.[17,18] Contact dermatitis to primrose has always been rare in North America, and a study by Mowad[19] yielded only one positive reaction out of 567 consecutively tested patients.

PHYTOPHOTODERMATITIS

Some families of plants contain psoralens or furocoumarins that trigger a phototoxic eruption when activated by exposure to ultraviolet A light after contact with the skin. This reaction is not immunologically mediated, and it affects anyone under appropriate circumstances. The plant chemicals loosely bind to DNA but, when photoexcited, become covalently bound to pyrimidine bases on DNA strands, leading to cell death.

Phytophotodermatitis is most often caused by contact with plants of the Apiaceae, or Umbelliferae, family. They include weeds and edible plants, such as hogweed, cowbane, carrot, parsnip, dill, fennel, celery, and anise. Their common botanic characteristic is their inflorescence known as an umbel, an umbrella-like cluster of long stalks radiating from a central point (**Fig. 4**). Psoralens are also present in Rutaceae, a family that comprises shrubs and trees of the genus *Citrus*, the gas plant (*Dictamnus albus*), and rue (*Ruta graveolens*), an herb often used as a condiment. Amongst phototoxic Moraceae and Fabaceae are found, respectively, the fig tree (*Ficus carica*) and babchi (*Psoralea cordifolia*), from which psoralens were named.

The typical pattern of phytophotodermatitis is meadow-grass dermatitis, also known as dermatitis bullosa striata pratensis of Oppenheim. Lesions will appear within 8 to 24 hours of exposure to the sap of a psoralen-containing plant followed by sun exposure. Accompanied by a burning sensation, erythematous, irregular patches and streaks appear on areas that were exposed to both plant and light. Vesicles and large blisters may be present, but pruritus is not a major feature of the eruption, as opposed to allergic phytodermatitis. As the lesions heal, they are replaced by deeply pigmented macules that slowly fade in the course of weeks to months.

The juice of lime or other citrus fruits may flow around the mouth, spill over the hands, or drip on the body of vacationers lying around swimming pools, producing bizarre blotches and trickle-shaped streaks of pigmentation (**Fig. 5**). Contact with the cut ends of psoralen-containing celery caused an epidemic of phytophotodermatitis affecting the forearms of grocery store workers.[20]

TULIP FINGERS

Originating from central Asia, *Tulipa gesneriana* was introduced in Holland in the 16th century.[21] There are now more than 2500 modern tulip cultivars in the family Liliaceae, propagated by their onion-like bulbs. Growers and sorters handle

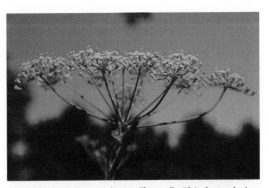

Fig. 4. *Foeniculum vulgare* (fennel). This lateral view shows the umbrella-shaped umbel bearing secondary umbellules.

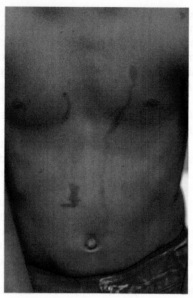

Fig. 5. Pigmentary stage of phytophotodermatitis caused by lime juice that trickled on the skin, producing a pattern reminiscent of berloque dermatitis.

them repeatedly, as they peel off dead tecta (outer skin) and bulblets from the main bulb. They often develop a severely fissured, hyperkeratotic dermatitis, at times accompanied by painful paronychia, involving the pulp of the first 3 fingers (Fig. 6).[22]

The allergen is tulipalin A, or α-methylene-γ-butyrolactone, an SL that does not cross-react with the SLs of the Asteraceae. It is hydrolyzed from tuliposide A, a glycoside present in all parts of the plant but more concentrated in the bulb. The same allergen also occurs in the stem, leaves, and petals of the Peruvian lily, Alstroemeria aurantiaca, a showy, trumpet-shaped flower with striped inner petals, which has become very popular in

flower arrangements (Fig. 7). Sensitized florists who handle the plant and cut leaves along the stem develop a pattern of dermatitis similar to tulip fingers.[23] The dermatitis, however, often extends to the entire volar surface of the second finger of the hand that holds the paring knife (Fig. 8).

Cooks who slice garlic bulbs occasionally develop an allergic contact dermatitis that mimics tulip fingers. The lesions are often unilateral, limited to the nondominant fingers that hold the clove that is being sliced with the other hand. The allergen in this case is diallyl disulfide, a molecule unrelated to SLs.

LESS COMMON PATTERNS OF PHYTODERMATITIS
Other Anacardiaceae and Ginkgoaceae

Mangoes, fruits of Mangifera indica, contain urushiol in their exocarp (outer skin). A mild to severe perioral dermatitis can occur when a sensitized individual bites into an unpeeled mango[24] (Fig. 9). Approximately 80% of Japanese cabinetmakers exposed to the varnish extracted from the lacquer tree, Toxicodendron verniciflua, develop a dermatitis that involves the hands and forearms.[25] Repeated low-grade exposure, however, induces some degree of tolerance, and the majority of lacquer workers can continue to ply their trade. Laundrymen in India, called dhobis, mark their customers' clothes with an urushiol-containing black oleoresin extracted from the nut of Semecarpus anacardium. The ink is unaffected by boiling and has caused numerous cases of "dhobi itch," allergic dermatitis at the site of contact, usually the nape of the neck[26] or around the waist. The closely related Brazilian cashew nut tree, Anacardium occidentale, bears reddish fruits that contain the kidney-shaped nut within a three-layered pericarp. The middle layer is filled with brownish oil rich in cardol and anacardic acid, chemically similar to urushiol. These

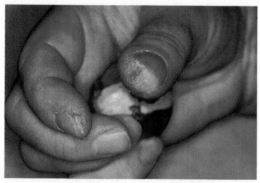

Fig. 6. Tulip fingers. Painful, fissured, and hyperkeratotic dermatitis of the pulp of the first 3 fingers.

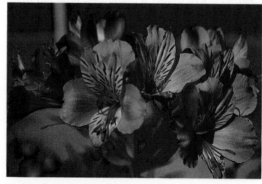

Fig. 7. Alstroemeria aurantiaca (Peruvian lily) displaying its striped inner petals.

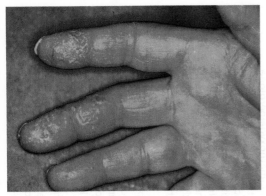

Fig. 8. Hand dermatitis in a florist sensitized to *Alstroemeria*.

catechols are destroyed when the nut is properly roasted and processed, but harvesters have developed occupational dermatitis from exposure to the oil. Cashew oil is also used in the production of phenolformaldehyde resins, varnishes, inks, and brake linings. Exposed workers can become sensitized and develop eczematous lesions on exposed parts of the body.[6]

Although unrelated to the Anacardiaceae, the *Ginkgo biloba* tree is also a source of urushiol-like catechols. The tree is dioecious, that is, divided into male and female individuals. The allergenic ginkgolic acid is present exclusively in the flesh of the drupe-like ovule. In 1963, an epidemic of allergic contact dermatitis affected 35 schoolgirls who presented with eczematous lesions on legs that had been splattered with the juice of trampled ovules.[27] Urban planners who use the ginkgo as ornamental tree along streets and avenues now recommend planting male specimens only.

Airborne Contact Dermatitis

The pattern of airborne contact dermatitis may be confused with photodermatitis, because both

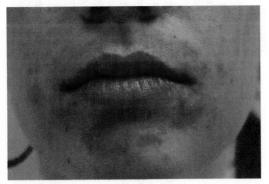

Fig. 9. Subacute perioral dermatitis in a poison ivy-sensitive patient, caused by biting into an unpeeled mango.

involve exposed areas. But photodermatitis spares the upper eyelids and the submental and retroauricular regions, which are areas that are affected by an airborne allergen or irritant.

The disease may be acute, with severe edema and blisters, as when a sensitized individual is exposed to the smoke of burning poison ivy, or chronic and lichenified from contact with SLs of windblown ragweed pollen or trichomes and dried particles of *Parthenium hysterophorus*, also known as "congress grass" or "the scourge of India." This plant, indigenous in the southern United States, was accidentally introduced in India in the 1950s and has rapidly spread throughout its country of adoption, sensitizing thousands in the rural population.

Sawmill workers, carpenters, cabinetmakers, and floor layers often work with indigenous and exotic woods from tropical areas. Pine, fir, and spruce softwood exudes a sticky resin from which are extracted turpentine and its solid residue, colophony, also known as rosin. These compounds are natural mixes of various terpenes, some of which are strong allergens in their oxidized form. Many tropical species contain allergenic quinones that are potent sensitizers (**Table 1**). Fine sawdust floating in the air sticks to the face and other exposed areas, giving rise to a true airborne contact dermatitis (**Fig. 10**). In addition, it infiltrates clothes and gets deposited in moist folds, hence the frequent involvement of antecubital fossae, axillae, waistline, and genitals.

Irritant Contact Dermatitis

Dieffenbachias and *Philodendrons* are tropical species of the Araceae family, grown as indoor plants for their shiny decorative foliage. Their sap is rich in needle-like calcium oxalate crystals, or raphides, that penetrate the skin and cause burning erythema, blisters, and, at times, necrosis on parts of the body, usually the hands and forearms, that come in contact with broken leaves or stems. Small children may chew the leaves and develop a severe stomatitis accompanied by abundant sialorrhea and aphonia, hence the name "dumb cane" given to some species of *Dieffenbachia*.[28]

The century plant, *Agave americana* or *tequilana*, of the Agavaceae family, is widely cultivated in Mexico. This succulent plant develops, almost at ground level, thick, broad, serrated, and sword-like leaves arranged in a rosette pattern.[29] Its sap contains not only inulin, which is hydrolyzed and fermented to produce mescal and tequila, but also various saponins and calcium oxalate raphides. Machete-wielding workers chop the leaves

Table 1
Some indigenous and tropical trees that cause allergic dermatitis

Family	Taxon	Vernacular Name	Allergens
Anacardiaceae, Ginkgoaceae, Magnoliaceae	*Anacardium occidentale* *Mangifera indica* *Schinus terebinthifolius* *Lithraea molleoides* *Ginkgo biloba* *Magnolia* spp	Cashew nut tree Mango tree Brazilian pepper tree Liter Ginkgo Magnolia	Various heptadecylcatechols and pentadecylcatechols, cardol, anacardic acid, etc
Bignoniaceae	*Tabebuia avellanedae*	Lapacho, ipe	Deoxylapachol Lapachenole Lapachol
Cupressaceae	*Thuya plicata*	Canadian red cedar, redwood	B-thujaplicin Thymoquinone
Fabaceae	*Dalbergia nigra* *Dalbergia latifolia* *Dalbergia melanoxylon* *Dalbergia retusa* *Dalbergia cearensis* *Machaerium scleroxylon* *Bowdichia nitida*	Brazilian rosewood Indian rosewood African blackwood Cocobolo Kingwood Jacaranda, pao ferro Sucupira	R-4-methoxydalbergione R-4-methoxydalbergione S-4-methoxydalbergione S-4-OH-4-methoxydalbergione S-4'-OH-4-methoxydalbergione R-4-methoxydalbergione Obtusaquinone Unspecified dalbergione R-3,4-dimethoxydalbergione 2,6-Dimethoxybenzoquinone Bowdichione
Meliaceae	*Khaya anthotheca* *Swietenia macrophylla*	African mahogany American mahogany	Anthothecol
Moraceae	*Chlorophora excelsa*	Iroko	Chlorophorin
Pinaceae	*Abies balsamea* *Picea glauca* *Pinus resinosa* *Pseudotsuga menzesii* *Tsuga Canadensis*	Balsam fir White spruce Red pine Douglas fir Eastern hemlock	Colophony, a natural mix that includes: D^3-carene hydroperoxides, abietic acid, dehydroabietic acid, dihydroabietic acid, pimaric acid, etc.
Sterculaceae	*Mansonia altissima*	Bete	Mansonon A
Verbenaceae	*Tectona grandis*	Teak	Deoxylapachol Lapachol

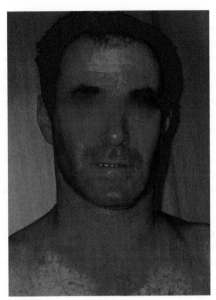

Fig. 10. Airborne allergic contact dermatitis in a woodworker.

to harvest the core of the plant. Sap is projected on exposed legs, hands, forearms, and face, quickly eliciting a burning sensation and a dermatitis referred to as "mal de agaveros."[30]

Calcium oxalate and possibly various alkaloids also play a role in the induction of occupational dermatitis in growers and handlers of daffodils and hyacinths. These perennial, bulbous, early-blooming plants belong, respectively, to the Amaryllidaceae (*Narcissus pseudonarcissus*) and Liliaceae (*Hyacinthus orientalis*) families. "Daffodil itch," or "lily rash," affects up to 50% of flower cutters whose hands and forearms come in contact with the sap.[21] Secondary involvement of the face and genital region occurs by transfer of the sap from contaminated hands. The dermatitis is usually mild but at times becomes chronic or generalized. Hyacinth bulbs contain up to 6% by weight calcium oxalate crystals. The outer skin of these bulbs is brittle and easily breaks down into dust or tiny sharp scales that become airborne and release raphides when deposited on the skin. Nearly all bulb handlers experience pruritus or dermatitis, known as "hyacinth itch" or "bulb scabies." Involved areas include the inner forearms, the face, thighs, anogenital region, and other areas where clothes rub on the skin.[21]

The so-called "sabra dermatitis" is another scabies-like condition, caused by mechanical rather than chemical irritation. It occurs in harvesters of prickle pears, the edible fruits of the cactus *Opuntia ficus-indica*. The dermatitis was first described in Israel and presents as an itchy, papular eruption of the hands, fingers, wrists, chest, buttocks, and genitals.[31] It is secondary to cutaneous implantation of fragments of fine bristles known as glochids.

Erythema Multiforme

Severe allergic contact dermatitis often becomes prone to autoeczematization and gives rise to disseminated lesions, distributed well beyond the initial site of contact. At times, these lesions display a concentric, target-shaped morphology. These targets are often atypical, being arciform or incomplete, lacking the dusky center of true erythema multiforme (EM). Histopathologic examination either reveals the characteristic interface dermatitis of EM or a spongiotic dermatitis, in which case the eruption is better called "EM-like."[32]

Allergens of plant origin are most often responsible for such eruptions. They include *Toxicodendron spp*;[33] numerous exotic woods, such as Brazilian rosewood, cocobolo, pao ferro, and so on; *Primula obconica*; plants of the Asteraceae family; and tea tree oil, extracted from the Australian tree *Melaleuca alternifolia*.[34,35]

Dermatitis from Plant Extracts and Botanicals

Plant extracts and products based on plant derivatives are ubiquitous in daily life and include gums, balsams, adhesives, textiles, wooden objects, paper, foods and spices, perfumes, cosmetics, and topical medicaments. Of the 65 allergens or mixes tested by the North American Contact Dermatitis Group in its standard series, 9 are of plant origin: colophony, some components of the fragrance mix I (cinnamic alcohol, cinnamal, eugenol, isoeugenol, and oak moss absolute) and of the fragrance mix II (coumarin, citronellol, and farnesol), *Myroxylon pereirae* (balsam of Peru), SL mix and Compositae mix, propolis, tea tree oil, and ylang-ylang. It is beyond the scope of this article to describe every pattern of reaction caused by contact with these plant derivatives, but some are worthy of mention.

Phytophotodermatitis caused by psoralen-containing perfumes is known as berloque dermatitis. This pattern is rarely seen nowadays, because most manufacturers have removed from their formulations the phototoxic bergapten, present in the oil of the bitter orange bergamot (*Citrus aurantiaca*). Women who sunbathed after applying these perfumes, such as the older version of Shalimar by Guerlain, developed pigmented, curvilinear, pendant-like streaks on the sides of the neck, the inner wrists and arms, back of hands, and so on.

Massage therapy has become popular in recent years. Practitioners use a wide variety of fragrant essential oils, believed to possess stress relieving or other medicinal properties. Numerous therapists have become sensitized to lavender, eucalyptus, ylang-ylang, sandalwood, or jasmine and suffer from occupational hand eczema involving mostly the palms and the volar aspect of the fingers.

Botanic extracts are increasingly added to cosmetic and therapeutic preparations and, not surprisingly, the incidence of allergic contact dermatitis to these compounds has risen. Kiken and Cohen[36] published an extensive review of herbal extracts reported to cause contact allergy. *Arnica montana*, or mountain tobacco, an SL-producing member of the Asteraceae family, is probably the most common offender.[37] It is often used as a tincture or ointment for the treatment of sprains, bruises, and other musculoskeletal ailments. Belonging to the same family, Roman chamomile, *Anthemis nobilis*, and its slightly less allergenic German counterpart, *Matricaria chamomilla*, are often brewed as herbal tea, and the decoction is used as soothing compresses for burns and other skin irritations or infections. Both have been reported to cause allergic contact dermatitis.[38,39] In recent years, tea tree oil has seen its popularity increase as a cure-all for psoriasis, acne, eczema, and warts, and numerous reports of allergic contact dermatitis have been published.[35,40,41] Other allergenic extracts include lavender oil (*Lavandula angustifolia*), peppermint oil (*Mentha piperita*), Asiatic pennywort (*Centella asiatica*), rosemary (*Rosmarinus officinalis*), sage (*Salvia officinalis*), witch hazel (*Hamamelis virginiana*), and cucumber (*Cucumis spp.*).[36]

The principle behind homeopathy is to fight evil with infinitesimal dilutions of evil. Manufacturers of homeopathic remedies have marketed phytotherapeutic preparations containing toxicodendron extracts, as lip balms for the purported relief of herpes labialis and as salves for treatment of muscle pains. These products may contain up to 392 mg/g of urushiol, well above the 0.05 to 0.005 mg that are needed to elicit a positive patch test reaction.[42] These preparations have caused allergic contact dermatitis in sensitized individuals when introduced in North America, and patch testing with them has actively sensitized some subjects.[43]

SYSTEMIC CONTACT DERMATITIS

Numerous botanic extracts, ingested as foods or medicaments, have the potential to induce widespread cutaneous reactions through allergic or toxic mechanisms. Systemic contact dermatitis is described in greater detail elsewhere in this issue, and may present with the following patterns of reaction in subjects previously sensitized by cutaneous exposure: (a) widespread eczematous or maculopapular eruption, (b) recall of the original dermatitis, (c) localized hand and foot dyshidrosis, and (d) the baboon syndrome.

Hamilton and Zug[44] reported a representative example of the baboon syndrome. Their patient had a past history of poison ivy dermatitis and suffered 2 episodes of pruritic dermatitis characterized by brightly erythematous plaques covering the buttocks, inner thighs, and axillary regions. These lesions occurred within 36 hours of eating raw cashews. In a series of 31 Korean patients, sensitized to *T. verniciflua*, who ingested the lacquer to treat gastrointestinal problems, maculopapular eruptions ensued in 65%, whereas EM and erythroderma were also seen.[45] Herbal teas, such as chamomile, have also triggered widespread eruptions and anal pruritus in individuals sensitized to SLs in Asteraceae.[39]

Ingestion of large amounts of psoralen-containing plants has resulted in enhanced phototoxicity during PUVA therapy.[46,47] Cattle that feed on St. John's wort, or *Hypericum perforatum*, develop phototoxic eruptions. Human consumption of extracts of this member of the family Clusiaceae has increased since the scientific demonstration of the antidepressant properties of hyperforin, one of its constituents.[48] A few human cases of cutaneous phototoxicity have been reported from its ingestion.[49–51]

SUMMARY

The characteristic pattern of allergic phytodermatitis is an intensely pruritic papulovesicular eruption, featuring irregular plaques and crisscrossing linear streaks. Similar lesions may be seen in the initial stage of phytophotodermatitis, but their resolution into darkly pigmented macules sign the diagnosis. Allergic contact dermatitis to Asteraceae simulates photodermatitis and presents as subacute to chronic eczema with marked lichenification. It is important for the clinician to be aware of these classic modes of presentation and also of the less common patterns, such as "tulip fingers," "hyacinth itch" and "sabra dermatitis," herein reviewed. Botanic extracts are ubiquitous and may cause dermatitis from cosmetics or topical medicaments. Their ingestion may at times cause widespread eruptions in previously sensitized individuals, and cutaneous exposure may give rise to erythema multiforme. The cutaneous manifestations of adverse reactions to plants thus cover a wide range of clinical patterns that the informed clinician will be able to recognize.

REFERENCES

1. Benezra C, Ducombs G, Sell Y, Foussereau J. Plant contact dermatitis. Toronto: BC Decker; 1985.
2. Lovell CR. Plants and the skin. Oxford (UK): Blackwell Science; 1993.
3. Sasseville D. Phytodermatitis. J Cutan Med Surg 1999;3(5):263–79.
4. Guin JD, Gillis WT, Beaman JH. Recognizing the toxicodendrons (poison ivy, poison oak, and poison sumac). J Am Acad Dermatol 1981;4(1):99–114.
5. Marks JG Jr, DeLeo VA. Contact and Occupational Dermatology. 2nd edition. St. Louis (MO): Mosby; 1997. p. 254.
6. Rietschel RL, Fowler JF Jr. Allergic sensitization to plants. In: Fisher's Contact Dermatitis. 6th edition. Hamilton (Canada): BC Decker; 2008. p. 405–53.
7. Baer H, Watkins RC, Kurtz AP, et al. Delayed contact sensitivity to catechols. III. The relationship of side chain length to sensitizing potency of catechols chemically related to the active principles in poison ivy. J Immunol 1967;99(2):370–5.
8. Stoner JG, Rasmussen JE. Plant dermatitis. J Am Acad Dermatol 1983;9(1):1–15.
9. Reynolds NJ, Burton JL, Bradfield JWB, et al. Weed wacker dermatitis. Arch Dermatol 1991;127(9):1419–20.
10. Warshaw EM, Zug KA. Sesquiterpene lactone allergy. Am J Contact Dermatitis 1996;7(1):1–23.
11. Mitchell JC, Dupuis G. Allergic contact dermatitis from sesquiterpenoids of the compositae family of plants. Br J Dermatol 1971;84(2):139–50.
12. Roed-Petersen J, Hjorth N. Compositae sensitivity among patients with contact dermatitis: value of compositae oleoresins in a standard test series. Contact Dermatitis 1976;2(5):271–81.
13. Arlette J, Mitchell JC. Compositae dermatitis: current aspects. Contact Dermatitis 1981;7(3):129–36.
14. Mitchell JC, Schofield WB, Singh B, et al. Allergy to Frullania: allergic contact dermatitis occurring in forest workers caused by exposure to Frullania nisquallensis. Arch Dermatol 1969;100(1):46–9.
15. Storrs FJ, Mitchell JC, Rasmussen JE. Contact hypersensitivity to liverwort and the Compositae family of plants. Cutis 1976;18(5):681–6.
16. Hjorth N. Seasonal variations in contact dermatitis. Acta Derm Venereol 1967;47(6):409–18.
17. Zachariae C, Engkilde K, Johansen JD, et al. Primin in the standard patch test series for 20 years. Contact Dermatitis 2007;56(6):344–6.

18. Connolly M, Mc Cune J, Dauncey E, et al. Primula obconica – is contact allergy on the decline? Contact Dermatitis 2004;51(4):167–71.
19. Mowad CM. Routine testing for Primula obconica: is it useful in the United States? Am J Contact Dermatitis 1998;9(4):231–3.
20. Seligman PJ, Mathias CGT, O'Malley MA, et al. Phytophotodermatitis from celery among grocery store workers. Arch Dermatol 1987;123(11):1478–82.
21. Bruynzeel DP. Bulb dermatitis. Dermatological problems in the flower bulb industries. Contact Dermatitis 1997;37(2):70–7.
22. Gette MT, Marks JG Jr. Tulip fingers. Arch Dermatol 1990;126(2):203–6.
23. Thiboutot DM, Hamory BH, Marks JG Jr. Dermatoses among floral shop workers. J Am Acad Dermatol 1990;22(1):54–8.
24. Zakon SJ. Contact dermatitis due to mango. JAMA 1939;113:1808.
25. Pusey WA. Lacquer dermatitis. Arch Dermatol Syph 1923;7:91–2.
26. Livingood CS, Rogers AM, Fitz-Hugh T. Dhobie mark dermatitis. JAMA 1943;123:23–6.
27. Sowers WF, Weary PE, Collins OD, et al. Gingko tree dermatitis. Arch Dermatol 1965;91(5):452–6.
28. Behl PN, Captain RM. Skin irritant and sensitizing plants found in India. New Delhi: S Chand, Ram Nagar; 1979. p. 53.
29. High WA. Agave contact dermatitis. Am J Contact Dermatitis 2003;14(4):213–4.
30. Salinas ML, Ogura T, Soffchi L. Irritant contact dermatitis caused by needle-like calcium oxalate crystals, raphides, in Agave tequilana among workers in tequila distilleries and agave plantations. Contact Dermatitis 2001;44(2):94–6.
31. Shanon J, Sagher F. Sabra dermatitis. An occupational dermatitis due to prickly pear handling simulating scabies. Arch Dermatol 1956;74(3):269–75.
32. Lachapelle JM. Dermatites aux plantes: confrontation anatomo-clinique. In: Avenel-Audran M, editor. Progrès en dermato-allergologie - Angers 2008. Montrouge: Editions John Libbey Eurotext; 2008. p. 221–30 [in French].
33. Werchniak AE, Schwarzenberger K. Poison ivy: An underreported cause of erythema multiforme. J Am Acad Dermatol 2004;51(Suppl 5):S87–8.
34. Goon A, Goh CL. Noneczematous contact reactions. In: Frosch PJ, Menné T, Lepoittevin JP, editors. Contact dermatitis. 4th edition. Berlin: Springer; 2006. p. 349–62.
35. Khanna M, Qasem K, Sasseville D. Allergic contact dermatitis to tea tree oil with erythema multiforme-like id reaction. Am J Contact Dermatitis 2000;11(4):238–42.
36. Kiken DA, Cohen DE. Contact dermatitis to botanical extracts. Am J Contact Dermatitis 2002;13(3):148–52.

37. Hausen BM. Identification of the allergens of *Arnica Montana* L. Contact Dermatitis 1978;4(5):308.

38. Bossuyt L, Dooms-Goossens A. Contact dermatitis to nettles and camomile in "alternative" remedies. Contact Dermatitis 1994;31(2):131–2.

39. Rodríguez-Serna M, Sánchez-Motilla JM, Rámon R, et al. Allergic and systemic contact dermatitis from *Matricaria chamomilla* tea. Contact Dermatitis 1998;39(4):192–3.

40. Bhushan M, Beck MH. Allergic contact dermatitis from tea tree oil in a wart paint. Contact Dermatitis 1997;36(2):117–8.

41. Knight TE, Hausen BM. Melaleuca oil (tea tree oil) dermatitis. J Am Acad Dermatol 1994;30(3):423–7.

42. Epstein WL. Allergic contact dermatitis to poison oak and ivy. Feasibility of hyposensitization. Dermatol Clin 1984;2(4):613–7.

43. Sasseville D, Nguyen K. Allergic contact dermatitis from *Rhus toxicodendron* in a phytotherapeutic preparation. Contact Dermatitis 1995;32(3):182–3.

44. Hamilton TK, Zug KA. Systemic contact dermatitis to raw cashew nuts in a pesto sauce. Am J Contact Dermatitis 1998;9(1):51–4.

45. Park SD, Lee SW, Chun JH, et al. Clinical features of 31 patients with systemic contact dermatitis due to ingestion of *Rhus* (lacquer). Br J Dermatol 2000;142(5):937–42.

46. Boffa MJ, Gilmour E, Ead PD. Celery soup causing severe phototoxicity during PUVA therapy. Br J Dermatol 1996;135(2):334.

47. Puig L, de Moragas JM. Enhancement of PUVA phototoxic effects following celery ingestion: cool broth can also burn. Arch Dermatol 1994;130(6):809–10.

48. Laakmann G, Schule C, Baghai T, et al. St. John's wort in mild to moderate depression: the relevance of hyperforine for the clinical efficacy. Pharmacopsychiatry 1998;31(Suppl 1):54–9.

49. Golsch S, Vocks E, Rakoski J, et al. Reversible increase in photosensitivity to UV-B caused by St. John's wort extract. Hautarzt 1997;48(4):249–52.

50. Cotterill JA. Severe phototoxic reaction to laser treatment in a patient taking St. John's wort. J Cosmet Laser Ther 2001;3(3):159–60.

51. Lane-Brown MM. Photosensitivity associated with herbal preparations of St. John's wort (*Hypericum perforatum*). Med J Aust 2000;172(6):302.

Factors Associated with Textile Pattern Dermatitis Caused by Contact Allergy to Dyes, Finishes, Foams, and Preservatives

David S. Brookstein, ScD

KEYWORDS

- Formaldehyde • Dermatitis • Textile allergies

Allergic contact dermatitis because of textiles is most severe in areas of perspiration and friction where garments have greatest skin contact, such as the axillary lines, medial thighs, posterior neck, and antecubital and popliteal folds. Because there are only a few textile finish resins that are widely used, sensitized patients are usually exposed from many of their garments and tend to have chronic dermatitis. There are many more textile dyes, and sensitized patients may be allergic to only a single item of clothing causing a more acute presentation. Allergic contact dermatitis because of textiles in furniture usually presents on the posterior thighs and forearms.

Essentially all textile materials used in apparel and furniture products contain dyes and finishes to impart color and a wide range of performance attributes. These textile materials can be natural or nature-based, like cotton, wool, silk, cellulosic and cellulose acetate; or synthetic like nylon, polyester, and acrylic. As a result of the chemical nature of these materials and the essentially infinite palette of colors desired by the consumer, there are a substantial number of dyestuffs available to impart the desired coloration.

A dye is an organic compound composed of a chromophore, the colored portion of the dye molecule, and an auxochrome, which slightly alters the color. The auxochrome makes the dye soluble and is a site for bonding on to the textile material (fiber). Dyes are molecules that can either be dissolved in water or some other carrier so that they will penetrate into the fiber. Any undissolved particles of dye remain on the outside of the fiber, where they can bleed and are sensitive to surface abrasion.

Dyes are classified by chemical composition or method of application. **Table 1** lists major dye classes along with the fibers that they are used to color.[1]

Hatch reported that as early as 1869 dyes were suspected to be a cause of dermatitis when Wilson suggested that a French soldier's foot lesion was because of his red aniline dyed socks.[2,3] Since that time there has been a substantial body of research that connects dermatitis to textile dyes exposure.

Hatch presented a table of early references from 1869 to 1950 for dermatitis caused by dyes on clothing and this work continues to the present by many researchers.

Recently, Lazorov and colleagues[4] looked at 286 consecutive dermatitis patients in Israel (190 females and 96 males) and found a significant number of patients' allergy to the following commonly used textile dyes and permanent press finishes: 12 to Disperse Blue 106, 21 to Disperse Blue 124, 9 to ethylene urea melamine

Pennsylvania Advanced Textile Research and Innovation Center, Philadelphia University, Philadelphia, PA 19144, USA
E-mail address: brooksteind@philau.edu

Dermatol Clin 27 (2009) 309–322
doi:10.1016/j.det.2009.05.001

Table 1
Major dye classes

Dye Class	Fabrics
Acid (anionic)	Wool, silk, modified rayon, modified acrylic, and polyester
Azoic or Azo	Cotton and polyester
Cationic (basic)	Acrylics, polyester, nylon, and direct prints on acetate and discharge prints on cotton
Developed (direct)	Cellulosic fibers including cotton
Direct (substantive)	Cellulosic fibers including cotton
Disperse	Most synthetic fibers including nylon and polyester
Mordant	Wool, silk, modified rayon, modified acrylic, and polyester
Reactive	Cotton and other cellulosics, wool, silk and nylon
Sulfur	Heavyweight cotton fabrics (mostly used for black color)
Vat	Cotton and cotton/polyester blends

formaldehyde, 7 to urea formaldehyde, and 7 to melamine formaldehyde.

EXPOSURE OF SKIN TO TEXTILE DYES AND FINISHES

Many clothing items are in direct contact with the skin. During contact there can be perspiration which involves moisture transport between the skin and the dyed and finished clothing items. Although modern dyes and finishes are chemically bound to the fibers in the clothing, there is always the possibility that residual dye (dye bleed) and finish are released and contact the skin. Degree of colorfastness can be a measure of dye bleed.

Textile materials are a capillary and porous material with different pore sizes, and can be saturated with both liquid and gaseous water during wear. The transportation of perspiration through this material at different temperatures is a very complex process, which can involve convection, capillary flow, penetration, molecular diffusion, evaporation, and solidification.

The transport of perspiration through clothing from the surface of human body is shown in **Figs. 1** and **2**. This process includes mass and heat transfer, as a temperature difference during the moisture (perspiration) transfer through the clothing exists. During the heat and mass (perspiration) transfer through the clothing medium, there generally exist 2 states of water phase, gaseous and liquid, and consequently several different interfaces between perspiration and clothing.[5]

These phenomena of moisture transfer and subsequent release of dyes from the textile material can be quantified and characterized as colorfastness. Colorfastness is commonly measured according to the American Association of Textile Chemist and Colorists (AATCC) standard test method 15 "Colorfastness to Perspiration."[6] The principle involves a specimen of dyed textile in contact with other fibrous materials. For color transfer, the test specimen is wetted out in

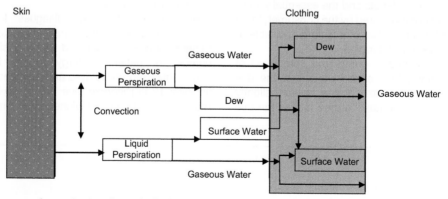

Fig. 1. Transport of perspiration through clothing.

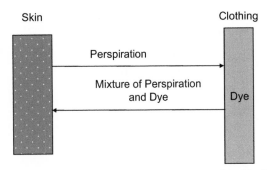

Fig. 2. Equilibrium mixing of perspiration and residual dye.

simulated acid perspiration solution, subjected to a fixed mechanical pressure and allowed to dry slowly at a slightly elevated temperature. After conditioning, the specimen is evaluated for color change and other fiber materials are evaluated for color transfer. An excellent review of the relationship between dye structure and fastness properties is provided by Giles and colleagues.[7]

DYE CLASSES OF CLINICAL INTEREST

Hatch and Maibach conducted a seminal clinical review of textile dye dermatitis.[8] It was found that the incidence of dye dermatitis varied from 1% to 15.9% depending on the country, patient sample, and number of dyes in the patch test series. Disperse Blue 106 and Disperse Blue 124 were the strongest clothing dye sensitizers. Disperse dyes with azo and anthraquinone structures were the most common dye sensitizers.

Today, worldwide there are 2 classes of dyes that are widely recognized as having the potential to cause allergic contact dermatitis and possibly cancer. These 2 dye classes are azoic (azo) and disperse dyes. In the European Union their use is regulated by law; in the United States, at this time, there exists only voluntary regulation by those companies agreeing to regulate their use.

Azo Dyes

Azo dyes are characterized by a chromophoric azo group $-N=N-$, whose nitrogen atoms are linked respectively to sp^2-hybridized carbon atoms. At least 1 of these carbon atoms belongs to an aromatic carbocycle (usually a benzene or naphthalene derivative) or the terocycle (eg, pyrazolone, thiazole), whereas the second carbon atom adjoining the azo group may also be part of an enolizable aliphatic derivative (eg, acetoacetic acid). The most common types of azo dyes can be summarized as follows:
aryl$-N=N-R$, where R can be an aryl, heteroaryl, or $-CH=C(OH)-$alkyl

As a result of the simple nature of the synthesis, usually in aqueous medium, and the almost unlimited choice of starting products, an extremely wide variety of azo dyes is obtainable. The number of combinations is further increased by the fact that a dye molecule can contain several azo groups. This diversity of inexpensively produced azo dyes permits a wide spectrum of shades and fastness properties suitable for use on a variety of textile substrates.

Depending on the number of azo groups, the azo dyes are called monoazo, disazo, trisazo, tetrakisazo dyes and so on, and those with 3 or more azo groups, polyazo dyes. The structure of an azo dye can be described by means of typical azo structural formulas such as those shown in **Figs. 3 and 4.**

Most azo dyes contain only one azo group, but some contain two (disazo), three (trisazo) or more. In theory, azo dyes can supply a complete rainbow of colors. However, commercially they tend to be used to produce more yellows, oranges and reds than any other colors.

Mechanism of Azo Dye Allergic Reaction

Hatch and Maibach reported that individuals who develop clothing dye dermatitis are rarely sensitized to the dye by repeated wearing of garments containing the dye.[8] Rather the skin is sensitized by either repeated exposure to the same dye in another product (primary sensitizer) or to a closely related chemical compound (cross sensitizer). Thus, sensitization and the latent or incubation period in the development of allergic contact dermatitis may have occurred before the wearing of the offending garment. Hatch and Maibach conclude that for individuals who are sensitive to azo dyes, paraphenylenediamine (PPD), a compound chemically related to azo dyes, is often the sensitizer. They further conclude that most of the positive reactions were from the disperse dyes with monoazo symmetric structures. Saunders and colleagues[9] reported a patient that developed a textile dye allergy following sensitation to PPD from a temporary tattoo. It was reported that PPD can be added to a temporary tattoo to produce a darker than normal color and this is often referred to as "black henna." Mayer, in his seminal papers, provided an explanation of

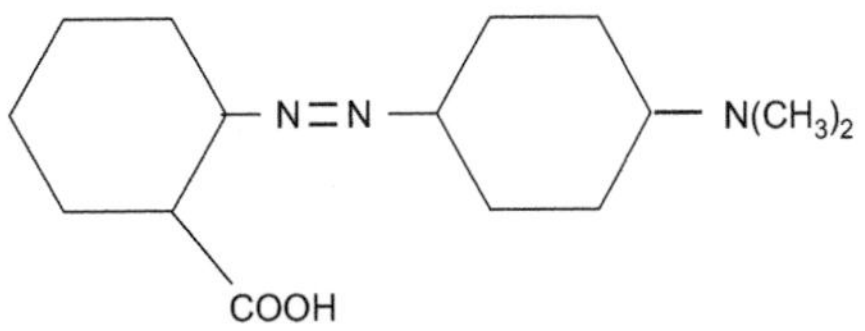

Fig. 3. Chemical structure of Methyl Red (MR).

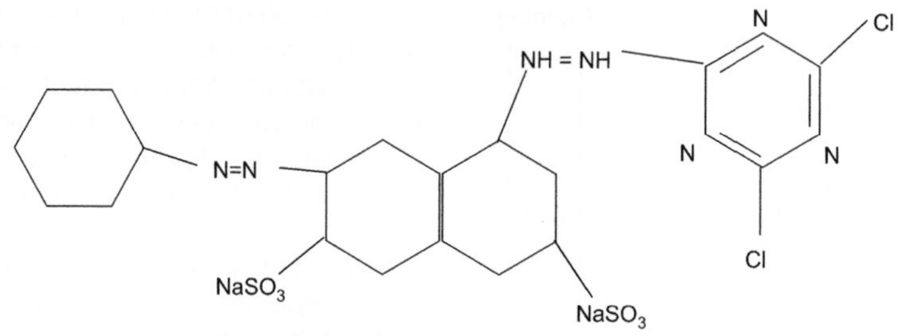

Fig. 4. Chemical structure of Procion Red Mx-5B.

cross hypersensitivity of PPD to azo dyes and the results were translated by Dobkevitch and Baer.[10–13] The common chemical basis is the quinine structure. It was hypothesized that PPD can be oxidized at skin cells to quinonediimine. Further, some azo dyes are converted to quinonediimines by way of metabolism to PPD. The mechanism of conversion from a typical azo dye (4-aminoazobenzene) to aniline and PPD and then the conversion from PPD to quinonediimine is depicted in **Fig. 5**.

The azo dye is reduced to 2 amines at the azo linkage, the resulting amines depending on the structure of the original compound. The split amines then undergo further reaction (ie, oxidation) and are then converted into quinonediimines. This reduction mechanism to aromatic amines is also sometimes referred to as cleavage and azo cleavage is suspected as causing some azo dyes to be carcinogenic.

Su and colleagues[14] report that the finding of multiple azo dye sensitivities may represent concomitant sensitization or cross-reactivities. Four groups of azo dyes have been described, based on their chemical structure: (1) aminoazobenzenes, (2) PPD, (3) thiazol-azolyl-PPD,

and (4) benzothiazol-azolyl-PPD. Cross-sensitivity between the aminoazobenzene Disperse Orange 3 and its metabolite PPD is common. Although cross-sensitivity between Disperse Orange 3 and the aminoazobenzenes Disperse Red 1 and Disperse Red 17 has been described, PPD does not generally cross react with these latter 2 aminoazobenzenes.

There is substantial worldwide concern, and in some cases standards and regulations, associated with the use of azo dyes in textiles, apparel, and home furnishings. In 1992 the European Union published a Directive (2002/61/EC) to restrict the marketing and use of certain dangerous substances and preparations (azo colorants) in textile and leather products.[15] The legislation is relevant for all products made of textile and leather, or in which textile and leather is used, and which come into direct and prolonged contact with the skin and mouth. These include producers of textiles and garments, leather goods, shoes, toys, furniture, decorative articles, jewelry and accessories. The concern has not been directed at acute contact dermatitis but instead the carcinogenic nature of certain azo dyes. Many of the

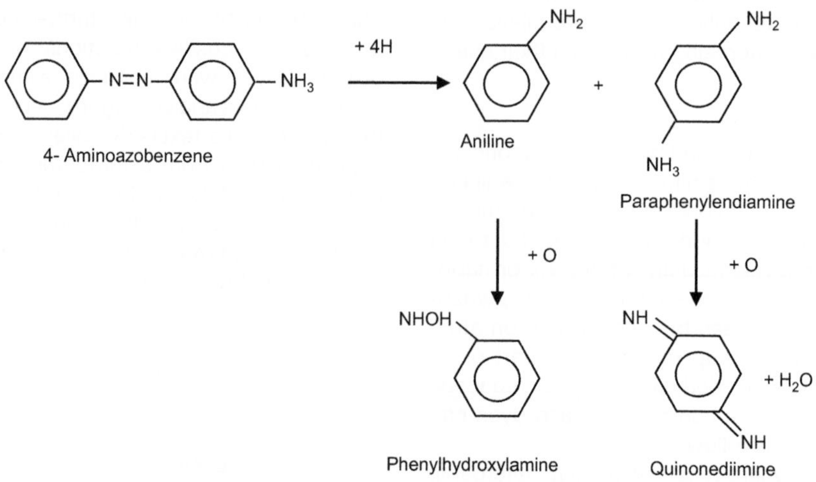

Fig. 5. Conversion of azo dye (aminoazobenzene) to quinonediimines.

same azo dyes that are now banned in the European Union for carcinogenic considerations are the same ones that have the potential for eliciting allergic responses. In the Directive it is stated "Textile and leather articles containing certain azo dyes have the capacity to release certain arylamines, which may pose cancer risks."

The standards required in the Directive state:

1. Azo dyes which, by reductive cleavage of 1 or more azo groups, may release 1 or more of the aromatic amines listed in the appendix, in detectable concentrations, of above 30 ppm in the finished articles or in the dyed parts thereof, according to the testing method established in accordance with Article 2a of this Directive, may not be used in textile and leather articles which may come into direct and prolonged contact with the human skin or oral cavity, such as:
   — clothing, bedding, towels, hairpieces, wigs, hats, nappies and other sanitary items, sleeping bags,
   — footwear, gloves, wristwatch straps, handbags, purses/wallets, briefcases, chair covers, purses worn round the neck,
   — textile or leather toys and toys which include textile or leather garments,
   — yarn and fabrics intended for use by the final consumer.
2. Furthermore, the textile and leather articles referred to in point 1 may not be placed on the market unless they conform to the requirements set out in that point. By way of derogation, until 1 January 2005, this provision will not apply to textile articles made of recycled fibers if the amines are released by residues derived from previous dyeing of the same fibers and if the listed amines are released in concentrations of less than 70 ppm.

The list of azo dyes covered by Directive (2002/61/EC) is provided in **Table 2**.

European Standards 14,362-1:2203 (Part 1) and 14,362-2:2003 (Part 2) provide the worldwide accepted method for determining certain aromatic amines derived from azo colorants. Although they are worldwide standards, at this time they are only enforced in the European Union. Part 1 is focused on detection of the use of certain azo colorants accessible without extraction and Part 2 is focused on the detection of certain azo colorants accessible by extracting the fibers.[16,17]

Although the Directive has authority in the European Union, the United States consumer market has no current regulations associated with azo dyes. Nonetheless, the American Apparel and Footwear Association (AAFA), the leading trade group for the industry, has published a Restrictive Substance List (RSL) that calls for voluntary acceptance by its members.[18] The AAFA RSL lists azo dyes which, by reductive cleavage of 1 or more azo groups, may release 1 or more of the following aromatic amines listed in **Table 3**.

Disperse Dyes

Disperse dyes are slightly water-soluble compounds whose fixation properties to fibers depend on their particle size and uniformity and on the nature of the dye disbursing agent.[19] The vast majority of chemical types of disperse dyes that are used are monoazo (essentially azo dyes), anthraquinone, and disazo that are shown in **Fig. 6**.[20] The widely accepted standard for determining the presence of disperse dyes in textile is German Standard DIN 54,321: Textiles - Detection of disperse dyestuffs.[21]

Disperse dyes were developed in the 1920s for dyeing nature-based cellulose acetate and cellulose triacetate fibers. Today these dyes are mostly used for dyeing polyester and polyester blends. They are also used for dyeing nylon, acrylic and modacrylic fibers.[22] Dye carriers are used for fixing disperse dyes to polyester and cellulose triacetate fibers. The other types of synthetic fibers that are colored with disperse dyes do not require carriers or other auxiliaries.

Allergic Dermatitis Reactions to Disperse Dyes

Pratt and Tanaka showed the allergenic nature of Disperse Blue 106 and Disperse Blue 124.[23] They advanced the concept that these dyes can be screening agents for subjects reacting to textile dyes (**Figs. 7** and **8**). Giusti and Seidenari subsequently added Disperse Orange 3 to the list.[24]

The International Oeko-Tex Association has determined that those disperse dyes listed in **Table 4** are allergenic.[25] Some are also suspected of carcinogenicity. For a textile product to obtain Oeko-Tex 100 certification these disperse dyes cannot be used. It is interesting to note that Disperse Blue 1 and Disperse Yellow 3 are recognized as both allergens and carcinogens (**Figs. 9** and **10**).

The AAFA RSL (2008) identifies the disperse dyes in **Table 5** as restricted on a voluntary basis for US manufacturers and distributors of clothing.[18] The International Oeko-Tex Association also lists these as allergenic.[25]

Basic Dyes

Hatch and Maibach reported that some basic dyes are common allergens. They are mainly used to dye wool, silk, cotton cellulosics, and

Table 2
Restricted azo colorants

	CAS Number	Index Number	EC Number	Substances
1	92-67-1	612-072-00-6	202-177-1	biphenyl-4-ylamine 4-aminobiphenyl xenylamine
2	92-87-5	612-042-00-2	202-199-1	benzidine
3	95-69-2		202-441-6	4-chloro-o-toluidine
4	91-59-8	612-022-00-3	202-080-4	2-naphthylamine
5	97-56-3	611-006-00-3	202-591-2	o-aminoazotoluene 4-amino-2', 3-dimethylazobenzene, 4-o-tolylazo-o-toluidine
6	99-55-8		202-765-8	5-nitro-o-toluidine
7	106-47-8	612-137-00-9	203-401-0	4-chloroaniline
8	615-05-4		210-406-1	4-methoxy-m-phenylenediamine
9	101-77-9	612-051-00-1	202-974-4	4,4'-methylenedianiline 4,4'-diaminodiphenylmethane
10	91-94-1	61 2-068-00-4	202-109-0	3,3-dichlorobenzidine 3,3-dichlorobiphenyl-4 ~ 4-ylenedia-mine
11	119-90-4	61 2-036-00-X	204-355-4	3,3-dimethoxybenzidine o-dianisidine
12	119-93-7	612-041-00-7	204-358-0	3,3'-dimethylbenzidine 4,4-bi-o-toluidine
13	838-88-0	612-085-00-7	212-658-8	4,4-methylenedi-o-toluidine
14	120-71-8		204-419-1	6-methoxy-m-toluidine p-cresidine
15	101-14-4	612-078-00-9	202-918-9	4,4-methylene-bis-(2-chloro-aniline) 2,2-dichloro-4,4-methylene-dianiline
16	101-80-4		202-977-0	4,4-oxydianiline
17	139-65-1		205-370-9	4,4-thiodianiline
18	95-53-4	612-09 1-00-X	202-429-0	o-toluidine 2-aminotoluene
19	95-80-7	612-099-00-3	202-45 3-1	4-methyl-m-phenylenediamine
20	137-17-7		205-282-0	2,4.5-trimethylaniline
21	90-04-0	612-035-00-4	201-963-1	o-anisidine 2-methoxyaniline
22	60-09-3	61 1-008-00-4	200-453-6	4-amino azobenzene

Table 3
Azo colorants on AAFA RSL

4-Amino azobenzene	3,3'-Dimethoxybenzidine
O –Aminoazotoluene	3,3'-Dimethylbenzidine
Aminodiphenyl	3,3'-Dimethyl-4,4'-diamino-diphenylmethane
2-Amino-4-nitrotoluene	4,4'-Methylene-bis-(2-chloroaniline)
O –Anisidine, Benzidine	2-Naphthylamine
P –Chloroaniline	4,4'-Oxydianiline
4-Chloro-o –toluidine	4,4'-Thiodianiline
p –Cresidine	2,4-Toluenediamine
2,4-Diaminoanisole	o-Toluidine
4,4'-Diamino-diphenylmethane	2,4,5-Trimethylaniline
3,3'-Dichlorobenzidine	2,4-Xylidine

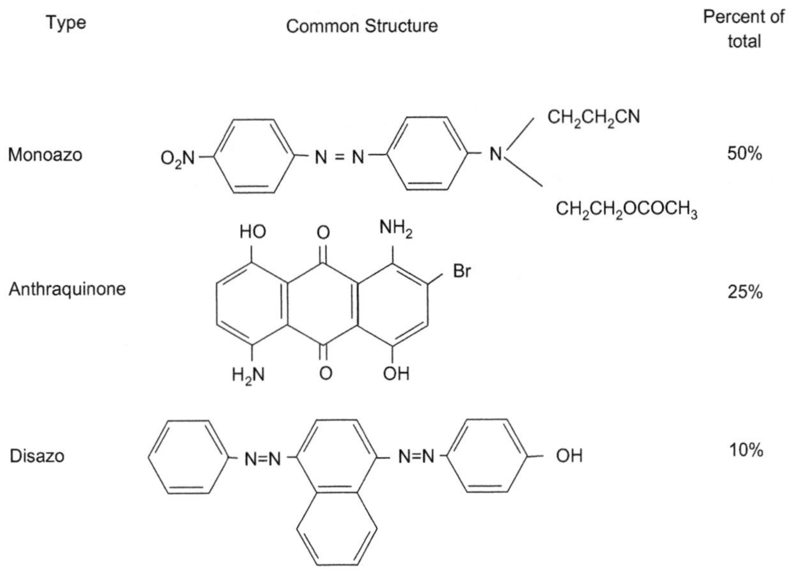

Fig. 6. Major types of disperse dyes used in commercial dyeing.

polyacrylonitriles. Basic Red 46, Basic Brown 1, Basic Black 1, Brilliant Green and Turquoise have been reported to cause textile dermatitis (Fig. 11).[8]

FORMALDEHYDE AS A SKIN ALLERGEN

Formaldehyde treatment of cellulosic fibers such as cotton was first taught in an invention by the British inventors Foulds, Marsh and Wood in US Patent 1,734,516.[26] The inventors claimed that "one of the greatest defects of a fabric composed entirely of cotton has been the ease with which such fabric is creased or crumpled when crushed or folded under pressure in the hand." The invention was to use a mixture of chemicals including formaldehyde to cause a chemical reaction with the cellulose that would cause cross-linking and thus render the fabric wrinkle free.

Substantial commercial interest developed as inherently wrinkle-free fabrics were commercialized and by the 1950s the family fabric caretaker (mostly women) were enlightened by the potential of wrinkle-free fabrics to reduce some of their homemaking chores. And as more and more women joined the workforce the entire family became interested in easy-care clothing. In addition to being used to produce wrinkle-free fabrics,

formaldehyde based compounds are also found in glues, adhesives in shoes, and as an auxiliary for creating flame retardant fabrics.

Prior to the 1960s formaldehyde resins for textiles were based on urea formaldehyde (dimethylol urea) and melamine and treated fabrics contained relatively high levels of free formaldehyde.[27] Although the earliest health concern was that which involved contact during textiles and clothing manufacturing, dermatitis often occurs from wearing permanent press apparel. In 1959, Marcussen (Denmark) reported a study from 1934–1958 in which there were 26 cases (11% of studied cases) of garment formaldehyde dermatitis.[28] A study in which 1%–3% of 36,000 eczematous patients from 1934–1955 showed formaldehyde sensitivity was also reported.[29] In 1964 Berrens and colleagues[30] reported that 200 ppm of free formaldehyde was less than the estimated reaction threshold for most formaldehyde-allergic individuals reported in earlier studies. In 1965, US dermatology researchers O'Quinn and Kennedy reported contact dermatitis caused by formaldehyde in clothing.[31] Hatch published a complete review of references to clothing-based formaldehyde sensitivity.[2] Lazorov and colleagues[4] found significant sensitivities to a range of formaldehyde resins used in textiles.

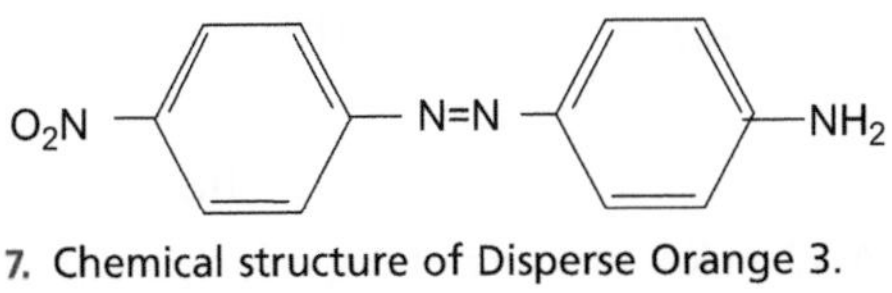

Fig. 7. Chemical structure of Disperse Orange 3.

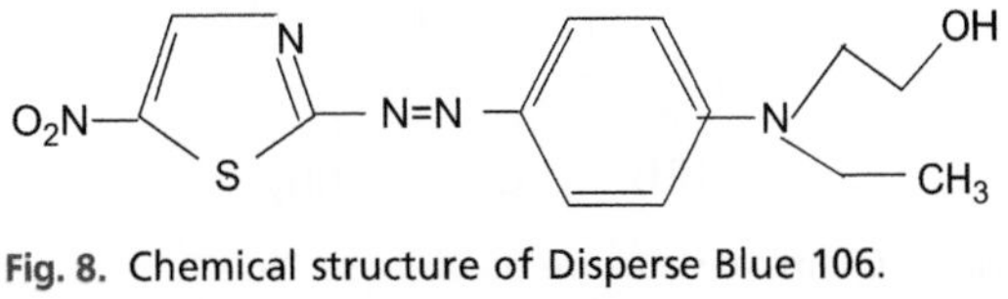

Fig. 8. Chemical structure of Disperse Blue 106.

Table 4
Oeko-Tex 100 list of textile allergens

C.I. Generic Name	C.I. Structure Number	CAS-Number	Carcinogenic
C.I. Disperse Blue 1	C.I. 64 500	2475-45-8	x
C.I. Disperse Blue 3	C.I. 61 505	2475-46-9	
C.I. Disperse Blue 7	C.I. 62 500	3179-90-6	
C.I. Disperse Blue 26	C.I. 63 305		
C.I. Disperse Blue 35		12,222-75-2	
C.I. Disperse Blue 102		12,222-97-8	
C.I. Disperse Blue 106		12,223-01-7	
C.I. Disperse Blue 124		61,951-51-7	
C.I. Disperse Brown 1		23,355-64-8	
C.I. Disperse Orange 1	C.I. 11 080	2581-69-3	
C.I. Disperse Orange 3	C.I. 11 005	730-40-5	
C.I. Disperse Orange 37	C.I. 11 132		
C.I. Disperse Orange 76	C.I. 11 132		
C.I. Disperse Red 1	C.I. 11 110	2872-52-8	
C.I. Disperse Red 11	C.I. 62 015	2872-48-2	
C.I. Disperse Red 17	C.I. 11 210	3179-89-3	
C.I. Disperse Yellow 1	C.I. 10 345	119-15-3	
C.I. Disperse Yellow 3	C.I. 11 855	2832-40-8	x
C.I. Disperse Yellow 9	C.I. 10 375	6373-73-5	
C.I. Disperse Yellow 39			
C.I. Disperse Yellow 49			

Dimethylol dihydroxy ethylene urea (DMDHEU) and modified DMDHEU are compounds which contain N-methylol and mainly N-alkoxymethyl groups and are extensively used in textile industry as durable press finishes.

Voncina and colleagues reported that during the finishing process the N-methylol compounds can react with hydroxyl groups of cellulose, which is the most preferable reaction. These compounds may also react with themselves or with reactive NH groups. These latter 2 reactions are not desirable, because some reaction places on cross-linking reagents are lost, and the formaldehyde can be simply released from the N-methylol compounds. Splitting of acetalic bonds is catalytically accelerated by acids and by bases as well (see **Fig. 12**).[32]

In 1993 Espada found that since the 1970s, most manufacturers have moved to the use of glycolated or methylated DMDHEU resins, which yielded fabrics with less than 300 ppm free formaldehyde and today fabrics treated with the latest modified DMDHEU resins predictably contain less than 75 ppm free formaldehyde.[33] There are resins available that do not employ formaldehyde, however, these resins are quite expensive and they found popularity primarily in the infant and children's clothing market.

Scheman and colleagues[34] looked at contact dermatitis response to subjects exposed to glycolated DMDHEU, the predominant resin currently used in textiles as a wrinkle free or permanent press resin. It was found that reactions to DMDHEU are the cause of most reports of contact dermatitis. Reactions to low-formaldehyde resins and non-formaldehyde resins were much less common, and generally of lesser intensity, than

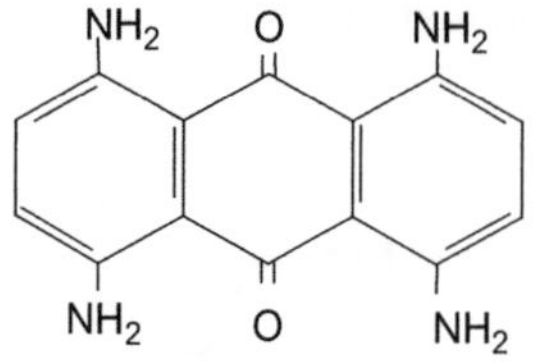

Fig. 9. Chemical structure of Disperse Blue 1.

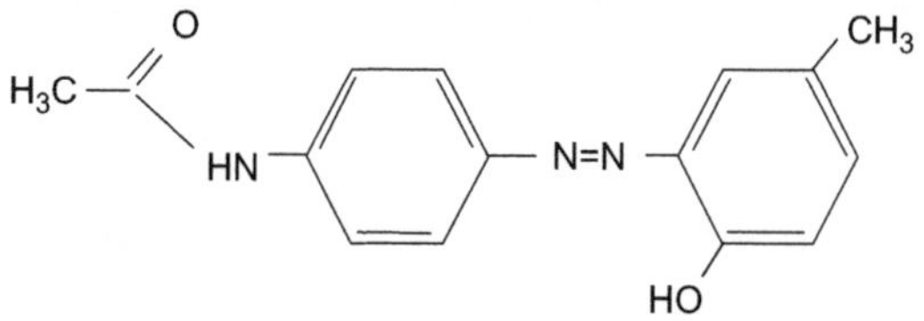

Fig. 10. Chemical structure of Disperse Yellow 3.

Table 5
AAFA Restricted Textile Dyes (Voluntary Compliance)

CAS Number	
2475-45-8	Disperse Blue 1
56,524-77-7 or 56,524-76-6	Disperse Blue 35
12,223-01-7	Disperse Blue 106
61,951-51-7	Disperse Blue 124
730-40-5	Disperse Orange 3
13,301-61-6	Disperse Orange 37/76
2872-52-8	Disperse Red 1
2832-40-8	Disperse Yellow 3

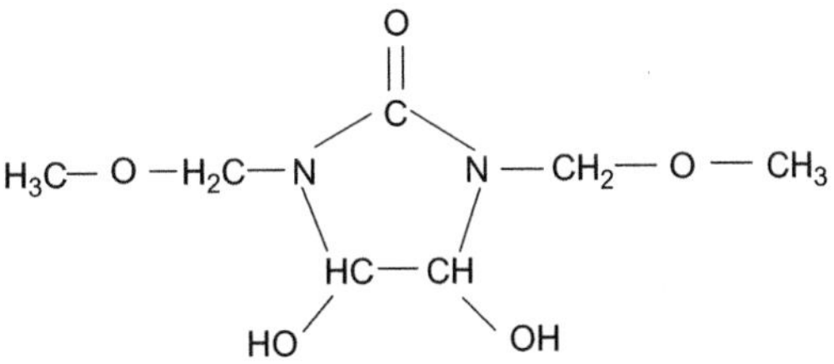

Fig. 12. Chemical structures of DMDHEU and modified DMDHEU.

reactions to the older formaldehyde resins, which release greater amounts of free formaldehyde.

Bille reported that there are a number of compounds which are capable of accepting the formaldehyde released from formaldehyde treated textiles.[35] For instance, urea, N-ethylurea and 1H-benzotriazole can form stable monomethyl compounds (**Fig. 13**).

Voncina showed that formaldehyde acceptors such as urea reduce the free formaldehyde value greatly and at the same time maintain dimensional stability of the treated clothing item.[32]

Wu and Yang indicated that it is necessary to use a cross-linking agent to bond a flame retarding hydroxyl-functional organophosphorus oligomer (FR) to cotton so that the flame resistance of the treated cotton fabric can be durable to multiple home laundering. Both (DMDHEU) and melamine–formaldehyde (M-F) have been used as the binding

agents between FR and cotton. Their data show not only that DMDHEU is much more effective for binding FR to cotton than M-F, but that the bonding between FR and cotton formed by DMDHEU is more durable to multiple home laundering than that formed by M-F.[36]

Formaldehyde is also found in glues and adhesive used to bond materials such as in layers of shoes. In particular, para-tertiary butylphenol (PTBP) formaldehyde resin is sometimes used. Zimerson and colleagues[37] have reported cases of contact dermatitis among some subjects exposed to PTBP.

The current medical literature is replete with many studies showing the adverse dermatologic effects of formaldehyde. An excellent current review of this subject has been written by Fowler.[27] Carlson, Smith and Nedorost found that textile dermatitis is more common in retired or current machine operators compared with other occupations, suggesting primary sensitization from formaldehyde-related biocides in coolants.[38]

As of yet, there are no formaldehyde restrictions or standards for clothing and other textile items that are distributed and sold in the United States. Nonetheless, in the recently passed Consumer Product Safety Commission Modernization Act of 2008 (H.R. 4040), there is a provision for the Consumer Product Safety Commission (CPSC) to conduct a study of the use of formaldehyde in textiles and apparel. More and more nations are adopting standards for formaldehyde in clothing and textiles. In Japan, textile fabrics are required

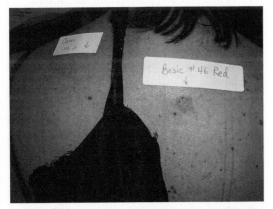

Fig. 11. Patient reaction to Basic Red 46 on right side. Dermatitis caused by the camisole shown (fiber content, 95% polyester, 5% spandex). (*Courtesy of S. Nedorost, MD, Cleveland, OH.*)

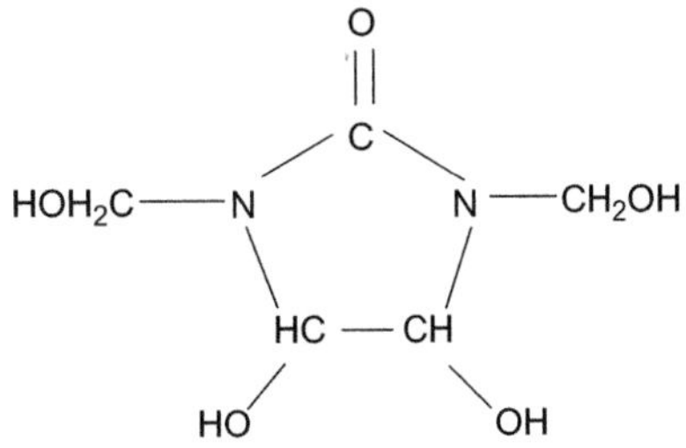

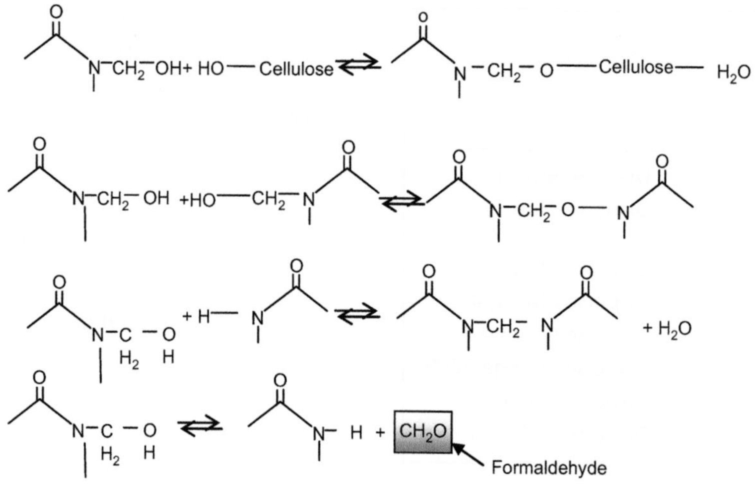

Fig. 13. Equilibrium reactions of N-methylol compounds of hydroxyl groups of cellulose, with themselves, with reactive NH groups and the formaldehyde release.

Table 6
Status of International Formaldehyde Regulations

Country	Regulations/Requirements	Objection Limit/Limit
Germany	Gefahrstoffverordnung, (Hazardous Substances Ordinance), Annex III, No. 9, 26.10.1993	Textiles that normally come into contact with the skin and release more than 1500 mg/kg formaldehyde must bear the label "Contains formaldehyde. Washing this garment is recommended before first time use to avoid irritation of the skin."
France	Official Gazette of the French Republic, Notification 97/0141/F	The regulations apply to products that are intended to come into contact with human skin, including textiles, leather, shoes, etc. Textiles for babies: 20 mg/kg, textiles for direct skin contact: 100 mg/kg, textiles not in direct skin contact: 400 mg/kg
Netherlands	The Dutch (Commodities Act), Regulations on Formaldehyde in Textiles (July 2000)	Textiles in direct skin contact must be labeled "Wash before first use" if they contain more than 120 mg/kg formaldehyde and the product must not contain more than 120 mg/kg formaldehyde after wash.
Austria	Formaldehydverordnung, BGBL Nr. 194/1900	Textiles that contains 1500 mg/kg or above must be labeled.
Finland	Decree on Maximum Amounts of Formaldehyde in Certain Textiles Products (Decree 210/1988)	Textiles for babies under 2-years-old: 30 mg/kg Textiles in direct skin contact: 100 mg/kg Textiles not in direct skin contact: 300 mg/kg
Norway	Regulations Governing the Use of a Number of Chemicals in Textiles (April 1999)	Textiles for babies under 2 years: 30 mg/kg Textiles in direct skin contact: 100 mg/kg Textiles not in direct skin contact: 300 mg/kg
China	Limits of Formaldehyde Content in Textiles GB18401-2001	Textiles for infants and babies: $\leq$20 mg/kg, Textiles in direct skin contact: $\leq$75 mg/kg, Textiles not in direct skin contact: $\leq$300 mg/kg
Japan	Japanese Law 112	Textiles for infants: not detectable, textiles in direct skin contact: 75 ppm

by law to contain less than 75 mg/kg free formaldehyde, as measured by the method described in Japan Law 112/ISO EN 14,184.[39] No free formaldehyde is tolerated for infant clothing. The Hong Kong Standards and Testing Center produced in **Table 6** shows the status of formaldehyde regulations in countries that are currently addressing this situation.[40]

The International Oeko-Tex Association which represents a group of 14 worldwide textile research institutes has developed the Oeko-Tex 100 standards. These standards, which are voluntary, place limitations on free formaldehyde in clothing and textiles.[25] For formaldehyde, the Oeko-Tex 100 standard requires no detectable formaldehyde for infant clothing (0-36 months), more than 36 months with direct skin contact (75 ppm) and more than 36 months with no direct skin contact (300 ppm).

While currently there are no US standards or regulations associated with formaldehyde in clothing and textiles, the AAFA published a 2008 RSL and requested that its members abide voluntarily to the standards listed.[18] For formaldehyde, the RSL suggests no detectable formaldehyde for infant clothing (0-36 months), more than 36 months with direct skin contact (75 ppm) and more than 36 months with no direct skin contact (300 ppm).

Brookstein, Barndt and Pierantozzi reported on a recent study of the presence of formaldehyde in some children's clothing.[41] Testing for free formaldehyde was conducted using a MORAPEX Extractor/Formaldimeter system. It was shown that the average free formaldehyde measured in accordance with ISO EN 14,184 ranges from essentially less than 20 ppm to 136 ppm for young men's khaki pants and from less than 20 ppm to 126 ppm for young men's dress shirts. Three of the pants and 1 of the shirts had average free formaldehyde in excess of the 75 ppm value suggested by the AAFA RSL, Oeko-Tex 100 and some countries with a 75 ppm allowable limit. Nonetheless, the data also indicate that it is possible to have a durable press finish with relatively low amounts of free formaldehyde.

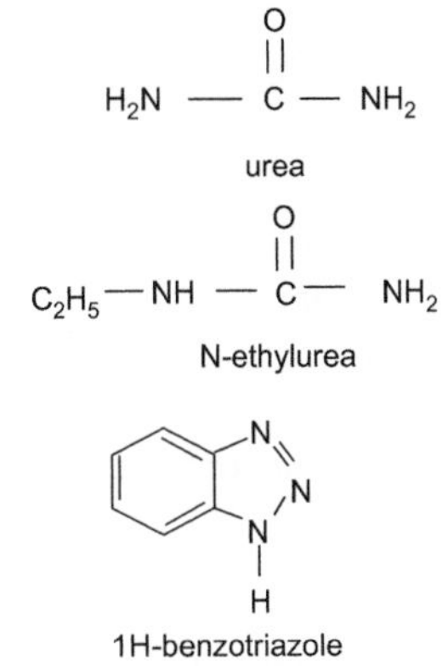

FURNITURE DERMATITIS
Isocyanates

Isocyanates can be combined with other polymers to enhance adhesion performance of textile fibers. Isocyanates are often used with polyurethanes and epoxides to make textile treatments. In some instances, isocyanates can be used alone to bond textiles or to bond textiles to other materials such as thermoplastic polyurethane foams

Fig. 14. Chemical structures of formaldehyde acceptors.

which are found in upholstered furniture. Isocyanates are also a constituent in the process to produce thermoplastic polyurethane foam. All isocyanates are characterized by the chemical formula shown in **Figs. 14** and **15**.

One of the key reactive materials required to produce polyurethane foams are diisocyanates. Diisocyanate (OCN-R-NCO) is reacted with a diol (HO-R-OH). The first step of this reaction results in the chemical linking of the 2 molecules leaving a reactive alcohol (OH) on one side and a reactive isocyanate (NCO) on the other side. These compounds are characterized by an (NCO) group, which are highly reactive alcohols. The most widely used isocyanates employed in polyurethane production are toluene 2,4 diisocyanate (TDI) and polymeric isocyanate (PMDI). TDI reacts with polyols to form polyurethanes. TDI is produced by chemically adding nitrogen groups on toluene, reacting these with hydrogen to produce a diamine, and separating the undesired isomers. PMDI is derived by a phosgenation reaction of aniline-formaldehyde polyamines (**Figs. 16** and **17**).

Bello and colleagues[42] published an excellent review of skin exposure to isocyanates and they indicated that unreacted isocyanates can cause skin problems.

Researchers have shown that based on patch testing, a few cases of allergic contact dermatitis have been reported with the use of consumer products made from isocyanates and

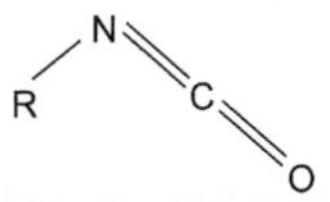

Fig. 15. Isocyanate chemical structure.

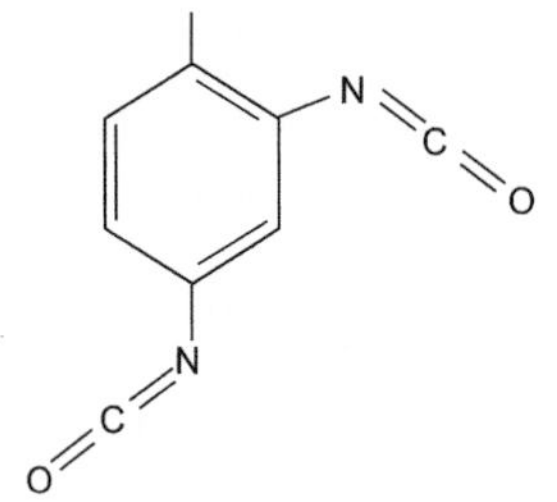

Fig. 16. Chemical structure of toluene 2,4 diisocyanate (TDI).

polyurethanes.[43–45] Items that elicited dermatitis included watch bands and eyeglass frames.

Thermoplastic polyurethane foams are regularly used to provide cushioning in furniture items such as sofas. On occasion the isocyanate compounds that were reacted with polyol to form the foam did not fully react. Accordingly, it is speculated that residual isocyanate vapor can permeate the foam's fabric covering or when a person is sitting on the sofa, perspiration can permeate through the fabric, mix with the unreacted isocyanate and then come in contact the person's skin.

In 2006 a series of previously unreported cases of dermatitis appeared in Finland. Rantanen reported that by 2007 "tens of cases from all over the country" were reported in the Internet discussion forum of the Finnish Dermatologic Society. After an extensive investigation it was found that the cases were as a result of exposure to dimethylfumarate (DMF) (**Figs. 18** and **19**).[46]

It was reported by British newspaper accounts that sachets of DMF were put in thousands of Chinese manufactured furniture items to prevent mold when in storage or when being transported.[47] Rantanen reported that the patients showed strong positive patch test reactions to upholstery fabric samples and to DMF, down to a level of 1 ppm. in the most severe case. It was concluded that the cause of the Chinese sofa chair dermatitis epidemic was likely to be contact allergy to DMF, a novel potent contact sensitizer.

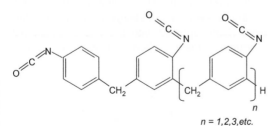

Fig. 17. Chemical structure of polymeric isocyanate (PMDI).

$n = 1,2,3,\text{etc.}$

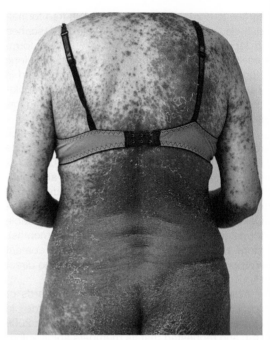

Fig. 18. Patient with allergic contact dermatitis from exposure to dimethylfumarate. (*Courtesy of* T. Rantanen, MD, Lahti, Finland.)

Although furniture fabrics themselves might not be allergenic, there could be release of allergenic agents from the foam cushioning.

SUMMARY

From as early as 1869, textile dyes and subsequently finishes have been reported to cause various manifestations of contact dermatitis, from mild to severe and debilitating. The European Union, through Directive (2002/61/EC) to restrict the marketing and use of certain dangerous substances and preparations (azo colorants) in textile and leather products, has taken the worldwide lead in restricting some dyes because of their carcinogenic nature. Some of the dyes listed in the directive are also responsible for contact dermatitis. The International Oeko-Tex Association, which is a worldwide voluntary standard and the corresponding voluntarily accepted AAFA RSL provides guidance on the use of dyes and formaldehyde. Many countries have now adopted regulations regarding the use of formaldehyde in textile and apparel products. The U S Congress

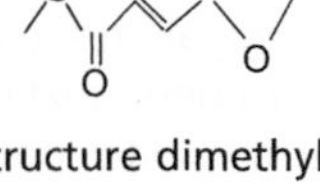

Fig. 19. Chemical structure dimethylfumarate (DMF).

has recently passed HR 4040 which modernizes the CPSC. In that Act there is a section calling for a study of the use of formaldehyde in textile and apparel products. Finally, given the recent discovery of the new route to contact dermatitis from the Finnish sofas, it is important to continue to be vigilant for new and unexpected sources of allergens from textile, apparel, and furniture items.

ACKNOWLEDGMENTS

I greatly appreciate the cooperation, advice, and consultation of Susan Nedorost, MD, during the preparation of this paper. The support of the Commonwealth of Pennsylvania Department of Community and Economic Development for their financial support and Institute of Textile and Apparel Product Safety at Philadelphia University is acknowledged.

REFERENCES

1. Radolph JA, Langford AL. In: Textiles 9th edition. Upper Saddle River (NJ): Prentice Hall; 2002. p. 317
2. Hatch KL. Chemicals and textiles, part I: dermatological problems related to fiber content and dyes. Textile Res J 1984;54:664–82.
3. Wilson E. Des stries et des Macules Atrophiques au Fausses Cicatrices de la Peau. Ann Dermatol Syphiligir 1869;141–2.
4. Lazorov A, Trattner A, Abraham D, et al. Frequency of textile dye and resin sensitization in patients with contact dermatitis in Israel. Contact Dermatitis 2002;46:119–20.
5. She FH, Kong LX. Theoretical investigation of heat and moisture transfer through porous textile materials. Research Journal of Textiles and Apparel 2004;4(1):37–42.
6. American Association of Textile Chemists and Colorists. Colorfastness to Perspiration, AATCC Test Method 15-2007. Raleigh (NC): American Association of Textile Chemists and Colorists; 2007.
7. Giles CH, Duff DG, Sinclair RS. The relationship between dye structure and fastness properties. Review of Progress in Coloration 1982;12:59–65.
8. Hatch KL, Maibach HI. Textile dye dermatitis. J Am Acad Dermatol 1985;12:1079–92.
9. Saunders H, O'Brien T, Nixon R. Textile dye allergic contact dermatitis following paraphenyldiamine sensitization from a temporary tattoo. Australas J Dermatol 2004;45:230–1.
10. Mayer RL. Die Ueberempfindlichkeit Gegen Koerper von Chinonstruktur. Arch Dermatol Syph 1928;156: 313–54.
11. Mayer RL. Ueber die Hautueberempfindlishkeit Gegen Koerper von Chinonstruktur. Klin Wochenschr 1928;7:1958.
12. Mayer RL. Untersuchungen uber die Durch Aromatische Amine Bedington Gewerblichen Erkrankungen. Arch Gewerbepathol 1930;1:436.
13. Dobkevitch S, Baer RL. Eczematous cross- hypersensitivity to azo dyes in nylon stockings and to paraphenylenediamine. J Invest Dermatol 1947;9:203–11.
14. Su JC, Horton JJ, et al. Allergic contact dermatitis from azo dyes. Australas J Dermatol 2007;39(1): 48–9.
15. Directive 2002/61/EC of the European Parliament and of the Council of 19 July 2002 amending for the nineteenth time Council Directive 76/769/EEC relating to restrictions on the marketing and use of certain dangerous substances and preparations (azocolourants). 2002.
16. European Committee for Standardization. Textiles – Methods for determination of certain aromatic amines derived from azo-colorants – Part 1: detection of the use of certain azo colorants accessible without extraction. EN 14362–1 [UK]: 2003.
17. European Committee for Standardization. Textiles – Methods for determination of certain aromatic amines derived from azo-colorants – part 2: detection of the use of certain azo colorants accessible by extracting the fibres. EN 14362–2 [UK]: 2003.
18. American Apparel and Footwear Association. Restricted Substance List, 2008.
19. Vigo TL. Textile processing and properties – preparation, dyeing and finishing. Amsterdam: Elsevier; 1994.
20. Gulrajani ML. Disperse dyes; mechanism of dyeing. In: Gulrajani ML, editor. Dyeing of polyester and its blends. New Delhi: Indian Institute of Technology; 1987.
21. Deutsches Institut für Normung, Textiles - Detection of disperse dyestuffs, DIN 54231, Germany.
22. Dawson JF. Fifty years of disperse dyes (1934-1984). Review of Progress in Coloration 1984;14: 90.
23. Pratt M, Tanaka V. Disperse blue dyes 106 and 124 are common causes of textile dermatitis and should serve as screening allergens for this condition. Am J Contact Dermatitis 2000;11:30–41.
24. Giusti F, Seidenari S. Disperse dye dermatitis: clinical aspects and sensitizing agents. Exog Dermatol 2003;2:6–10.
25. International Oeko-Tex Association. Limit values and fastness. Oeko-Tex 100. Switzerland: International Oeko-Tex Association; 2008.
26. Foulds PR, Marsh JT, Wood FC. Textile material and the production thereof. 1929, US Patent 1,734,515.
27. Fowler JF. Formaldehyde as a textile allergen. Basel, Karger. In: Elsner P, Hatch K, Wigger-Alberti W, editors. Textiles and the skin. Curr Probl Dermatol 2003;31:156–65.
28. Marcussen PV. Contact dermatitis due to formaldehyde in textiles, 1934–1958, preliminary report. Acta Derm Venereol 1959;39:348–56.

29. Marcussen PV. Dermatitis caused by formaldehyde resins in textile. Dermatologica 1962;125:101–11.

30. Berrens L, Young E, Jansen LH. Free formaldehyde in textiles in relation to formalin contact sensitivity. Br J Dermatol 1964;76:110–5.

31. O'Quinn SE, Kennedy CB. Contact dermatitis due to formaldehyde in clothing textiles. JAMA 1965;194: 593–6.

32. Voncina B, Bezek, le Marechal AM. Eco-friendly durable press finishing of textile interlinings. Fibers and Textiles in Eastern Europe July/Septmeber 2002;68–71.

33. Espada B. Recent developments in low-formaldehyde and non-formaldehyde resin finishing. Charlotte (NC): Report for BASF Corporation; 1993.

34. Scheman AJ, Carroll CA, Brown KH, et al. Formaldehyde-related textile allergy: an update. Contact Dermatitis 1998;38:332–6.

35. Bille H. Paper presented at the Society of Dyers and Colourists meeting in Handford. Cheshire, UK; August 1983.

36. Wu W, Yang CQ. Comparison of DMDHEU and melamine-formaldehyde as the binding agents for a hydroxy-functional organophosphorus flame retarding agent on cotton. J Fire Sci 2004;22(2):125–42.

37. Zimerson E, Bruze M, et al. Contact allergy to phenol-formaldehyde resins. In: Kanerva L, Elsner P, Wahlberg JE, et al, editors. Handbook of occupational dermatology. Berlin: Springer Verlag; 2000.

38. Carlson RM, Smith MC, Nedorost ST. Diagnosis and treatment of dermatitis due to formaldehyde resins in clothing. Dermatitis 2004;15(4):169–75.

39. International Organization for Standardization. Textiles – Determination of formaldehyde – part 1: free and hydrolyzed formaldehyde (water extraction method). ISO EN 14184–1. Switzerland: International Organization for Standardization; 1998.

40. Hong Kong Standards and Testing Centre. Formaldehyde Requirements in Textiles. Available at: http://202.66.77.118/UserFiles/File/Newsletter/TMD/Flormaldehyde_2004.pdf. Accessed September 1, 2008.

41. Brookstein DS, Barndt HJ, Pierantozzi J. On current research associated with textile and apparel product safety. Proceedings of the 86th Textile Institute World Conference, Hong Kong, 2008.

42. Bello H, Herrick CA, Smith TJ, et al. Skin exposure to isocyanates: reason for concern. Env Health Persp 2007;14(3):328–34.

43. Alomar A. Contact dermatitis from a fashion watch. Contact Dermatitis 1986;15:44–5.

44. Morgan CJ, Haworth AE. Allergic contact dermatitis from 1,6-hexamethylene diisocyanate in a domestic setting. Contact Dermatitis 2003;48(4):224.

45. Vilaplana J, Romaguera C, Grimalt F. Allergic contact dermatitis from aliphatic isocyanate on spectacle frames. Contact Dermatitis 1987;16(2): 113.

46. Rantanen T. The cause of the Chinese sofa/chair dermatitis epidemic is likely to be contact allergy to dimethylfumarate, a novel potent contact sensitizer. Br J Dermatol 2008;159:218–21.

47. Brown D. Thousands injured by toxic gas from Chinese sofas. UK: The Times; July 21, 2008.

Patient Education to Enhance Contact Dermatitis Evaluation and Testing

Mary C. Smith, RN, MSN

KEYWORDS
- Patient education • Patch testing • Allergen avoidance
- Contact dermatitis

Patients presenting for evaluation of possible allergic contact dermatitis (ACD) have many educational needs. They come with preconceived notions of what is causing their rash, often have seen many other health care professionals, and may be frustrated. Their condition may have caused interruption of sleep, stress on personal relationships, or jeopardized their jobs. Health care professionals face the limitations of time because of the limited number of specialists in this area, and quality patient education for patch test patients becomes a challenge.

BACKGROUND OF PATIENT EDUCATION

Florence Nightingale emphasized teaching Civil War soldiers the importance of fresh air, nutrition, exercise, and personal hygiene to improve well-being. In 1993, the Joint Commission on Accreditation of Health care Organizations (JCAHO) came out with standards that identified the need for health care professionals to educate patients to "enhance their knowledge, skills, and those behaviors necessary to fully benefit from the health care interventions provided by the organizations."[1] In 1996, JCAHO added additional standards to include that patient education must be provided by an interdisciplinary healthcare team, with consideration given to the client's literacy level, educational level, and language. This education must be understandable and "culturally appropriate" to the patient and/or significant other.[1]

Often in contact dermatitis clinics, the immunologic basis of ACD, avoidance of allergens, and the proper use and side affects of corticosteroids need to be explained to patients. Nurses can play a vital role in assessing, planning, and implementing patient education to empower patients with ACD.

However, learning more about a disease process does not necessarily bring about change in behavior. Knowledge that sunburns were associated with skin cancer did not improve adolescent sun protection behavior.[2] Educational programs in elementary schools did not sustain impact on sun protective behavior.[3] However, college students showed improved intention to practice sun protective behaviors when shown photographs depicting underlying sun damage to skin.[4]

If simply providing information about the disease process does not automatically change behavior, then where should patient education focus? "Stages of Change Model" was introduced by Prochaska and DiClemente,[5] who originally looked at the stages cigarette smokers went through as they were trying to quit. The theory has been adapted for use with stroke patients,[6] smoking cessation programs,[7,8] weight reduction programs,[9] and other lifestyle changes.[10] Being aware of the patient's stage of change, building on existing knowledge, and collaboration with other healthcare providers are found to be significant factors in empowering patients to make healthy choices.

University Hospitals Case Medical Center, Department of Dermatology, 11100 Euclid Avenue, Cleveland, OH 44106, USA
E-mail address: mary.smith@UHhospitals.org

Dermatol Clin 27 (2009) 323–327
doi:10.1016/j.det.2009.05.011
0733-8635/09/$ – see front matter © 2009 Elsevier Inc. All rights reserved.

So with limited time and resources, what can healthcare professionals do to affect ACD patients' behaviors to reach healthy outcomes? According to Prochaska and DiClemente,[5] patients trying to quit smoking went through 5 stages of change. These stages could be seen in ACD patients also:

1. The first stage, the precontemplation stage, identifies individuals who are not aware of the health implications for their actions. For ACD patients, this translates into lack of knowledge regarding the exposure that leads to their dermatitis.
2. The second stage, the contemplative stage, is when the patient starts to seriously think about changing behavior, but no action is taken. This stage often takes place for ACD patients when the final reading is done and when they learn about avoiding their allergens. Together with the healthcare professional, they identify which allergens are relevant, and what items or products need to be avoided for a cure.
3. The third stage is labeled as the preparation stage; it is when the individual is orienting to or attempting the target behavior. This stage may include experimenting with small changes. This stage often starts when the patient with ACD is at the drugstore and is selecting personal care products that do not contain their allergen. Then they "try" different products to see if their condition improves. One study in 2007 reports that patients with fragrance allergies smelled the products as a strategy for determining safe products.[11]
4. The fourth stage is the action stage, when the action is taken. An example of this stage would involve using products from the allergy-free list generated from the Computerized Allergen Replacement Database (CARD) for 1 month to test for relevance. It is during this stage that patients develop health beliefs about their treatment. In the 2007 study mentioned earlier, Noiesen and colleagues[11] found that almost half of the study population did not trust the labels of ingredients, with one explanation being that patients experienced eczema eruptions even when they attempted avoidance of allergens by reading the labels.
5. The fifth stage is known as the maintenance stage and is reached when the individual has performed the behavior for 6 months. In this model, patients can progress, regress, or remain in any stage for a period of time. Six months after patch testing could be a good time for a follow-up visit or phone call. With the ACD patients, a "flare" is often seen about 1 year after patch testing. They have been rash free for a while and "forget" to check the labels on products.

ASSESSING LEARNING NEEDS

Some simple questions can be efficient and provide valuable clues to the patient education needs (Table 1). When rooming patients for the consultation, nurses can ask, "What do you think is causing your rash?" Depending on their answer, explaining the delayed reaction to contact allergens that a dermatologist patch tests for as compared with the immediate type I response to the allergens that an allergist tests with scratch testing can be beneficial to the patient. The concept that what touches their skin today can cause a rash that starts in 2 to 7 days and lasts a month, helps patients include a more complete exposure history to include products they may use infrequently or that feel good on application.

Table 1
Questions to ask to facilitate patient education

When to Ask Questions	Questions to Ask
Before consultation	Would you like us to send you information about contact dermatitis?
At consultation visit intake	What do you think is causing your rash? What do you hope comes from patch testing? How familiar are you with contact dermatitis?
At the final reading, after avoidance education	What did the doctor tell you? How confident are you that you can avoid your allergens?
One-month follow up	What advice would you give to a patient who just found out they are allergic to your allergens?

When patch testing is scheduled, nurses can also ask, "What do you hope comes from patch testing?" Depending on their answer, nurses might stress the need to avoid contact allergens for a month before seeing improvement. And immediately following the dermatologist's discussion of the patient's patch test results and avoidance instructions, the nurse can ask, "What did your patch testing show?" It provides a great way to evaluate the patient's understanding of what they just heard. Some patients reply that they are allergic to A, B, and C, and now they have to use their list to go shopping, whereas others reply that they are allergic to chemicals that have such long names that they cannot pronounce them, and they "don't know what to do"!

Each patient comes to the clinic with different health literacy abilities, different support systems, and different allergens. Low educational levels attributed to increased difficulty reading cosmetic labels. In one qualitative study, participants with hand eczema and at least one nonoccupational contact allergen were interviewed to examine their strategies for selecting personal care products. Those in the higher social status were able to read and pronounce ingredients. Participants in the middle social status could not pronounce the chemical names of the allergens, so strategies such as comparing the first syllable of the allergen with the first syllable of the ingredients on the label were used. This group doubted their "decoding" ability. The lowest social position rarely read the ingredients on the labels, but their strategies included counting the number of letters in the allergen to compare with the number of letters on the ingredient list or asking sales personnel for help counting or reading.[11]

INITIATING PATIENT EDUCATION

Who do you teach? In a clinic situation, you usually teach the ones in the examination room. When a family member or friend answers many of the questions during intake interview or a teaching session, it can be an indication that they can play an important role in managing the patient's care. When an elderly man's initial reading indicates a positive patch test to textile resins, inviting a daughter or spouse to the final reading is a good idea. The "shopper" of the personal care products and clothing is often the relative or friend who is the driver for appointments and sitting in the waiting room; with the patient's permission, this person can be a great support at the final reading.

When do you teach? Teaching should start before the first consult visit. Information can be mailed to the home or a telephone call can be made before the appointment, informing the patient to bring in a shopping bag filled with their personal care products. By listening to the patient's questions and providing answers about the consult visit or even directions to the office, the nurse can begin to develop a teaching relationship. A handout can be given to the patient in the waiting room, informing them of the delayed onset of symptoms following the exposure to allergens. This can facilitate the intake interview. During the patch test application, there is an opportunity to discuss expectations of resolution of the rash that follows prolonged avoidance and to answer patient's questions. Many patients are more relaxed with the nurse and reveal their questions and misconceptions.

At the one-month follow-up visit, reinforcement of allergen avoidance is usually needed. Identifying the areas that have cleared and linking this to the patient's avoidance behaviors is an important element in empowering patients. The nurse should acknowledge what they did to improve their condition and stress the need to maintain 100% avoidance to remain clear. Sometimes all the avoidance information given at the final reading needs to be repeated. This is especially true for patients who take a month to stop itching and get some sleep, restoring cognitive function and concentration.

What should be taught? That depends on the patient, their readiness to learn, their allergens, and other conditions. For example, because of the multifactorial nature of hand dermatitis, skin care for the underlying diagnosis of irritant dermatitis may also be important for the patient to understand. The distinction between minimizing irritant exposure to prevent hand dermatitis from getting worse and 100% avoidance of an allergen to prevent an allergic reaction is very important for patients with hand dermatitis to understand (**Table 2**).

For example, a hand dermatitis patient, who is the mother of young children, who patch tests positive to cocamidapropyl betaine should be instructed to use the CARD printout to choose shampoos and soaps that are free of this surfactant, for her personal use and for use when shampooing her children. It should be stressed that 100% avoidance is needed for approximately 1 month before significant improvement of her current dermatitis is expected. Patient education for this patient at risk for irritant dermatitis should also include instruction on using alcohol-based hand sanitizers, to decrease the number of wet-to-dry cycles when possible, to use mild soaps when needed, and to apply moisturizers to hands immediately after each washing, while skin

Table 2
Irritant versus contact dermatitis

	Irritant Dermatitis	Allergic Contact Dermatitis
Onset	Few hours	2–7 d
Duration	Few hours to few days	4–6 wk
Exposure	Strong soaps or frequent hand washing	Allergens like nickel, fragrance, preservatives
Occupation	Mother of small children Health care workers	Hairdressers, mechanics, assemblers
Atopy	History of asthma, hay fever, or childhood eczema	No history of childhood eczema

is still damp. Also, wearing cotton gloves under vinyl or rubber gloves when doing wet work or using irritating household cleaners serves to avoid contact with the irritating chemicals and to decrease the number of wet-to-dry cycles when cotton gloves absorb any perspiration and are changed to a dry pair when needed.

EMPOWERING PATIENTS FOR HEALTHY OUTCOMES

By giving patients the knowledge, tools, confidence, and support they need to engage in healthy behaviors, the health care provider empowers patients to become active participants in their health care. For ACD patients, at the final patch test reading, relevant allergens need to be discussed, and their avoidance needs to be outlined. Often, the amount of information that needs to be transferred to the patient and family is challenging.

How should the information be taught? Handouts, discussion, and return demonstrations can all be used to make information available. Handouts can be effective transfers of valuable information. They can be referred to at a later date or shared with family members. Handouts used in patient education should be written at a sixth grade reading level or below. Many of the allergens that are included in patch testing handouts have complex chemical names and quickly elevate reading levels.

The American Contact Dermatitis Society has a Web site, www.contactderm.org, where CARD can provide a list of personal care products that do not contain the identified allergens and education handouts available to its members. These handouts are specific to many allergens.[12] Discussion that highlights the allergens that are relevant to the individual and ends with a summary with a 2- or 3-point action plan can be very helpful. For example, a hand dermatitis patient with multiple allergens might be given a glove order

form, handouts for each of their allergens, and a CARD printout. A discussion of the relevance of each allergen, and proper use of the CARD printout could be summarized with a plan to:

(1) Purchase 1 product from each category on the CARD list and use until they return for their one-month follow-up,
(2) Avoid allergens 100% of the time by bringing "own soap" in travel bottle for use at work or in a public restrooms, and
(3) Purchase cotton gloves for use under vinyl gloves as directed.

Return demonstrations can also enhance patient education by providing immediate individual guidance.[1] The nurse can demonstrate the health behavior and then ask the patient to do the same. It provides an opportunity for the patient to practice and for the nurse to evaluate the patient's understanding of the patient education that was done. For example, various samples of the hand cream, daily facial cleanser, body lotion, and gentle skin care soap made by the same manufacturer can be lined up on the counter in the examination room to offer the nurse a chance to demonstrate how he could use the CARD list to select products free from their allergens. Patients are then asked to use their CARD printout to select the products in front of them that would be safe for them to use. This return demonstration can simulate the patient's upcoming experience at the drug store and prepare them for selection of their allergen-free personal care products. Reinforcing what they do right, identifying what they need help with, and offering suggestions for conquering obstacles, are important.

One patient, when given his CARD list and a lineup of samples was asked if this was the selection at the drugstore, "which products would you pick?" He stated that he would probably just pick the one that was on sale. After repeating how using products containing his allergens could cause his rash to return, he was able to identify the 2 appropriate products from his CARD list. Another man who was asked for the same demonstration, admitted that he was feeling overwhelmed with trying to make the selection. He was given a wallet card that listed his allergens and samples of the soap, shampoo, and cream that he could use for 1 month, which were highlighted on his CARD list. He was instructed to inform his pharmacist that because of allergies, he needed help with obtaining these exact products.

DOCUMENTING AND EVALUATING PATIENT EDUCATION

Patient education is an important aspect of patient care in the contact dermatitis clinic, but often underdocumented. At the final patch test reading and the one-month follow-up visit, specific patient teaching should be documented. Ideally, time spent on teaching, handouts given, questions answered, and return demonstrations done should be included.

Finally, patient education needs to be continuously evaluated. The nurse should verify what the patient understood and what more they need to learn. The one-month follow-up appointment is a great time to ask what worked for the patient and what questions they still have. Also ask, "What helped you avoid your allergens?" or "What advice would you give someone who just found out that they are allergic to the same allergens that you are?"

As patients are empowered, they can teach practitioners how to better teach future patients. Patients help to help others by informing what products are no longer offered, updating contact lists, and offering solutions to problems that present to individuals with contact dermatitis.

ACKNOWLEDGMENT

The author would like to express gratitude to Susan T. Nedorost, MD, for her content and editorial contributions made to this article.

REFERENCES

1. Bastable SB. Patient education. Sudbury (MA): Jones and Bartlett Publishers; 2006.
2. Robinson J, Rademaker A, Cook B. Summer sun exposure: knowledge, attitudes, and behaviors of Midwest adolescents. Prev Med 1997;26(3): 364–72.
3. Milne E, Jacoby P, Giles-Corti B, et al. The impact of the kidskin sun protection intervention on summer suntan and reported sun exposure: was it sustained? Prev Med 2006;42(1):14–20.
4. Mahler H, Kulik J, Butler H, et al. Social norms information enhances the efficacy of an appearance-based sun protection intervention. Soc Sci Med 2005;67(2):321–9.
5. Prochaska J, DiClemente C. Stages and processes of self-change of smoking: toward an integrative model of change. J Consult Clin Psychol 1983; 51(3):390–5.
6. Green T, Haley E, Eliasziw M, et al. Education in stroke prevention: efficacy of an educational counseling intervention to increase knowledge in stroke survivors. Can J Neurosci Nurs 2007;29(2):13–20.
7. Patten CA, Decker PA, Dornelas EA, et al. Changes in readiness to quit and self-efficacy among adolescents receiving a brief office intervention for smoking cessation. Psychol Health Med 2008; 13(3):326–36.
8. Prochaska JO, DiClemente CC. Standardized, individualized, interactive, and personalized self-help programs for smoking cessation. Health Psychol 1993;13:39–46.
9. Turner SL, Thomas AM, Wagner PJ, et al. A collaborative approach to wellness: diet, exercise, and education to impact behavior change. J Am Acad Nurse Pract 2008;20(6):339–44.
10. van Weel-Baumgarten E. Patient-centered information and interventions: tools for lifestyle change? Consequences for medical education. Fam Pract 2008;403(1–3):34–58. [Epub 2008 15].
11. Noiesen E, Munk MD, Larsen K, et al. Difficulties in avoiding exposure to allergens in cosmetics. Contact Dermatitis 2007;57(2):105–9.
12. El-Azhary RA, Yiannias J. A new patient education approach in contact allergic dermatitis: the Contact Allergen Database (CARD). Int J Dermatol 2004; 43(4):278–80.

Relevance and Avoidance of Skin-Care Product Allergens: Pearls and Pitfalls

Steven A. Nelson, MD, James A. Yiannias, MD*

KEYWORDS
• Allergic contact dermatitis • Relevance • Avoidance
• Skin-care • Fragrance • Preservative

Patch testing can be particularly rewarding when skin-care product allergens are identified. Careful determination of relevance, followed by careful education regarding allergen avoidance, can result in dramatic clinical improvement. Several common clinical scenarios are reviewed with a focus on pragmatic solutions to heighten positive patient outcomes.

CLINICAL SCENARIOS
Scenario 1

A patient with fragrance mix I (FM I) allergy returns to your office asking if she can use fragrance-containing lotion, rinse-off soap, and laundry detergent. None of the ingredients specifically list the FM I allergens. Which of these products will you recommend that she use, if any?

Scenario 2

A young father with an allergy to balsam of Peru wants to know about using tea tree oil skin-care products, Hawaiian Bath and Body Pineapple Soap, and Vicks VapoRub cream on his child. What are your recommendations?

Scenario 3

A patient allergic only to quaternium-15, who tested negative to formaldehyde, has been faithfully avoiding the allergen but continues to experience eruptions of dermatitis. Patch testing did not include dimethyl-dimethyl (DMDM) hydantoin or bromonitropropane. Would her eczema improve if the patient avoided all formaldehyde-releasing preservatives?

Fragrances and preservatives found in skin-care products are major culprits in skin-care product allergic contact dermatitis (ACD). Relevance and avoidance of these allergens can be tricky when one considers the choices of available personal care products on the market today and the impressive number of products each person uses on a daily basis. The average woman uses 12 personal care products on a daily basis, which encompass a total of 168 unique ingredients.[1] The average man uses 6 personal care products daily with a total of 85 unique ingredients.[1] Not surprisingly, the rates for positive patch test reactions for skin-care product ingredients are rising.[2] Clinicians involved in the diagnosis and treatment of ACD must be prepared to answer questions from patients concerning the relevance and avoidance of skin-care product allergens.

Patch testing remains the most useful objective tool used by physicians to discover allergens causing ACD. Patch testing involves more than just applying allergens to the patient's back and reading the results. The process of patch testing involves obtaining a thorough history and physical examination, choosing the correct allergens to test, conducting the patch test properly,

Mayo Clinic Arizona, 13400 East Shea Boulevard, Scottsdale, AZ 85259, USA
* Corresponding author.
E-mail address: yiannias.j@mayo.edu (J.A. Yiannias).

Dermatol Clin 27 (2009) 329–336
doi:10.1016/j.det.2009.05.009
0733-8635/09/$ – see front matter © 2009 Elsevier Inc. All rights reserved.

interpreting the results, determining the relevance of the results, and educating the patient by translating the findings into helpful and practical avoidance strategies. Often, the most challenging steps are determining relevance, educating the patient, and follow-through with allergen avoidance education. We review several pearls and pitfalls of this process, with an emphasis on avoidance of the most common allergens found in skin-care products.

SET EXPECTATIONS EARLY

Before committing to patch testing, patients should know what to expect and why the test is being recommended. Identification of the allergen based only on history and physical examination has been shown to be inadequate, only discovering the allergen in 29% to 54% of cases.[3] Overall, however, patch testing has been shown to be cost effective. In 1989, the cost of hypothetically patch testing everyone in the United States with dermatitis/eczema was estimated to save approximately $40 to $90 million a year when compared with cost of treatment.[4] Studies suggest that early patch testing also improves quality of life in patients with chronic ACD.[5] Furthermore, patch testing is a safe and effective process, and most patients perceive a benefit in skin treatment.[6]

From the outset of discussing the performance of patch testing, patients should be counseled that the testing may not reveal a specific allergen as the cause of their dermatitis. Because patch testing is a time-consuming and labor-intensive process, patients should know the time required and the cost of the patch test before it is undertaken. The price ranges from $4 to $29 per allergen patch, depending on the insurance carrier and the type of patch test used. Setting realistic expectations early is important to prevent dissatisfaction among patients in whom no relevant allergens are found. Clinicians should also consider providing general avoidance strategies of common allergens rather than immediately proceeding to patch testing, especially in limited eczema or of short duration.

ALLERGENS: FIRST BECOME FAMILIAR

Clinicians interpreting patch tests should become familiar with the allergens of the patch test series they administer. This knowledge is critical because it increases the likelihood of determining potential relevance. Optimally, primary care dermatologists and other health care providers who manage allergic contact eczema should know the sources of skin-care product allergens to facilitate allergen avoidance. It is the unfortunate patient who has gone to the trouble of having undergone patch testing, but does not have a thorough understanding of the known allergens or how to avoid them.

An excellent resource for clinicians who desire to learn overview concepts about common allergens is found in *Contact Allergy: Alternatives for the 2007 NACDG Standard Screening Tray*.[7] Avoidance of skin-care product allergens specific to a given patient can be readily accomplished by using only those products recommended by the customized shopping list generated by the Contact Allergen Replacement Database (CARD, discussed later).

Studies over the years have identified the most common allergens causing ACD.[2,8] The North American Contact Dermatitis Group (NACDG) and the Mayo Clinic have published the largest series analyzing patch testing results for North America. A comparison of the most recent top 10 allergens causing ACD, published by the NACDG and the Mayo Clinic, is listed in **Table 1**. Many of the top allergens identified by the Mayo Clinic Contact Dermatitis Group (MCCDG) and the NACDG are found in skin-care products and cosmetics.

The allergens can be categorized into functional groups of similar allergens (**Box 1**). Fragrances and preservatives encompass a large percentage of relevant allergens overall, and are the most common skin-care product related causes of ACD.[8] The following sections serve as a brief review of several common fragrance and preservative allergens, including helpful avoidance tips.

Fragrances

Fragrances are a common ingredient in skin-care products, with about 3,000 different fragrances used in cosmetics.[9] Specific fragrance formulas are not required to be written on the ingredients list of cosmetic products, because the Fair Packaging and Labeling Act consider them trade secrets.[7] Frequently, they are only listed as "perfumes," "colognes," "aroma chemicals," "masking fragrance," "essential oils," or "toilet water."[10] The lack of information regarding fragrances can be a sizable frustration for any patient suffering from ACD. Furthermore, labels such as "unscented" and "hypoallergenic" and even "fragrance-free" do not guarantee that the product is truly free of all fragrances. "Unscented products" may still contain masking fragrances. Some companies label their products as "fragrance-free" despite containing natural fragrances, or containing a fragrance that is also acting as a preservative or emulsifier.[7] The main

Table 1
Top 10 Allergens from the North American Contact Dermatitis Group (NACDG) and the Mayo Clinic Contact Dermatitis Group (MCCDG)

10 Most Common Allergens NACDG	10 Most Common Allergens MCCDG
Nickel sulfate	Nickel sulfate
Neomycin	Balsam of Peru
Balsam of Peru	Gold sodium thiosulfate
Fragrance mix	Neomycin
Thimerosal	Fragrance mix
Gold sodium thiosulfate	Thimerosal
Quaternium-15	Cobalt chloride
Formaldehyde	Formaldehyde
Bacitracin	Benzalkonium chloride
Cobalt chloride	Bacitracin

screening tools used to evaluate for fragrance allergy are balsam of Peru (BOP), fragrance mix I (FM I), and fragrance mix II (FM II). Some patch test providers offer specialized series such as a cosmetics series, botanic series, or fragrance series, all of which may detect additional fragrance allergens.

BOP is an aromatic fluid that comes from a tree native to El Salvador.[7] It is a natural mixture of resins and essential oils, consisting of 6 components (**Box 1**). BOP is not found in skin-care products today, but any of the 6 components can be used individually as fragrances and flavorings in foods and oral preservatives.[11] BOP has many synonyms, including China oil, Peruvianum, Peruvian balsam, Indian balsam, Honduras balsam, Black balsam, balsamum, and Surinam balsa.[10] Uses of BOP in skin-care products and potential cross-reacting substances are summarized in **Table 2**.

Certain foods have chemical ingredients identical to the components of BOP, and case reports have shown a flare of dermatitis in BOP-sensitive patients.[12] These foods include citrus fruits, tomatoes, sweets, alcoholic beverages, vermouth, dark-colored sodas, and spices (cinnamon, cloves, curry, vanilla).[7] Continued dermatitis in a patient with sensitivity to BOP, despite avoidance of its topical components, warrants a trial of dietary restriction of such food.

FM I is another screening tool, made up of the 8 fragrances and an emulsifier listed in **Box 1**. Historically, FM I was able to identify 70% to 80% of individuals allergic to fragrances.[13] Furthermore, the 2 main screening tools for fragrances, FM I and BOP, have been estimated in the past to have detected approximately 90%

of fragrance allergies.[14] With a rising number of new fragrance formulas being produced, the current estimates for the screening ability of BOP and FM I is much lower, only around 60%.[7] As a result, new screening allergens are being tested for more accurate detection of fragrance sensitivity. FM II is thus being incorporated into many standard series, adding 6 fragrance antigens, as listed in **Box 1**.

Ideally, patients with fragrance allergies should avoid any product that lists any fragrances and potential cross-reactors, or a product with an incomplete listing of the ingredients such as "other ingredient," or only listing active ingredients. In addition to using traditional allergen avoidance sheets to guide patients on allergen avoidance, use of a computer-generated shopping list free of the patient's allergens can ease the process, especially when facing the broad allergen category of "fragrance." Specifically, the Contact Allergen Replacement Database (CARD) generates a list of skin-care products free of known patient allergens. For example, on entering "fragrance" into CARD, the default programming eliminates all fragrances and potential cross-reactors of fragrance. However, botanicals and other fragrance-related allergens without a high risk for potential cross-reaction with fragrance are able to be optionally included.

Two of the scenarios given at the beginning of the article are examples of patients allergic to specific fragrance allergens but who are reluctant to give up all fragrances. Scenario 1 illustrates a patient with trunk, arm, and leg dermatitis in a setting of FM I allergy. This patient wishes to use other products with fragrances (eg, tea tree oil and ylang ylang) that are not included in FM I.

Box 1
Groupings of common allergens

Most Common Allergen Groups

Metals

- Nickel
- Gold sodium thiosulfate
- Cobalt chloride

Topical antibiotic preparations (Neomycin and Bacitracin)

Fragrances

Balsam of Peru

- Cinnamic acid
- Benzoyl cinnamate
- Benzoyl benzoate
- Benzoic acid
- Vanillin
- Nerodilol

Fragrance Mix I

- α-Amyl cinnamic alcohol
- Cinnamic alcohol
- Eugenol
- Cinnamic aldehyde
- Hydroxycitronellal
- Geraniol
- Isoeugenol
- Oak moss absolute
- Sorbitan sesquioleate (emulsifier)

Fragrance Mix II

- Hydroxyisohexyl 3-cyclohexene carboxaldehyde
- Citral
- Farnesol
- Coumarin
- Citronellol
- α-Hexyl cinnamal

Preservatives

Formaldehyde

Formaldehyde releasers

- Quaternium-15
- 2-Bromo-2-nitropropane-1,3-diol
- Diazolidinylurea
- Imidazolidinylurea
- DMDM hydantoin

Benzalkonium chloride

Thimerosal

Table 2
Balsam of Peru

Balsam of Peru Uses
Cleansing cloths
Antiperspirants/deodorants
Hair sprays, gels, tonics, and lotions
Hair colorants/"permanents-relaxers"
Soaps/cleansers
Shampoos/conditioners
Moisturizers
Make-up
Sunscreens
Perfumes/colognes/aftershaves
Flavorings
Cross-reactants
Balsam of Tolu
Benzoin
Benzyl acetate
Benzyl alcohol
Cinnamic alcohol /cinnamic aldehyde
Cinnamon oil
Clove oil
Diethylstillbestrol
Essential oils of orange peel
Eugenol
Propolis

Several approaches may be taken: If the patient is recovering from moderate to severe ACD, then guiding the patient away from all fragrances while she recovers is the best option. It is tempting to simplify management by counseling the patient that rinse-off products may be less likely than leave-on products to cause ACD. However, this patient's products, including the rinse-off soap, may contain allergens to which the patient is highly sensitive, but that simply have not been identified. Additional patch testing to the product in question or to a broad cosmetic/botanic or fragrance supplemental series could be considered if any of the product ingredients are contained in the supplemental series. If the patient has fully recovered from the dermatitis, a trial-and-error method can be performed by applying the product (in this case, just the lotion) to the forearm in the same small area twice daily for 1 week. If no dermatitis develops, the product may be considered safe to use.

In scenario 2, a patient with hand eczema and allergy to BOP wishes to use Hawaiian Bath and Body Pineapple Soap and tea tree oil skin products for himself, and wants to apply Vick's VapoRub to his son's chest when he gets a cold. This patient needs to know that he is at an increased risk for flares of his dermatitis on exposure to any fragrance-containing product. Ideally, all fragrances should be avoided. Although none of these products has the ingredients contained in BOP, the soap contains orange peel oil, which has been shown to cross-react with BOP. Tea tree oil cross-reactivity with BOP is less predictable, and thus, optimally, the patient would be patch tested to tea tree oil to understand more fully the safety of its use. Alternatively, he could employ a use test on his forearm as described above. Vick's VapoRub cream contains several ingredients including menthol, cedarleaf oil, eucalyptus oil, and nutmeg oil. The patient could use gloves while applying it to his son's chest; however, the most conservative course of action would simply be to avoid all fragrance-containing skin-care products.

Formaldehyde-Releasing Preservatives

Formaldehyde-releasing preservatives (FRP) are found in many cosmetic products and are the second most common allergen in skin-care products.[7] There are 5 main FRPs: quaternium-15, diazolidinyl urea, DMDM hydantoin, imidazolidinyl urea, and 2-bromo-2-nitropropane-1,3-diol (bromonitropropane).[7] Individuals allergic to formaldehyde may also be allergic to any of the FRPs. Formaldehyde-sensitized individuals can experience an exacerbation of ACD with certain foods, such as aspartame, coffee, cod fish, caviar, maple syrup, shiitake mushrooms, and smoked ham.[7] Of note, quaternium-15 does not cross-react with other "quaterniums" or quaternary ammonium salts. The patient in scenario 3 continues to suffer from ACD despite avoiding quaternium-15, yet the patient was not tested to all of the FRPs. Most clinicians recommend that any patient allergic to one FRP should avoid all of them. Of note, CARD eliminates all FRPs if formaldehyde or any FRP is entered as an allergen to which the patient is allergic. Physicians may optionally permit inclusion of the FRPs of their choice if they feel comfortable liberalizing patient exposure.

ALLERGENS: CHOOSE CAREFULLY

For patch tests to identify relevant allergens and act as a gold standard, the clinician must decide which allergens to test. With more than 2,800 known allergens available for patch testing,[15] it is impractical and ineffective to test for every one. To help clinicians, standard screening series have been created based on studies showing the most common allergens responsible for ACD. The challenge with "standard" series is that the number and types of allergens vary widely from practice to practice, and they are continuously being updated.[2] For example, the thin-layer rapid use epicutaneous test (TRUE test) is a commercial patch test used by 74% of dermatologists who perform patch tests.[16] The manufacturer of the TRUE test recently expanded the number of allergens tested, bringing the total to 29. In comparison, the NACDG uses 65 allergens and the MCCDG uses 74 allergens in the screening tray.[8]

Clinicians who perform patch testing must choose practical screening series that do not miss relevant allergens. Very large series can be expensive, difficult to maintain, and impractical to place on the patient's skin. However, smaller screening series have been shown to miss relevant allergens and may not adequately evaluate the patient.[2] For instance, the TRUE test only identifies about two-thirds of relevant allergens and is more likely to give false-negative reactions when compared with the Finn Chambers.[7,17] Broad-standard series, such as that used by the NACDG, may not always detect all allergens (16.7% of patients had relevant allergic patch test reactions to supplemental allergens not identified in the NACDG standard series).[8] The TRUE test is used by the majority of general dermatologists and allergists who patch test, because it is a good starting point, more affordable, and conveniently produced on ready-to-use chambers.

When patients continue to struggle with dermatitis after initial patch testing, they may also need expanded patch testing of contact allergens outside the standard series based on history, occupation, or location of the dermatitis. For example, a cosmetic/botanic supplemental series typically contains additional fragrances found in cosmetics and other skin-care products. This series may be indicated in patients using a variety of make-up products or for those who use botanic or "all natural" products.

IS IT REALLY RELEVANT?

Relevance assesses the likelihood that the test-positive allergen is the culprit causing the patient's dermatitis. Relevance reactions are divided into the following categories: no relevance, past relevance, or current relevance. Past relevance describes a positive patch-test result that explains a previous, unrelated episode of ACD. Positive patch tests to nickel and neomycin often present as illustrations of past-relevant reactions, where the patient recalls a prior episode of dermatitis on exposure to an allergen and has subsequently avoided it. For example, patients may recognize that costume jewelry/belt buckles or an over-the-counter antibiotic ointment once induced a rash and they ceased using the product. Current relevance may be further subdivided into 3 categories (definite, probable, and possible relevance) based on the likelihood that the patch-test positive allergen is causing the ACD. Definite relevance is determined if the patient has a positive patch-test reaction to the suspected object or compound.[8] Relevance is declared probable if the positive patch test identifies a substance that is a known skin contactant of the patient and the clinical distribution is consistent.[8] The relevance is possible if the patient was exposed to circumstances in which skin contact with materials known to contain the suspected allergen likely occurred.[8]

Determining the relevance of a positive reaction can be the most difficult part of patch testing and should be approached as a physician-patient team. A detailed list of the occurrences of the allergen in the patient's home and work environments should be studied with the patient. Reviewing the history (including exposures, time course, relapses, and location of the patient's current dermatitis) may aid in the investigation.[18] In addition to the initial encounter, many clinicians have patients complete a worksheet containing detailed information regarding all cosmetics and skin-care products, occupation, and hobbies. Relevance can be verified if the dermatitis clears after the patient removes the patch-test-positive allergen from his or her environment and then reappears after the allergen is reintroduced.

HAVE RESOURCES READILY AVAILABLE

Allergen avoidance resources are vital to a successful outcome with patch testing. They can turn complication and aggravation into compliance and appreciation. One of the greatest pitfalls a clinician could make after a positive patch test is simply handing the patient an allergen information sheet (many available at www.contactderm.org or via allergen vendors) as a substitute for practical face-to-face patient education. This approach may seem quicker in the short term, but it may leave the patient feeling overwhelmed, especially if the allergen is ubiquitous or carries a difficult name with many synonyms. Avoidance begins with thoroughly educating the patient.

Relevant allergens should be discussed in detail, and practical avoidance strategies must be tailored to the patient. Unless the patient has skill sets akin to those of a biochemist, the names of most allergens are foreign and difficult to remember. On average, 50% of relevant patch-test-positive allergens could not be recalled by patients.[6] Even if the patient remembers the names, finding and avoiding the products that contain the allergens can be a daunting task. Reviewing 10 to 20 unfamiliar ingredients on every skin-care product can be tedious (especially in patients with presbyopia, given the small print found on most package labels).

Avoidance resources include a general dermatitis handout designed to empirically avoid common allergens (shotgun approach), allergen avoidance handouts specific to a given allergen, and a CARD shopping list or similar product recommendation list.

A general dermatitis handout can serve as a foundation of avoidance strategies for clinically suspected allergic and irritant contact dermatitis patients. The handout should include a selection of specific suggestions for most personal skin-care products and give general recommendations on gentle skin-care measures. If the dermatitis is mild, of short duration, or if the patient is unwilling or unable to pursue patch tests, many clinicians will start with strict adherence to the handout for several months before considering patch testing. The dermatitis handout that is used at Mayo Clinic Arizona is shown in the **Fig. 1** as one of many possible examples. Additionally, CARD can generate a shopping list free of the MCCDG and NACDG top 10 most common allergens, thereby providing "virtual" patch testing. This is particularly helpful for empiric selection of truly hypoallergenic make-up.

Specific allergen avoidance information given in traditional handouts should be provided to the patient, even in the era of computer-generated skin-care-product shopping lists. These allergen sheets normally include the name of the allergen with a brief description of its uses, synonyms, and suggestions on how to avoid it. The physician should demonstrate to the patient the use of these definitional handouts. For example, if the patient is sensitive to methylchloroisothiazolinone/methylisothiazolinone (MCI/MI), the physician should read the patient's liquid soap and shampoo bottles to determine if they contain MCI/MI. If there is no skin-care product identified during the final patch test reading that contains MCI/MI, then the patient should be asked to keep a log of skin-care products and compare this list with the allergen information sheets. Indeed, if this task is overwhelming to the patient, he or she should be instructed to bring all of his or her skin-care products to a subsequent visit for physician review. Since the turn of the 21st century, many clinicians have turned alternatively to a computer-generated shopping list, detailing products that are free of the patient's know allergens and cross-reactors.

CARD, an extensive database comprising 65 skin-care product categories, is a practical

Introduction

Eczema, also known as Dermatitis, is an inflammation of the skin due to dryness irritation or possible external allergy. Eczema/Dermatitis is not contagious.

Some skin care products contain fragrance even though the package says "fragrance free" or "unscented." Therefore, please choose the skin care products as listed below by their exact brand name.

Suggestions

Soaps/Cleansing

- Vanicream Cleansing Bar®
- Free and Clear Liquid Cleanser®
- Aveeno® Moisturizing Bar for Dry Skin, Fragrance Free or Aveeno ® Eczema Care Body Wash
- Oilatum Unscented Soap®
- Neutrogena Original Formula® Fragrance-Free® (bar or liquid)
- Any of the shampoos listed in this brochure may be used as your hand or body soap
- Aveeno ® Therapeutic shave gel or Edge® unscented shave gel

Moisturizers

- Vanicream ® , Vanicream Lite®
- Aveeno ® Daily Moisturizing Lotion, Fragrance Free or Aveeno ® Eczema Care Moisturizing Cream
- Plain Vaseline®
- DML unscented®
  - ᴘ Use moisturizers twice daily
  - ᴘ All of the above are OK to use on face
  - ᴘ To assist with your applying the cream after shower, just blot water off with hand and apply cream. Do not use a towel to dry off.
- Robathol Bath Oil®

Deodorants

- Almay® unscented antiperspirants
- Mitchum® unscented cream antiperspirant and deodorant
- May use plain cornstarch from grocer

Shampoo

- Free and Clear Shampoo ® and Conditioner
- DHS Clear Shampoo ® and DHS Conditioner®
- If you have dandruff, use DHS Sal Shampoo or Neutrogena T-SAL Shampoo (*not* T-Gel)
- Conditioners can be used as "leave on" hair gel

Hairspray

- Fragrance-Free hairspray such as Free and Clear® Hairspray
  (Caution: Hairsprays labeled as "un-scented" may not be fragrance free.)

Laundry and Home Care

- Unscented laundry detergents (Tide Free ®, Cheer Free and Gentle®, All Free and Clear ®, Arm & Hammer Unscented ®, Wisk Free®, Purex Unscented®)
- Wash all new clothes and linens five times before using.
- Old clothes and fabrics are preferred.
- White vinegar in rinse cycle help to remove soap, and may be used as a general household cleaner.

Hand, Nail & General Skin Care Tips

- Wear cotton gloves under rubber/vinyl gloves for any activities where hand-wetting is expected.
- Trim nails short. Long nails are dangerous to skin especially when sleeping.

Sunscreens

- Vanicream Sunscreen # 30 or 60®

Avoid

Soaps/Cleansing

- No hot water (use lukewarm).
- Avoid hot tubs.
- No rubbing alcohol.

Moisturizers

- No creams, lotions, oils or powders other than those recommended in this brochure.
- No Neosporin ® products.

Fragrances

- No perfumes, colognes, after-shave, pre-shave on any part of body / clothing.

Laundry and Home Care

- No fabric softener in washer.
- No fabric softener sheets in dryer.
- No washing machine water softener such as Calgon® (in-house water softeners are acceptable).

Hand, Nail & General Skin Care Tips

- No wetting of hands more than 5 times a day.
- No tight fitting clothes
- No scrubbing! No Loofa! No pumice stone!
- Do not pull off dead skin. Snip with scissors instead.

Fig. 1. Mayo Clinic General Dermatitis Hanout.

tool to help physicians search through more than 2,500 topical products and more than 6,500 ingredients for skin-care products. CARD is available as an online tool for members of the American Contact Dermatitis Society at www.contactderm. org. The database allows clinicians to enter any number of allergens to generate a printable "shopping list" of skin-care products free of the entered allergens. It eliminates products containing not only the entered allergens, but also those known to have cross- or co-reactions. The main philosophy of CARD is to err on the side of caution. For example, in scenarios 1 and 2 at the beginning of the article, CARD would generate a list of products free from all fragrance-related allergens, not just those in FM I or BOP. For patient 1, the fragrance lotion, rinse-off soap, and laundry detergent would be disqualified from the shopping list. All 3 products mentioned by patient 2 would also be excluded. Fortunately, the database provides hundreds of alternatives that both patients could use. CARD would do the same for the formaldehyde-releasing preservatives by eliminating all 5 of them if 1 allergy was detected on patch test. The physician has the option of allowing many of the prohibited "questionable" cross-reactors to be included in the shopping list. For example, the physician can override CARD's default action of eliminating all formaldehyde releasers if the patient is only allergic to formaldehyde or a limited number of formaldehyde releasers.

Although use of CARD has not shown a statistically significant difference in clinical disease activity, it has been shown to correspond with much higher level of patient satisfaction while decreasing mean counseling time by the physician.[19]

SUMMARY

Evaluating a patient with ACD can be particularly rewarding for both the patient and clinician if the recommendations result in substantial clinical improvement. Clinicians should maintain a high suspicion for personal skin-care products as allergen culprits during such evaluations, and become especially familiar with top skin-care product allergens, including fragrance- and formaldehyde-related allergens. On the clinician's development of a thorough understanding of the allergens included in their patch test series, patients will be able to have greater trust in the therapeutic recommendations provided. Patient satisfaction and compliance will also increase if meaningful resources, such as specific lists of "safe" personal skin-care products, are provided.

REFERENCES

1. Available at: http://www.cosmeticsdatabase.com/research. Accessed April 1, 2009.
2. Davis MD, Scalf LA, Yiannias JA, et al. changing trends and allergens in the patch test standard series: a Mayo clinic 5-year retrospective review, January 1, 2001, through December 31, 2005. Arch Dermatol 2008;144:67–72.
3. Mowad CM. Patch testing: pitfalls and performance. Curr Opin Allergy Clin Immunol 2006;6:340–4.
4. Rietschel RL. Is patch testing cost-effective? J Am Acad Dermatol 1989;21:885–7.
5. Kadyk DL, McCarter K, Achen F, et al. Quality of life in patients with allergic contact dermatitis. J Am Acad Dermatol 2003;49:1037–48.
6. Scalf LA, Genebriera J, Davis MD, et al. Patients' perceptions of the usefulness and outcome of patch testing. J Am Acad Dermatol 2007;56:928–32.
7. Scheman A, Jacob S, Zirwas M, et al. Contact allergy: alternatives for the 2007 NACDG standard screening tray. Dis Mon 2008;54(1–2):7–156.
8. Scheman A, Jacob S, Zirwas M, et al. North American Contact Dermatitis Group Patch-Test Results, 2001–2002 Study Period. Dermatitis 2004;15:176–83.
9. Devos SA, Constandt L, Tupker RA, et al. Relevance of positive patch-test reactions to fragrance mix. Dermatitis 2008;19(1):43–7.
10. Marks JG, Elsner P, DeLeo V. Contact and occupational dermatology. 3rd Edition. Mosby, Inc.; 2002.
11. Api AM. Only Peru balsam extracts or distillates are used in perfumery. Contact Derm 2006 Mar;54(3):179.
12. Ortiz K, Yiannias J Contact dermatitis to cosmetics, fragrances, and botanicals. Dermatol Ther 2004;17(3):264–271.
13. Larsen WG. Perfume dermatitis. J Am Acad Dermatol 1985;12(1 pt 1):1–9.
14. Larsen W, Nakayama H, Lindberg M, et al. Fragrance contact dermatitis: a worldwide multicenter investigation (Part 1). Am J Contact Dermat 1996;7(2):77–83.
15. De Groot AC. Patch testing: test concentrations and vehicles for 2800 allergens. Amsterdam, New York, Oxford: Elsevier; 1986.
16. Warshaw EM, Moore JB, Nelson D. Patch testing practices of American contact dermatitis society members: a cross-sectional survey. Am J Contact Dermatitis 2003;14(1):5–11.
17. Larking A, Rietschel RL. The utility of patch tests using larger screening series of allergens. Am J Contact Dermatitis 1998;9:142–5.
18. Frosch PJ, Menne T, Lepoittevinet JP. Contact Dermatitis. 4th Edition. New York: Springer; 2006. p. 201–14.
19. Kist J, el-Azhary RA, Hentz JG, et al. The contact allergen replacement database and treatment of allergic contact dermatitis. Arch Dermatol 2004;140(12):1448–50.

Acute and Recurrent Vesicular Hand Dermatitis

Niels K. Veien, MD, PhD

KEYWORDS
- Pompholyx • Dyshidrosis • Dyshidrotic eczema
- Systemic contact dermatitis • Nomenclature

INTRODUCTION AND NOMENCLATURE

The nomenclature of recurrent, vesicular hand dermatitis, including pompholyx and dyshidrotic eczema, is confusing. In 1873, Tilbury Fox[1,2] described dyshidrosis as an eruption of deep-seated vesicles on the sides of the fingers and on the palms with little or no clinical sign of inflammation. Three years later, in 1876, Hutchinson described the same features in characterizing cheiropompholyx.[3]

Initially, when such eruptions were seen in association with hot weather, they were thought to be a manifestation of abnormal sweating, or were associated with "nervousness." It became clear; however; that the vesicles were in no way connected to the sweat ducts, and the condition has since by most authors been considered to be a morphologic variant of hand eczema.

Kutzner and colleagues[4] examined 93 biopsies of vesicles from patients with vesicular hand dermatitis and found spongiotic dermatitis and no relationship to the acrosyringia. Simons[5] and Shelley[6] had similar findings.

Storrs[7] has reviewed the nomenclature and stresses that in the strictest sense, the term *pompholyx* refers to a rare, severe eruption of vesicles and bullae on the palms and occasionally also on the soles. Rather than recurrent vesicular hand eczema, she prefers "chronic vesicular hand eczema." She concludes, however, that this spectrum of dermatitis is probably best described as acute and recurrent vesicular hand dermatitis as suggested in a review by Veien and Menné.[8]

The morphologic diagnosis of recurrent, vesicular hand eczema does not have 1 distinct etiology. There may be several causes of this morphology, including allergic contact dermatitis, other types of contact dermatitis, dermatophytid, other id reactions, and other endogenous skin diseases such as atopic dermatitis. For a considerable number of patients, it is not possible to establish an etiology.

In this review, the terminology used in the individual papers will be cited. Suggestions for descriptive nomenclature are given in the final section.

CLINICAL APPEARANCE

Among the authors who have dealt with this condition, there is reasonable agreement that vesicular hand eczema is primarily located on the palms, the palmar aspects of the fingers, and the sides of the fingers and that the condition is eruptive. There is less agreement on how common it is, whether or not there may be dermatitis on areas of the body other than the palms and soles, and whether inflammatory lesions should be included.

Fox[1] includes more than just a palmar eruption in his description of dyshidrosis. He includes "more or less dermatitis" in his description and states that "I have seen the back of the hand and the palm with bullae." He also writes that "the eruption about the hand or hands may be complicated by a rash, more or less general over the body" and that "sometimes awfully painful surface is left behind and becomes chronic." The condition is described as being of common occurrence. A patient with palmar dyshidrosis as well as lesions on the forearms and upper arms is also described.[2]

Dermatology Clinic, Vesterbro 99, DK-9000 Aalborg, Denmark
E-mail address: veien@dadlnet.dk

Dermatol Clin 27 (2009) 337–353
doi:10.1016/j.det.2009.05.013
0733-8635/09/$ – see front matter

Hutchinson[3] describes less severe forms of the disease cheiropompholyx as "tolerably common, while severe forms are rare." In his words, "the hands are the first part affected; the feet come next, and in a few instances, a rash appears over the whole body." Two of the 3 patients had lesions on parts of the body other than the hands.

The author of the current review considers the severe forms of acute vesicular palmar dermatitis to be rare. When they do occur, a cause is seldom found. Morphologically, the condition may present only on the skin of the palms with sharp delineation toward the skin of the forearms and the dorsal aspects of the hands. The palmar skin has an unexplained, curious ability to produce lesions that do not extend to dorsal or forearm skin (**Fig. 1**).

Acute vesicular, palmar dermatitis may present as large, vesicular and/or bullous lesions on non-inflamed skin (**Figs. 2** and **3**), but inflammation is often seen during the course of the eruption. The question of inflammation is, therefore, only of interest in early lesions.

A very pruritic vesicular eruption of limited intensity is a much more common clinical manifestation. It is often seen most clearly on the sides of the fingers, either without inflammation (**Fig. 4**) or with slight inflammation (**Fig. 5**). If frequent vesicular eruptions occur, for example on the palms, the lesions do not have time to heal completely between attacks. Residual scaling may, therefore, be seen and the skin may become visibly inflamed (**Fig. 6**). Careful inspection with a magnifying glass

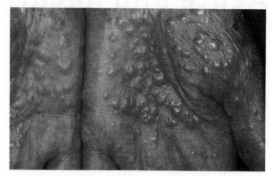

Fig. 2. Vesicular and bullous hand dermatitis.

may be necessary to detect the vesicles (**Fig. 7**). At a casual glance, the dermatitis may look like chronic hand eczema. As described by Hutchinson[3]; a similar eruption may be seen on the soles, although less often than on the palms.

In some patients sensitized to nickel, cobalt, or chromate, the vesicular response can be reproduced experimentally by oral challenge with the hapten in a placebo-controlled fashion (**Figs. 8** and **9**). Time for response is also revealed in such experiments, with vesicular eruptions seen 24 to 48 hours after ingestion of the hapten. A severe, bilateral, vesicular, and bullous eruption was seen in 1 woman with nickel allergy after patch testing with nickel (**Fig. 10**).

Palmar eruptions may be the only manifestation. However, many patients who are contact sensitized to the aforementioned metals will, on contact with the metals, experience a vesicular flare on the hands as well as a flare-up at the sites of recent, previously positive patch tests to the metals. Patients sensitive to nickel may experience flares at sites of contact with nickel.[9]

DIFFERENTIAL DIAGNOSIS

Superficial peeling of the skin—dyshidrosis lamellosa sicca or recurrent, palmar peeling—may

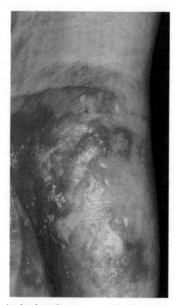

Fig. 1. Vesicular hand eczema with the involvement of palmar skin but not the skin of the forearms.

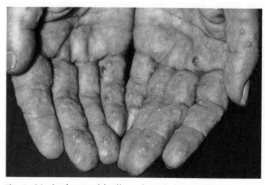

Fig. 3. Vesicular and bullous hand dermatitis.

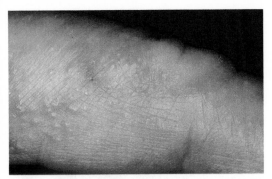

Fig. 4. Vesicular hand dermatitis without inflammation on the side of a finger.

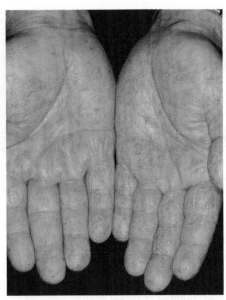

Fig. 6. Vesicular hand dermatitis with inflammation and scaling mimicking chronic hand dermatitis.

mimic recurrent, vesicular hand eczema. This superficial peeling does not have fluid-containing vesicles. It is so superficial that initially small dry scales are seen. The individual scales break and become discrete annular scaling (**Figs. 11** and **12**). If multiple eruptions occur over a short period of time, the stratum corneum thins, resulting in erythema and thin, sensitive skin on the palms.

Pustular eruptions like palmoplantar pustulosis may have an early vesicular stage, but pustules usually develop within a few days.[9] Palmoplantar pustulosis may present with pruritus at onset, but the pruritus is mild and transient, as opposed to the intensely pruritic vesicles associated with recurrent vesicular hand eczema.

Infantile acropustulosis is a vesiculopustular dermatosis that may be seen on the palms, soles, and also on the dorsa of the feet of infants.[10,11]

As in allergic contact dermatitis caused by direct contact with the hapten, vesicular eruptions seen in protein contact dermatitis are limited to the areas of contact with the offending item.

Bullous pemphigoid may have a vesicular palmar and/or plantar eruption as the presenting symptom.[12,13] The lesions may be hemorrhagic.[14,15] Similar findings have been made in linear IgA diseases and in herpes gestationis.[16,17]

THE MECHANISM AND SPECIFICITY OF VESICULAR ERUPTIONS ON THE HANDS AND FINGERS IN RELATION TO SYSTEMIC CONTACT DERMATITIS

The pathomechanism involved in vesicular palmar eruptions is largely unknown. Dermatopathology has shown that the vesicles are part of a spongiotic type of dermatitis, and it is assumed that the vesicles remain intact because of the thick stratum corneum of palmar skin. In other areas of the

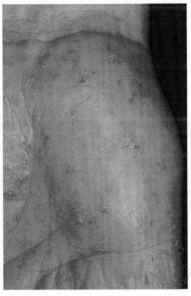

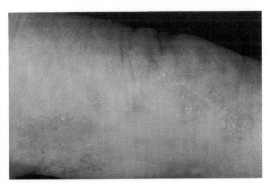

Fig. 5. Vesicular hand dermatitis with moderate inflammation on the side of a finger.

Fig. 7. A close-up view of the patient in Fig. 6. Note vesicles.

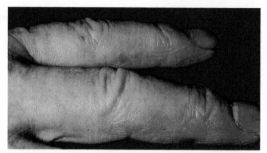

Fig. 8. Sides of the fingers of a chromate-allergic man before placebo-controlled oral challenge with 2.5 mg of chromium given as 7.1 mg potassium dichromate.

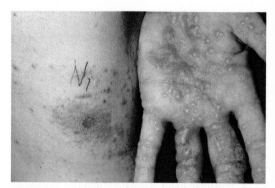

Fig. 10. A woman with nickel allergy developed a symmetric, bullous eruption on the palms after patch testing with nickel.

skin, spongiotic vesicles would break after minimal trauma.

Deliberate exposure to nickel either by immersion of a finger in a nickel solution or patch testing on the fingers resulted in a vesicular eruption in a limited number of nickel allergic patients.[18]

In placebo-controlled trials, oral challenge with nickel in patients sensitive to nickel with recurrent, vesicular hand eczema reproduced the hand eczema on a regular basis.[19] In another study, a flare-up of dermatitis was often seen at the site of a previous, positive patch test to nickel or at the site of current or previous nickel dermatitis.[20] De novo vesicular hand eczema has been seen in patients sensitive to nickel or cobalt treated for chronic alcoholism with disulfiram.[21] Disulfiram is known to mobilize nickel and initially causes a high serum level of nickel.[22,23] De novo vesicular hand eczema has also been seen in persons with contact sensitivity to neomycin who take oral neomycin in spite of the fact that neomycin is very poorly absorbed.[24,25]

This evidence leaves little doubt that vesicular eruptions on the hands can be a specific phenomenon and an example of systemic contact dermatitis in contact-sensitized persons. A similar, unknown mechanism may explain vesicular

dermatophytid of the hands. A positive trichophytin test should be required for making this diagnosis.

To clearly define a vesicular palmar eruption, it is probably necessary to look more specifically at the immune reactions when such an eruption occurs, for example in oral challenge experiments. Which cells are present, and what is the cytokine profile in lesional tissue during an eruption? Comparison of the immune reactions in the palm when a vesicular palmar eruption occurs and events that might be taking place in the neighboring forearm skin could explain why vesicular eruptions seen after oral challenge, for example in patients sensitive to nickel, occur only on palmar skin with no clinical evidence of immune response in the adjacent skin of the forearm or on the dorsum of the hands (see **Fig. 1**).

DETERMINATION OF SEVERITY

Several instruments have in recent years been developed to assess the severity of hand eczema. Coenraads and colleagues[26] have developed a photographic guide with images of the various stages of hand eczema: (1) clear, (2) almost clear, (3) moderate, (4) severe, and (5) very severe.

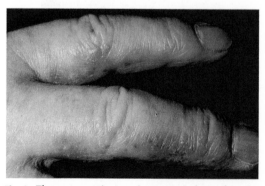

Fig. 9. The same patient as in **Fig. 8**, 2 days after the oral challenge.

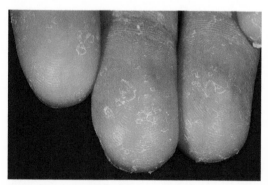

Fig. 11. Dyshidrosis lamellosa sicca or recurrent palmar peeling.

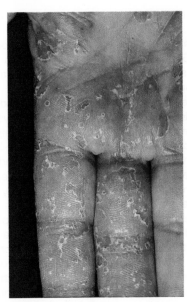

Fig. 12. Dyshidrosis lamellosa sicca or recurrent palmar peeling. Note annular scaling.

Expert dermatologists evaluated 28 patients with hand eczema in order to validate the guide. There was good interobserver reliability and reproducibility on retesting. A modified photographic guide for use by patients with hand eczema has been developed by Hald and colleagues.[27]

A point-based score system, the hand eczema severity index (HECSI), includes a score for the number of vesicles.[28] The severity of vesicular hand eczema can be evaluated with the HECSI, something that is not possible using the photographic guide.

In the Dyshidrotic Eczema Area and Severity Index (DASI) developed by Vocks and colleagues,[29] scores are given for number of vesicles, erythema, desquamation, and itching. The index was found to be useful in 2 clinical trials.

REVIEWS

Menné and Hjorth[30] reviewed pompholyx-dyshidrotic eczema defined as an acute or chronic vesicular eruption on the hands and feet. Based on twin studies, no genetic factors were found to be an important cause of the eczema. Allergic contact dermatitis, in particular systemic contact dermatitis, was found to be an important cause.

Lambert[31] used the term *dysidrose palmo-plantaire* and distinguished between dermatitis with (1) a known etiology such as an id reaction caused by dermatophytes or other microorganisms, allergic contact dermatitis, or drug reactions and (2) essential dyshidrosis associated with atopy and possibly with sweat retention.

Veien and Menné[8] introduced the term *acute and recurrent vesicular hand dermatitis*. Patients who had dermatitis in areas other than the hands and feet were also included and it was stressed that the condition is a non-specific reaction pattern that may have many causes.

Lofgren and Warshaw[32] distinguished between pompholyx as a rare condition characterized by the explosive onset of large bullae on the hands and dyshidrosis or dyshidrotic eczema as a common, chronic, recurrent condition with 1 mm to 2 mm vesicles on the palms, soles, and/or lateral aspects of the fingers. Treatment options were reviewed extensively.

EPIDEMIOLOGY

Thelin and Agrup[33] examined a 1-year series of 68 patients with pompholyx in the outpatient clinic of the dermatology department at the University Hospital in Lund, Sweden. The 68 cases were an estimated 1 percent of all patients referred to the department. Unfortunately, no clear inclusion or exclusion criteria were provided.

As a part of a population-based investigation in Sweden, Agrup found that acrovesiculatio recidivans was present in 6% of the hand dermatoses examined.[34]

In a population-based study by Meding,[35] 5% of 1457 patients were diagnosed with pompholyx. Patients with allergic contact dermatitis, irritant contact dermatitis, and atopic dermatitis were excluded from the study.

Among 522 consecutive patients with hand eczema seen in a private dermatology clinic that serves as a secondary referral center, recurrent vesicular hand eczema was the most common morphologic diagnosis, irrespective of etiology in 54 men (31%) and 173 women (50%).[36]

It is obvious that the variation in frequency of vesicular hand eczema in the aforementioned studies is at least in part because of differences in the definition of the condition.

Other studies of patients with acute or recurrent vesicular hand eczema have typically dealt with series of patients seen in the outpatient clinics of hospital departments of dermatology.

CAUSES

Young[37] described 75 patients and compared them to 55 controls. He used the term *dysidrotic (endogen) eczema* and listed the synonyms *dysidrosis, dysidrosiform eruption, pompholyx, and cheiro-pompholyx* for describing a symmetric eruption, primarily of vesicles (or bullae) on the palms and soles.

Forty-five percent of Young's patients had 1 or more positive intracutaneous tests to inhalant or food allergens compared with 5.5% of the controls. Twenty-eight percent of the patients and 3.5 percent of the controls had a positive intracutaneous test and a family history of atopy. Similar findings among 68 patients with dyshidrosis were made by Shuppli.[38]

Twenty five of the patients (33%) in Young's study experienced seasonal variation in the frequency of eruptions. Nineteen of the patients had eruptions of vesicular hand eczema in the spring and summer months. Five of the 19, compared with 3 of 56 who did not experience flares during the spring and summer had a positive intracutaneous test to pollen. Vesicular hand eczema was provoked by the injection of a pollen extract in 2 patients.

Menighini and Angelini[39] examined 364 consecutive patients with pompholyx of the palms and/or soles. Pompholyx was defined as a recurrent or chronic eruption of deep-seated vesicles on non-erythematous skin of the palms and/or soles but a small proportion of patients had inflammatory skin changes. All 364 patients were patch tested, and for 213, intradermal tests with among other substances such as candidin, epidermophytin, or trichophytin were performed. Thirty percent had 1 or more positive patch tests, mostly to topical drugs. Only 7 patients reacted to nickel. Two hundred eighteen of the patients were men, and 146 were women. Skin testing with microbial antigens contributed little to a final etiologic diagnosis.

Lodi and coworkers[40] examined 104 patients with a clinical diagnosis of pompholyx defined as crops of clear, deeply seated, sago-like, often very itchy vesicles and/or bullae with no erythema. These patients were compared with 208 controls matched for age and sex who had no eczema. Fifty percent of the patients, compared with 11.5% of the controls, had a personal or family history of atopy. Forty-eight percent of the patients and 16% of the controls had 1 or more positive patch tests, most commonly to nickel (20%), whereas 6% of the controls had positive patch tests to nickel. Six of 83 patients with negative patch tests to nickel reacted to oral challenge with 5.6 mg nickel but not to a placebo. Biopsies obtained from all 104 patients showed spongiotic dermatitis with lymphocytes scattered throughout the epidermis.

Castelain[41] compared the results of his investigation of 145 patients with "Les Dysidroses" with the results of other similar studies. Twenty-six percent of the patients had what he described as atopic "dysidroses." Ten of Castelain's patients experienced flares of their dermatitis after oral challenge with nickel, cobalt, and/or chromate.

One patient reacted to oral challenge with balsam of Peru.

A likely etiologic diagnosis was made for 99 of the 145 patients included in Castelain's study, whereas for 46 patients, no specific diagnosis could be made.

Shelley[6] conducted experimental studies to determine the role of the sweat glands in dyshidrosis (pompholyx) and found no relationship. The condition defined as acute, recurrent, non-inflammatory vesicular eruption was strictly limited to the palms and/or soles and followed a non-specific reaction pattern that could be induced by drugs or id reactions or be psychosomatic.

Guillet and colleagues[42] examined 120 patients referred for pompholyx. There were no clear inclusion criteria, and the term allergic contact pompholyx was introduced as the most common cause of the eczema seen in 81 of the 120 patients. It is of concern that the most common, relevant positive patch test was to shower gel and the second most common was to shampoo.

Pitché and colleagues[43] performed a case-control study of 100 patients with pompholyx and 200 controls. In a multivariate analysis, atopy and tinea pedis were found to be the only factors statistically associated with pompholyx.

In a Chinese family, a gene associated with pompholyx was found on chromosome 18.[44]

RELATIONSHIP TO ATOPY

Schwanitz[45] performed a detailed study of 58 patients with dyshidrosis and coined the term "Das atopische Palmoplantarekzem." An association to smoking was found and considered the entity to be a variant of atopic dermatitis.

Lodi and colleagues[40] found personal and familial atopy in 50% of their patients with pompholyx compared with 11.5% in controls.

Norris and colleagues[46] observed pompholyx in 8 of 50 adult patients admitted to hospital for the treatment of atopic dermatitis. No explanation was found for the eruptions but speculated that the high temperature of the ward could have caused the condition.

Bryld found no statistical association between atopy and vesicular hand eczema in his study of twins[47] nor did Edman[48] among 153 patients with palmar eczema.

CONTACT DERMATITIS, DRUG REACTIONS, AND RECURRENT VESICULAR HAND ECZEMA

Allergic and irritant contact dermatitis caused by external contact with the offending items has also been described as the cause of vesicular hand eczema. An irritant reaction to soluble oil was the suspected cause in 1 series of patients.[49] In 1 patient an irritant reaction following contact with *Dieffenbachia* presented as a vesicular eruption on the palms.[50]

Meneghini and Angelini[39] found a number of cases of allergic contact dermatitis to topical drugs among their group of 364 patients with pompholyx.

Of 50 patients clinically suspected of having pompholyx, 20 had 1 or more positive patch tests, most commonly to nickel, potassium dichromate, phenylenediamine, nitrofurazone, and fragrance mix.[51,52]

De novo eruptions of vesicular hand eczema have been seen in contact-sensitized patients who have ingested the contact allergen. Ekelund and Möller[53] gave oral neomycin to 12 patients known to be sensitive to neomycin and saw pompholyx in 3 patients.

A patient sensitive to pyrazinobutazone had a vesicular palmar flare-up reaction when 300 mg of pyrazinobutazone was given orally twice daily for 3 days.[53] Oral piroxicam induced vesicular hand eczema in a contact-sensitized patient.[54]

In 1 study, 4 patients sensitive to preservatives in moistened toilet tissue had symmetric vesicular hand dermatitis.[55] Fungicides used on flowers caused erythematous vesicular palmar dermatitis in a florist.[56]

Eighteen of 20 patients with positive patch tests to sesquiterpene lactone mix had 1 or more positive patch tests to herbal teas. Seventeen of the patients were patch tested because they had long-standing hand eczema of pompholyx type.[57]

In another study of sesquiterpene lactone-sensitive patients, Möller and colleagues[58] patch tested 17 patients with ragweed, recently discovered in Sweden. Sixteen of the patients had chronic hand eczema of pompholyx type. Fifteen of the 17 reacted to ragweed. Fifteen of the 16 with pompholyx had a flare of the pompholyx after patch testing with ragweed.

An id-like vesicular eruption on the palms was seen in a patient with allergic contact dermatitis on the ankle as a result of a neoprene ankle support.[59]

Thyssen and Maibach[60] reviewed drug-elicited systemic contact dermatitis and noted that pompholyx, baboon syndrome, and a macular-papular rash occurred in the same patients, suggesting related pathomechanisms.

IMPLANTED METALS

Metals used for prostheses, wires, screws, and plates used to repair fractures or for orthodontic purposes have been suspected to have cutaneous side effects. The alloys used in these appliances have varied over time. Current usage does not seem to constitute a significant problem with regard to vesicular hand eczema.

In the older literature there are, however, rather convincing case reports of such side effects. For example, widespread dermatitis, including a vesicular palmar and plantar eruption, was seen in a chromate-sensitive patient after insertion of a metal dental plate. The dermatitis disappeared after the plate was removed and recurred when the plate was reinserted.[61]

A 14-year-old boy developed palmar and plantar eczema after orthodontic treatment with bands of stainless steel containing chromium and nickel. He had positive patch tests to nickel and cobalt. The dermatitis faded after discontinuation of the orthodontic treatment.[62]

Three girls who were seen by a dermatologist because of vesicular hand dermatitis wore steel wires as part of their orthodontic treatment. The wires contained nickel and chromium. One had a positive patch test to chromate and reacted to placebo-controlled oral challenge with 2.5 mg chromium given as potassium dichromate. Two were patch test negative. One of the 2 had a positive reaction to oral challenge with 2.5 mg nickel, the other to oral challenge with chromate. The dermatitis of 2 of the 3 girls faded after discontinuation of orthodontic treatment.[63]

Two patients sensitive to nickel developed vesicular palmar dermatitis after the use of infusion needles shown to release nickel.[64]

Three of 4 patients, sensitive to nickel developed pompholyx-like hand eczema when metal clips were used for closure after an operation. All 3 patients had positive reactions to patch tests with the clips.[65]

A man whose ankle fracture was repaired with a nickel-chromium steel plate developed vesicular hand eczema 1 month after the operation. Patch testing showed a +++ reaction to nickel and a +reaction to chromate. The hand eczema improved upon removal of the steel plate.[66]

A patient who developed vesicular hand eczema after a titanium plate and screws were used to repair a fractured hand had negative patch tests to titanium but a lymphocyte transformation test to titanium was positive.[67]

ORAL INGESTION OF METALS

After Christensen and Möller in 1975[68] found that 9 of 12 women sensitive to nickel had flares of vesicular hand eczema after an oral dose of nickel, numerous studies have confirmed their results.[20]

The flare-up of vesicular hand eczema in patients sensitive to nickel appears to be a specific clinical expression of their disease. This view is supported by a study of 202 patients with vesicular hand eczema and negative patch tests who were challenged orally with nickel, cobalt, and chromate. Flares of vesicular hand eczema after oral challenge with nickel were seen primarily in young women, whereas men reacted more often to chromate.[69] Some of the women who reacted to nickel had a history of nickel sensitivity, indicating that some of the patch tests may have been false negative. In contrast to this study, a similar study among patients who had dermatoses other than vesicular hand eczema had no vesicular flares after oral challenge with the metals nickel, cobalt, and chromium.[70]

After intoxication with nickel from a dialysis system, none of 23 patients developed vesicular hand eczema. The nickel concentration in plasma was approximately 3 mg/L.[71] None of 20 workers who accidentally ingested up to 2.5 g of nickel in drinking water developed vesicular hand eczema.[72] Symptoms of intoxication were nausea, abdominal pain, vomiting, diarrhea, coughing, and shortness of breath.

Whether or not patients sensitive to nickel react to oral challenge with nickel is probably a question of dose. Few patients react to 0.5 mg nickel, about half react to 2.5 mg nickel, whereas most patients react to 5 mg or more of nickel.[73]

A flare-up of vesicular hand eczema has also been seen after deliberate ingestion of food with high nickel content.[74]

The amount of nickel in serum in the general population is less than0.3 mg/L, and the upper limit is 1.1 mg/L.[75] In sweat from the arms, Omokhodion[76] found a concentration of 69.9 mg/L of nickel.

Among a group of 25 patients with pompholyx, the perspiration volume was found to be 2.5 times higher than age-matched controls without pompholyx. Among the patients sensitive to metal in this group, most had vesicular flare-ups on the hands after oral challenge with the metal.[77]

The studies mentioned earlier indicate that nickel excreted in sweat may reactivate vesicular hand eczema and that this response can be reliably reproduced by oral challenge with nickel.

NICKEL AND COBALT

Thirty-one of 49 patients with nickel allergy (63%) reacted to oral challenge with 2.24 mg of nickel in a controlled study. Fifteen of the patients who reacted to nickel had vesicular hand eczema.[78]

One patient developed a de novo pompholyx reaction after oral challenge with 3 mg of nickel. This patient was 1 of 30 patients who took part in a study of recall reactions of positive nickel patch tests after oral challenge with a placebo, 1 mg of nickel, and 3 mg of nickel. The study showed a correlation between the intensity of a previously positive patch test and the flare-up reaction.[79]

Veien and colleagues[80] performed a placebo-controlled study of oral challenge with 2.5 mg nickel and 1 mg cobalt in 144 patients with positive patch tests to nickel and/or cobalt and morphology of dermatitis for which a systemic cause of the dermatitis was suspected. Seventy-five of the 144 patients had flares of their dermatitis after challenge with nickel and/or cobalt.

Of 97 patients with positive patch tests only to nickel, 31 reacted only to oral challenge with nickel, 8 reacted to both nickel and cobalt and 8 reacted to cobalt.

Four of 34 patients with positive patch tests to both nickel and cobalt reacted to oral challenge with nickel, 5 reacted to nickel and cobalt and 10 to cobalt alone. Seven of 13 with positive patch tests to cobalt alone reacted only to oral challenge with cobalt, 1 reacted to nickel and cobalt and 1 reacted only to nickel.

This study indicates that cobalt may be of significance in maintaining the dermatitis of patients who have positive patch tests to both nickel and cobalt. These results are supported by animal experiments that showed increased reactivity following oral challenge with the hapten in guinea pigs that were sensitized to both nickel and cobalt than in non-sensitized animals.[81]

Fifty-three of the 144 patients in the afore mentioned study[80] had recurrent vesicular hand eczema. Of the 13 patients who had positive patch tests to cobalt alone, 6 had recurrent vesicular hand eczema. Three of the 6 reacted to oral challenge with cobalt.

The results prompted a study of patients who were sensitive only to cobalt. Four of 6 patients sensitive to cobalt with vesicular hand eczema had flares of their hand dermatitis after placebo-controlled oral challenge with 1 mg cobalt. Three of the 4 who reacted to cobalt experienced improvement of their dermatitis after following a low-cobalt diet.[82]

In a recent review of the literature on cobalt and dyshidrotic eczema and cobalt in food, Stuckert and Nedorost[83] provide a detailed low-cobalt diet.

A cobalt-sensitive patient who was treated with disulfiram for chronic alcoholism developed vesicular hand eczema 1 to 2 days after initiation of this therapy.[84]

Several case reports have supported the observation of flare-ups of nickel dermatitis after the initiation of disulfiram treatment of alcoholism in patients sensitive to nickel.[85] Such flare-ups have included vesicular hand dermatitis.[22]

The fact that disulfiram chelates nickel has been used therapeutically. Groups of patients sensitive to nickel with vesicular hand eczema have been treated with a daily dose from 50 mg to 300 mg of disulfiram. Most of the patients initially experienced flares of their dermatitis, but in several series of patients, the treatment proved effective.

Fowler found disulfiram to be effective in the treatment of 9 patients with hand eczema and nickel allergy in a double-blind, placebo-controlled, crossover study.[86] Kaaber and colleagues[87] found disulfiram to be marginally more effective than placebo in a placebo-controlled trial of 24 patients with nickel allergy and vesicular hand eczema.

Sharma treated 11 patients sensitive to nickel with vesicular hand eczema for 4 weeks with disulfiram as well as a low-nickel diet.[88] The hand eczema of 10 of the 11 patients cleared completely compared with 1 of 10 patients who received a placebo tablet and no dietary instructions.

Hepatic side effects have limited the use of disulfiram as a routine treatment. In a retrospective study, Kaaber and colleagues[89] studied 61 patients sensitive to nickel with hand eczema who had been treated in 63 treatment series with 50 mg to 400 mg disulfiram for 4 to 56 weeks. Eleven patients developed biochemical evidence of hepatotoxicity. Five had clinical evidence of hepatitis. For 4 of the patients this was verified by liver biopsy. In 29 treatment series, the dermatitis cleared, in 19 series it improved, and in 15 series no change was seen.

Pigatto[90] found that 1500 mg to 2000 mg of disodium cromoglycate given 3 times a day reduced vesicular palmar dermatitis in patients sensitive to nickel. He suggested that these patients be treated with a combination of diet treatment and disodium cromoglycate.

Nickel is one of the most common metals in the earth's crust, and it is present to a varying degree in foodstuffs derived from plants and also as a contaminant from the processing of some foods. In a modified meta-analysis of the data on experimental oral exposure to nickel in patients sensitive to nickel, Jensen[73] reviewed 17 studies of oral challenge with nickel in such patients. Nine of the studies were included in a dose-response model. Patients sensitive to nickel reacted to oral nickel in a dose-dependent manner, and a minority of these patients reacted to the amounts of nickel realistically present in food and in drinking water.

Nielsen and colleagues[74] asked 14 patients sensitive to nickel with vesicular hand eczema to ingest foods rich in nickel. Eleven of them experienced flares of their vesicular hand eczema. The patients were asked to follow a very special diet and consume large amounts of foods that would not normally be eaten, and the study showed the principle that it is possible for these patients to ingest sufficient amounts of nickel to reproduce their vesicular hand eczema.

It would, therefore, be tempting to try to reduce the nickel intake of such patients, in particular, those whose dermatitis does not clear when external contact with nickel is avoided and whose clinical picture is not easily explained by external contact with nickel.

The first of such diet trials was performed in the 1970s when limited knowledge of the nickel content in food was available. Of 28 patients with vesicular hand eczema and nickel allergy, 17 experienced flares of hand eczema after a single-blind, oral challenge with nickel.[91] Aggravation was determined clinically and by blinded evaluation of close-up photographs taken before and after the challenge. The dermatitis of 9 of the 17 patients improved after 6 weeks on a low-nickel diet. For 11 of the 14 patients for whom information on the level of nickel in urine was available after the 6 week period, urine excretion was reduced.

The diet phase of this study was open. It is extremely difficult to carry out long-term diet trials in a well controlled fashion. The determination of the urinary excretion of nickel compensates to some extent for the lack of controls.

A subsequent study by Veien and colleagues[92] included 216 patients sensitive to nickel whose dermatitis was suspected to be of endogenous origin. The patients were selected over a 5-year period from among 770 consecutive patients sensitive to nickel diagnosed after patch testing in a private practice of dermatology. The 216 patients were challenged orally with 2.5 mg of nickel given as nickel sulfate in a placebo-controlled, double-blind design. Of the 96 patients who reacted to nickel but not to the placebo, 90 agreed to follow a low-nickel diet for 1 to 2 months. After that period, the patients were seen again. Seventy-three of the 90 patients had obvious or some benefit from the diet. They were asked to continue the diet in a moderate form, to make it more socially acceptable and in order to avoid some of the less healthy effects of the diet.

A questionnaire was mailed to the patients 1 to 2 years after initiation of the diet to enquire about long-term results. Fifty-five of the 64 questionnaires returned could be evaluated. Forty of the 55 patients stated that they had long-term benefit of the diet. Thirty-one of the 55 patients had recurrent vesicular hand eczema. Twenty-one of the 31 had long-term benefit of the diet.

CHROMATE

In relation to hand eczema, chromate has attracted much less attention than nickel. Of 50 patients with pompholyx, Jain and colleagues[51] found that 8% had positive patch tests to potassium dichromate. Yokozeki[77] found that 25% of 25 patients with pompholyx had positive patch tests to chromate, 16% reacted to cobalt, and 28% to nickel. Oral challenge with 2.5 mg nickel, 1 mg cobalt, or 2.5 mg chromium resulted in flares of hand dermatitis in 4 of 6 patients.

Kaaber and Veien[93] challenged 31 patients who had positive patch tests to potassium dichromate with an oral dose of 2.5 mg chromium given as potassium dichromate in a double-blind, placebo-controlled trial. Close-up photographs taken before and 2 days after the challenge were evaluated blindly. Eleven of the 31 patients reacted to dichromate but not to the placebo. Nine of 14 of the patients who had vesicular hand dermatitis reacted to chromate, compared with 2 of 11 who did not have vesicular hand eczema.

A man and a woman challenged with 2.5 mg of chromium in a placebo-controlled study reacted to the challenge with flares of vesicular hand eczema as well as flares of scaly, keratotic eruptions on the elbows.[94]

After oral challenge with 2.5 mg of chromium, a man with vesicular hand eczema developed pruritus on the hands.[95] When 5 mg of chromium was given, a vesicular eruption was seen after 12 hours.

Thirty patients with positive patch tests to potassium dichromate were challenged orally with 2.5 mg of chromium in a double-blind, placebo-controlled study. Eight of 12 of the patients in the study who had vesicular hand eczema reacted to the oral challenge with chromate but not to the placebo.[96]

RECURRENT VESICULAR HAND ECZEMA AND FOOD INTAKE

Flood and Perry[97] found that the eczema of 30 patients with recurrent vesicular hand eczema improved after they had followed a strict diet, avoiding foods that were suspected of causing the eczema. The foods they avoided were tuna, tomato, pineapple, American cheese, milk, egg, wheat, lamb, chocolate, and chicken. The results of a trial with another 13 patients with eczematoid dermatitis were published in which they concluded that cutaneous testing was not dependable, and that the only reliable diagnostic test was to watch the reaction after the patients ingest the suspected food.[98]

Rowe[99] found that food played a role in the dermatitis of 82 of 182 patients with hand dermatitis. Recurrent, vesicular dermatitis in some of the patients was described, but exact number was not given. The dermatitis was referred to as atopic food allergy and cases caused by pollen were also seen.

Livingood and Pillsbury[100] described 26 patients in whom they were convinced food items played an important role in the eczema. Most of the patients had hand eczema, and judging from some of the illustrations accompanying the paper, some patients obviously had recurrent vesicular hand dermatitis.

The eczema of 21 coffee drinkers (>10 cups a day), 9 of whom had recurrent vesicular hand eczema, improved after coffee consumption was reduced. Five of the patients were challenged orally with caffeine without reaction.[101]

A man who had a positive patch test to garlic experienced vesicular hand eczema after the ingestion of garlic tablets. He also reacted with a flare of the eczema after placebo-controlled oral challenge with garlic.[102]

One of 4 patients with contact allergy to lettuce had a flare of vesicular hand eczema after oral challenge with lettuce.[103] Paulsen[104] described a similar situation in her thesis. One of 4 patients with contact allergy to lettuce developed vesicular hand eczema within 12 hours of oral challenge with lettuce. An oral challenge was performed with feverfew among 10 patients with contact allergy to feverfew. One of 7 with hand eczema had a positive reaction. No details were given of the type of hand eczema seen.

Dooms-Goossens and colleagues[105] described 3 patients with contact allergy to spices whose vesicular hand eczema flared after ingestion of various spices.

Hjorth[106] described a male physician whose vesicular hand eczema flared after ingestion of a large amount of orange marmalade. The patient had wanted to test the Hjorth's advice to avoid foods that might contain balsams after patch testing had resulted in a positive reaction to balsam of Peru.

In a placebo-controlled, double-blind study, 17 patients were challenged orally with balsam of Peru. Four of 4 patients who had recurrent vesicular hand eczema experienced flares of their hand eczema after challenge with balsam of Peru but not after the placebo.[107]

Niinimäki saw a reaction after oral challenge with 1 g balsam of Peru in 8 of 22 patients. A reaction was defined as an increase in the number of vesicles in the palms 1 day after the challenge. All the patients had positive patch tests to balsam of Peru.[108] In another study, pompholyx reaction was seen in 3 of 7 patients with hand eczema after 71 patients with positive patch tests to balsam of Peru participated in an oral challenge with spices.[109]

Pfützner and colleagues[110] described 3 patients with systemic contact dermatitis to balsam of Peru. One had dyshidrotic dermatitis on her hands as well as eczema in the armpits and groin.

Twenty-eight of 46 patients treated with long-term dietary restriction of balsams in food, selected from among 834 patients with positive patch tests to balsam of Peru, indicated in a questionnaire that diet treatment was helpful in the long-term control of their dermatitis. Diet treatment was effective for 10 of 16 with vesicular hand eczema.[111]

OTHER CAUSES OF VESICULAR HAND ECZEMA

Hansen and colleagues[112] considered the psychosomatic aspects of pompholyx in a study of 20 patients—most of who were women—and concluded that the pathogenesis might be a complication of (pregenital) conversion, with the hands as the affected body part. Ten of the 20 patients had positive patch tests, 6 of them to nickel.

In a speculative paper, Kellum[113] describes the "dyshidrotic personality" as serious-minded, conscientious, dependable, and with an almost compulsive approach to life. Means with which to handle daily tension are suggested.

Biofeedback training was successfully used in treating 5 patients with pompholyx. Three of the patients experienced flares of their dermatitis as a result of stress.[114]

Skin conductance conditioning by means of biofeedback was used in treating 33 patients with dyshidrotic eczema. Twenty-two of the patients were trained to decrease skin conductance and 11 to increase it. It appeared that training to decrease skin conductance improved the dermatitis.[115]

A patient with hyperhidrosis and long-standing palmar eczema who was treated with unilateral cervical sympathectomy experienced clearing of hyperhidrosis and eczema on the treated but not on the untreated side. No mention was made of whether the patient had vesicular eczema.[116]

In spite of the apparent success of biofeedback training, there is no recent literature dealing with the method in relation to patients with vesicular hand eczema.

Photo-induced pompholyx was seen in 5 patients after intense exposure to sunlight.[117] In 4 patients, all smokers, dyshidrotic eczema of the feet was followed by painful ulcerations at the sites of the eczema. Three of the patients also had dyshidrotic eczema on the hands.[118]

DERMATOPHYTID

A classical cause of vesicular hand eczema is a dermatophytid following tinea of the feet. There is a paucity of literature on this reaction.

Peck[119] described in great detail 23 cases of epidermophytid on the hands. Two types of id reactions were noticed; one that was indistinguishable from dyshidrosis or cheiropompholyx and a squamous form which appeared as dyshidrosis lamellosa sicca. The latter form was generally considered to be a sequela of the first.

Histologically, the 2 conditions were similar and had the appearance of dyshidrosis.

Kaaman and Tossander[120] described 9 patients with dermatophytid on the hands. Examination showed that 7 of the patients had vesicular hand dermatitis, and 2 had erythema and scaling.

Veien and colleagues[121] found 37 cases of dermatophytid. Twenty-seven of 78 patients (35%) with inflammatory Trichophyton (T.) mentagrophytes of the feet had a dermatophytid compared with 9 of 128 (7%) of those infected with T. rubrum.

A study of 398 individual twins who had fungal cultures made from material from the fourth interdigital space on the right foot showed that patients with tinea pedis had a statistically significant increased relative risk for vesicular hand eczema.[47]

TREATMENT

Current treatment options for dyshidrosis have been expertly reviewed by Lofgren and Warshaw[32] and details will, therefore, not be given here. The authors stress that pompholyx on the hands with explosive eruptions of large bullae is a different entity from dyshidrosis. The latter is described as a common eruption of symmetric vesicular eruptions on the palms, soles, and/or lateral aspects of the fingers with no eruptions elsewhere on the body. The vesicles are 1 mm to 2 mm in size and are deep-seated on a non-erythematous base.

One difficulty with this definition appears in the next sentence where it is stated that the course is frequently chronic. The author of the current review has seen these eruptions with no obvious inflammation and has seen them clear within a month. However, pompholyx, as it is defined by Lofgren and Warshaw, and the vesicular eruption for which they use the term dyshidrosis are not common conditions. The most common eruption is the repeated eruption at irregular intervals of vesicles that eventually causes inflammation and scaling.

Recurrent vesicular hand eczema is characterized by symmetric, very pruritic vesicular eruptions in the palms, on the palmar aspects and sides of the fingers, and occasionally on the plantar aspects of the feet.

Theoretically, a single, endogenous, vesicular eruption on the hands and fingers would clear spontaneously if the patients sat still and did not use their hands! In the real world, patients do use their hands, and contact with irritants or allergens will aggravate the dermatitis. Recurrent vesicular hand dermatitis is, therefore, most commonly an eczematous eruption and should be treated accordingly.

Topical steroids can suppress the symptoms of recurrent vesicular hand dermatitis and remain the cornerstone of the topical treatment of eczematous hand dermatoses.[122] There have been reports of the usefulness of calcineurin inhibitors, but their effect is generally limited.[123] A review by Wollina[124] identifies phototherapy as a cornerstone in the treatment of pompholyx.

Glucocorticoids can be a useful systemic treatment, but no studies of the treatment of vesicular hand dermatitis with glucocorticoids have been made. It has been suggested that patients with rare eruptions take 30 mg prednisolone daily for a few days and then stop treatment. This will frequently abort an eruption that it would otherwise take weeks to control with topical treatment.

In an open study of 5 patients with pompholyx, methotrexate was useful in doses from 12.5 mg to 20 mg per week.[125]

Azathioprine was found to be useful in doses from 50 mg to 150 mg per day in 6 patients with pompholyx.[126]

Alitretinoin is a new retinoid with anti-inflammatory properties. In a large controlled study of 1032 patients, it was shown to be effective in the treatment of chronic hand eczema. A group of the patients had pompholyx, and although the cure rate among these patients was not as high as for patients with keratotic hand eczema, the pompholyx of 37 of 111 patients cleared or had almost cleared after 12 weeks.[127]

Oral Psoralen Ultra-Violet A (PUVA) treatments have been shown to be effective in the treatment of vesicular hand dermatitis as have topical PUVA treatments.[128] Radiation therapy has been effective in small series of patients with vesicular hand eczema.[129]

Iontophoresis is an old treatment for hyperhidrosis. Although it has been shown that pompholyx is a vesicular dermatitis with no direct relationship to the sweat glands, patients with pompholyx often experience excessive sweating.[77] In a randomized, single-blind, right-left study, iontophoresis was shown to improve vesicular hand eczema.[130]

Botulinum toxin has been used successfully to treat palmar hyperhidrosis as shown in promising studies involving patients with dyshidrotic eczema.[131] Treatment of the palms is painful and requires a nerve block.

Other treatment modalities like biofeedback techniques, diet treatment, and hyposensitization are discussed throughout the issue. Details are presented in Lofgren and Warshaw's review.[32]

SUMMARY

It is difficult to extract meaningful conclusions about the incidence and prevalence of acute and recurrent hand eczema from the literature. This is largely because of the lack of a common definition.

Some authors use the terms *pompholyx* and *dyshidrosis* for the rare, explosive, vesicular, bullous eruptions and include only patients with this condition among those they consider to have vesicular hand dermatitis. Others include moderate types of eruptive vesicular hand dermatitis in their studies. This means that the latter have a much larger percentage of vesicular hand dermatitis in their cohorts of hand eczema patients than the former.

If the morphologic terms *vesicular* and/or *bullous* are used, and the dynamic term *eruptive* is added, it should be possible to define this intriguing eruptive condition on the palms and/or the sides of the fingers. There seems to be no reason to exclude patients who have dermatitis on parts of the body other than the palms and soles. Many of the patients included in the original description of dyshidrosis/cheiropompholyx had dermatitis at sites other than the palms and soles.

The author is of the opinion that the terms *dyshidrosis* and *dyshidrotic eczema* are best abandoned because all evidence points toward an eczematous reaction that is unrelated to the sweat ducts.

The term *pompholyx* has been used to describe the rare, severe, noninflamed, symmetric vesicular or bullous eruption on the palms and/or soles as well as other types of vesicular eczematous eruptions. *Pompholyx* is best used to describe only the rare, severe, eruptive variant of vesicular hand dermatitis.

Vesicular eczematous eruptions on the palms and sides of the fingers represent a spectrum ranging from

1. the rare, symmetric, acute, severely pruritic, and painful eruption of vesicles and bullae (see **Figs. 2** and **3**)

2. recurrent, usually symmetric eruptions of severely pruritic, non-inflamed vesicles seen on the palms with a distinct demarcation where palmar skin joins the skin of the forearm (see **Fig. 1**) and/or on the sides of 1 or several fingers of both hands (see **Fig. 4**) with recurrences so infrequent that the skin heals between attacks without the development of inflammation

3. an eczematous eruption similar to 2 but with recurrences so frequent that inflammation and scaling are seen. Unless studied through a magnifying glass, this eruption could easily appear to be chronic hand eczema (see **Figs. 6 and 7**). However, tiny clusters of vesicles may be seen, and the patient gives a history of bouts of severely pruritic vesicles. As a result of scratching, the vesicles on thin skin or the sides of the fingers are often broken and look like tiny erosions.

All 3 of the above entities can be described as acute and recurrent vesicular hand dermatitis. Since 1 is rare, the term *recurrent vesicular hand dermatitis* will encompass 2 and 3 and, thereby, most cases of this entity. Since there may be overlap between 2 and 3, there seems little reason to separate them. To make a diagnosis of acute and recurrent vesicular dermatitis, the dynamics in terms of an eruptive dermatosis should be added to the morphology.

Some patients, atopics for example, have dermatitis on parts of the body other than the palms, fingers and/or soles at the same time as recurrent, vesicular hand dermatitis. It seems unwarranted to exclude such patients from the workup used for patients with recurrent, vesicular hand dermatitis.

As Shelley has pointed out,[6] this morphology of hand dermatitis most likely represents a non-specific reaction pattern that may have many different causes. The background may be atopic dermatitis, a drug reaction, allergic contact dermatitis following external or internal challenge, protein contact dermatitis, a dermatophytid, a psychosomatic reaction, or may have some other as yet unknown source.

In the workup of the individual patient, it can be useful to keep in mind the experience gained in the numerous oral challenge experiments in patients with allergic contact dermatitis who have been challenged with the hapten to which they are allergic. These experiments have shown that vesicular eruptions on the hands develop approximately 24 hours after the challenge. Patients with vesicular eruptions should, therefore, be instructed to search for eliciting causes 1 to 2 days before the eruption of pruritic vesicles.

REFERENCES

1. Fox T. On dysidrosis. Am J Syphilol Dermatol 1873;1–7.
2. Fox T. Clinical lecture on dysidrosis (an undescribed eruption). BMJ 1873;365–6.
3. Hutchinson J. Cheiro-pompholyx. Notes of a clinical lecture on "a recurrent bullous eruption on the hands". Lancet 1876;1:630–1.
4. Kutzner H, Wurzel RM, Wolff HH. Are acrosyringia involved in the pathogenesis of "dyshidrosis"? Am J Dermatopathol 1986;8(2):109–16.
5. Simons RDGPh. Eczema of the hands. Investigations into dyshidrosiform eruptions. 2nd edition. Basel (Switzerland): S. Karger; 1966.
6. Shelley WB. Dysidrosis (pompholyx). Arch Dermatol Syph 1953;68:314–8.
7. Storrs FJ. Acute and recurrent vesicular hand dermatitis. Not pompholyx or dyshidrosis. Arch Dermatol 2007;143(12):1578–80.
8. Veien NK, Menné T. Acute and recurrent vesicular hand dermatitis (pompholyx). In: Menné T, Maibach HI, editors. Hand eczema. 2nd edition. Boca Raton (FL): CRC Press; 2000. p. 147–64.
9. Veien NK. Systemic contact dermatitis. In: Frosch PJ, Menné T, Lepoittevin J-P, editors. Contact dermatitis. 4th edition. Berlin: Springer; 2006. p. 295–307.
10. Uehara M. Pustulosis palmaris et plantaris: evolutionary sequence from vesicular to pustular lesions. Semin Dermatol 1983;2(1):51–6.
11. Vignon-Pennamen M-D, Wallach D. Infantile acropustulosis. A clinicopathologic study of six cases. Arch Dermatol 1986;122:1155–60.
12. Klein CE, Weber L, Kaufmann R. Infantile akropustulose. Hautarzt 1989;40:501–3.
13. Sugimura C, Katsuura J, Moriue T, et al. Dyshidrosiform pemphigoid: report of a case. J Dermatol 2003;30(7):525–9.
14. Patrizi A, Rizzoli L, Benassi L, et al. Another case of dyshidrosiform pemphigoid. J Eur Acad Dermatol Venereol 2003;17:370.
15. Barth JH, Rairris GM, Wojnarowska F, et al. Haemorrhagic pompholyx is a sign of bullous pemphigoid and an indication for low-dose prednisolone therapy. Clin Exp Dermatol 1986;11:409–12.
16. Duhra P, Ryatt KS. Haemorrhagic pompholyx in bullous pemphigoid. Clin Exp Dermatol 1988;13:342–3.
17. Duhra P, Charles-Holmes R. Linear IgA disease with haemorrhagic pompholyx and dapsone-induced neutropenia. Br J Dermatol 1991;125:172–4.
18. Barth JH, Venning VA, Wojnarowska F. Palmoplantar involvement in auto-immune blistering disorders – pemphigoid, linear IgA disease and herpes gestationis. Clin Exp Dermatol 1988;13:85–6.

19. Nielsen NJ, Menné T, Kristiansen J, et al. Effects of repeated skin exposure to low nickel concentrations: a model for allergic contact dermatitis on the hands. Br J Dermatol 1999;141:676–82.

20. Veien NK. Systemic contact dermatitis. In: Zhai H, Wilhelm K-P, Maibach HI, editors. Marzulli and Maibach's dermatotoxicology. 7th edition. Boca Raton (FL): CRC Press; 2008. p. 135–53.

21. Christensen OB, Lindström C, Löfberg H, et al. Micromorphology and specificity of orally induced flare-up reactions in nickel-sensitive patients. Acta Dermatovener (Stockholm) 1981;61:505–10.

22. Veien NK. Cutaneous side effects of antabuse® in nickel allergic patients treated for alcoholism. Boll Dermatol Allergol Prof 1987;2:139–44.

23. Christensen OB, Kristensen M. Treatment with disulfiram in chronic nickel hand dermatitis. Contact Dermatitis 1982;8:59–63.

24. Kaaber K, Menné T, Tjell JC, et al. Antabuse® treatment of nickel dermatitis: chelation – a new principle in the treatment of nickel dermatitis. Contact Dermatitis 1979;5:221–8.

25. Menné T, Weismann K. Hämatogenes Kontaktekzem nach oraler Gabe von neomyzin. Hautarzt 1984;35:319–20 [in German].

26. Coenraads PJ, Van Der Walle H, Thestrup-Pedersen K, et al. Construction and validation of a photographic guide for assessing severity of chronic hand dermatitis. Br J Dermatol 2005;152:296–301.

27. Hald M, Veien NK, Laurberg G, et al. Severity of hand eczema assessed by patients and dermatologists using a photograhic guide. Br J Dermatol 2007;156:77–80.

28. Held E, Skoet R, Johansen JD, et al. The hand eczema severity index (HECSI): a scoring system for clinical assessment of hand eczema. A study of inter- and intraobserver reliability. Br J Dermatol 2005;152:302–7.

29. Vocks E, Plötz SG, Ring J. The dyshidrotic eczema area and severity index – a score developed for the assessment of dyshidrotic eczema. Dermatology 1999;198:265–9.

30. Menné T, Hjorth N. Pompholyx – dyshidrotic eczema. Semin Dermatol 1983;2(1):75–80.

31. Lambert D. La dysidrose palmo-plantaire. [Palmoplantar dyshidrosis] [French]. Rev Pract 1984;34:2457–61.

32. Lofgren SM, Warshaw EM. Dyshidrosis: epidemiology, clinical characteristics, and therapy. Dermatitis 2006;17(4):165–81.

33. Thelin I, Agrup G. Pomphlyx – a one year series. Acta Derm Venereol (Stockh) 1985;65:214–7.

34. Agrup G. Hand eczema and other hand dermatoses in South Sweden [thesis]. Acta Derm Venereol 1969;49(Suppl 61):1–91.

35. Meding B. Epidemiology of hand eczema in an industrial city [thesis]. Acta Derm Venereol 1990;(Suppl 153):1–43.

36. Veien NK, Hattel T, Laurberg G. Hand eczema: causes, course, and prognosis I. Contact Dermtitis 2008;58:330–4.

37. Young E. Dysidrotic (endogen) eczema. Dermatologica 1964;129:306–10.

38. Schuppli R. Zur Ätiologie der Dysidrosis. [On the etiology of dyshidrosis] [German]. Dermatologica 1954;108:393–8.

39. Meneghini CL, Angelini G. Contact and microbial allergy in pompholyx. Contact Dermatitis 1979;5:46–50.

40. Lodi A, Betti R, Charelli G, et al. Epidemiological, clinical and allergological observations on pompholyx. Contact Dermatitis 1992;26:17–21.

41. Castelain P-Y. Les Dysidroses. Ann Dermatol Venereol 1987;114:579–85 [in French].

42. Guillet MH, Wierzbicka E, Guillet S, et al. A 3-year causative study of pompholyx in 120 patients. Arch Dermatol 2007;143(12):1504–8.

43. Pitché P, Boukari M, Tchangai-Walla K. Factors associated with palmoplantar or plantar pompholyx: a case-control study. Ann Dermatol Venereol 2006;133(2):139–43.

44. Chen JJ, Liang YH, Zhou FS, et al. The gene for a rare autosomal dominant form of pompholyx maps to chromosome 18q22.-18q22.3. J Invest Dermatol 2006;126(2):300–4.

45. Schwanitz HJ. Das atopische Palmoplantarekzem. Berlin: Springer-Verlag; 1986.

46. Norris PG, Levene GM. Pompholyx occurring during hospital admission for treatment of atopic dermatitis. Clin Exp Dermatol 1987;12:189–90.

47. Bryld LE, Agner T, Menné T. Relation between vesicular eruptions on the hands and tinea pedis, atopic dermatitis and nickel allergy. Acta Derm Venereol 2003;83(3):186–8.

48. Edman B. Palmar eczema: a pathogenetic role for acetylsalicylic acid, contraceptives and smoking? Acta Derm Venereol (Stockh) 1988;68:402–7.

49. De Boer EM, Bruynzeel DB, Van Ketel WG. Dyshidrotic eczema as an occupational dermatitis in metal workers. Contact Dermatitis 1988;19:184–8.

50. Corazza M, Romani I, Poli F, et al. Irritant contact dermatitis due to Dieffenbachia s.p.p. J Eur Acad Dermatol Venereol 1998;10:87–9.

51. Jain VK, Aggarwal K, Passi S. Role of contact allergens in pompholyx. J Dermatol 2004;31(3):188–93.

52. Ekelund A-G, Möller H. Oral provocation in eczematous contact allergy to neomycin and hydroxyquinolines. Acta Derm Venereol 1969;49:422–6.

53. Dorado Bris JM, Montanes M, Sols Candela M, et al. Contact sensitivity to pyrazinobutazone

(Carudol®) with positive oral provocation test. Contact Dermatitis 1992;26:355–6.

54. Piqué E, Pérez JA, Benjumeda A. Oral piroxicam-induced dyshidrosiform dermatitis. Contact Dermatitis 2004;50:382–3.

55. De Groot AC. Vesicular dermatitis of the hands secondary to perianal allergic contact dermatitis caused by preservatives in moistened toilet tissues. Contact Dermatitis 1997;36:173–4.

56. Crippa M, Misquith L, Lonati A, et al. Dyshidrotic eczema and sensitization to dithiocarbamates in a florist. Contact Dermatitis 1990;23:203–4.

57. Lundh K, Hindsén M, Gruvberger B, et al. Contact allergy to herbal teas derived from Asteraceae plants. Contact Dermatitis 2006;54:196–201.

58. Möller H, Spirén A, Svensson Å, et al. Contact allergy to the Asteraceae plant *Ambrosia artemisiifolia* L. (ragweed) in sesquiterpene lactone-sensitive patients in southern Sweden. Contact Dermatitis 2002;47:157–60.

59. Haapasaari K-M, Niinimäki A. Vesicular palmar eczema from theneoprene tongue of an ankle support. Contact Dermatitis 2000;42:248.

60. Thyssen JP, Maibach HI. Drug-elicited systemic allergic (contact) dermatitis—update and possible pathomechanisms. Contact Dermatitis 2008;59:195–202.

61. Hubler WR Jr, Hubler WR Sr. Dermatitis from a chromium dental place. Contact Dermatitis 1983;9:377–83.

62. Kerosuo H, Kanerva L. Systemic contact dermatitis caused by nickel in a stainless steel orthodontic appliance. Contact Dermatitis 1997;36(2):112–3.

63. Veien NI, Borchorst E, Hattel T, et al. Stomatitis or systemically-induced contact dermatitis from metal wire on orthodontic materials. Contact Dermatitis 1994;30:210–3.

64. Smeenk G, Teunissen PC. Allergische reacties op nikkel uit infusie-toedieningssystemen [in Dutch]. Ned Tijdscht Geneeskd 1977;121:4–9.

65. Oakley AMM, Ive FA, Carr MM. Skin clips are contraindicated when there is nickel allergy. J R Soc Med 1987;80:290–1.

66. Kanerva L, Förström L. Allergic nickel and chromate hand dermatitis induced by orthopaedic metal implant. Contact Dermatitis 2001;44:103–4.

67. Thomas P, Bandl W-D, Maier S, et al. Hypersensitivity to titanium osteosynthesis with impaired fracture healing, eczema, and T-cell hyperresponsiveness *in vitro*: case report and review of the literature. Contact Dermatitis 2006;55:199–202.

68. Christensen OB, Möller H. External and internal exposure to the antigen in the hand eczema of nickel allergy. Contact Dermatitis 1975;1:136–41.

69. Veien NK, Hattel T, Justesen O, et al. Oral challenge with metal salts. (I). Vesicular patch-test-negative hand eczema. Contact Dermatitis 1983;9:402–6.

70. Veien NK, Hattel T, Justesen O, et al. Oral challenge with metal salts (II). Various types of eczema. Contact Dermatitis 1983;9:407–10.

71. Webster JD, Parker TF, Alfrey AC, et al. Acute nickel intoxication by dialysis. Ann Intern Med 1980;92(5):631–3.

72. Sunderman FW Jr, Dingle B, Hopfer SM, et al. Acute nickel toxicity in electroplating workers who accidentally ingested a solution of nickel sulfate and nickel chloride. Am J Ind Med 1988;14(3):257–66.

73. Jensen CS, Menné T, Johansen JD. Systemic contact dermatitis after oral exposure to nickel: a review with a modified meta-analysis. Contact Dermatitis 2006;54:79–86.

74. Nielsen GD, Jepsen LV, Jørgensen PJ, et al. Nickel-sensitive patients with vesicular hand eczema: oral challenge wit a diet naturally high in nickel. Br J Dermatol 1990;122:299–308.

75. Templeton DM, Sunderman FW Jr, Herber RF. Tentative reference values for nickel concentrations in human serum, plasma, blood, and urine: evaluation according to the TRACY protocol. Sci Total Environ 1994;148(2–3):243–51.

76. Omokhodion FO, Howard JM. Trace elements in the sweat of acclimatized persons. Clin Chim Acta 1994;231(1):23–8.

77. Yokozeki H, Katayama I, Nishioka K, et al. The role of metal allergy and local hyperhidrosis in the pathogenesis of pompholyx. J Dermatol 1992;19(12):964–7.

78. Bedello PG, Goitre M, Cane D, et al. Nichel: aptene ubiquitario. [Nickel: a ubiquitous hapten] [Italian]. G Ital Dermatol Venereol 1985;120:293–6.

79. Hindsén M, Bruze M, Christensen OB. Flare-up reactions after oral challenge with nickel in relation to challenge dose and intensity and time of previous patch test reactions. J Am Acad Dermatol 2001;44:616–23.

80. Veien NK, Hattel T, Justesen O, et al. Oral challenge with nickel and cobalt in patients with positive patch tests to nickel and/or cobalt. Acta Derm Venereol (Stockh) 1987;67:321–5.

81. Lammintausta K, Pitkänen OP, Kalimo K, et al. Interrelationship of nickel and cobalt contact sensitization. Contact Dermatitis 1986;13(3):148–52.

82. Veien NK, Hattel T, Laurberg G. Placebo-controlled oral challenge with cobalt in patients with positive patch tests to cobalt. Contact Dermatitis 1995;33:54–5.

83. Stuckert J, Nedorost S. Low-cobalt diet for dyshidrotic eczema patients. Contact Dermatitis 2008;59:361–5.

84. Menné T. Flare-up of cobalt dermatitis from Antabuse® treatment. Contact Dermatitis 1985;12(1):53.

85. Lein LR, Fowler JF Jr. Nickel dermatitis recall during disulfiram therapy for alcohol abuse. J Am Acad Dermatol 1992;26(4):645–6.

86. Fowler JF Jr. Disulfiram is effective for nickel allergic hand eczema. Am J Contact Dermatitis 1992;3:175–8.

87. Kaaber K, Menné T, Veien N. Treatment of nickel dermatitis with Antabuse®; a double blind study. Contact Dermatitis 1983;9:297–9.

88. Sharma AD. Disulfiram and low nickel diet in the management of hand eczema: a clinical study. Indian J Dermatol Venereol Leprol 2006;72(2):113–8.

89. Kaaber K, Menné T, Veien NK, et al. Some adverse effects of disulfiram in the treatment of nickel-allergic patients. Derm Veruf Umwelt 1987;35(6):209–11.

90. Pigatto PD, Gibelli E, Fumagalli M, et al. Disodium cromoglycate versus diet in the treatment and prevention of nickel-positive pompholyx. Contact Dermatitis 1990;22:27–31.

91. Kaaber K, Veien NK, Tjell JC. Low nickel diet in the treatment of patients with chronic nickel dermatitis. Br J Dermatol 1978;98:197–201.

92. Veien NK, Hattel T, Laurberg G. Low nickel diet: an open, prospective trial. J Am Acad Dermatol 1993; 29:1002–7.

93. Kaaber K, Veien NK. The significance of chromate ingestion in patients allergic to chromate. Acta Dermatovener (Stockh) 1977;57:321–3.

94. Kaaber K, Sjølin KE, Menné T. Elbow eruptions in nickel and chromate dermatitis. Contact Dermatitis 1983;9:213–6.

95. Goitre M, Bedello PG, Cane D. Chromium dermatitis and oral administration of the metal. Contact Dermatitis 1982;8:208–9.

96. Veien NK, Hattel T, Laurberg G. Chromate-allergic patients challenged orally with potassium dichromate. Contact Dermatitis 1994;31(3):137–9.

97. Flood JM, Perry DJ. Recurrent vesicular eruption of the hands due to food allergy. J Invest Dermatol 1946;7:309–27.

98. Flood JM, Perry DJ. Role of food allergy in eczematoid dermatitis. Arch Derm 1947;55:493–506.

99. Rowe AH. Atopic dermatitis of the hands due to food allergy. Arch Derm 1946;54:683–703.

100. Livingood CS, Pillsbury DM. Specific sensitivity to foods as a factor in various types of eczematous dermatitis. Arch Derm 1949;60:1090–115.

101. Veien NK, Hattel T, Justesen O. Dermatoses in coffee drinkers. Cutis 1987;40:421–2.

102. Burden AD, Wilkinson SM, Beck MH, et al. Garlic induced systemic contact dermatitis. Contact Dermatitis 1994;30:299–300.

103. Oliwiecki S, Beck MH, Hausen BM. Compositae dermatitis aggravated by eating lettuce. Contact Dermatitis 1991;24(4):318–9.

104. Paulsen E. Compositae-dermatitis på Fyn. Ph.D thesis. Odense, Denmark: University of Southern Denmark; 1996. p. 139.

105. Dooms-Goossens A, Fubelloy R, Degreef H. Contact and systemic contact-type dermatitis to spices. Dermatol Clin 1990;8(1):89–93.

106. Hjorth N. Eczematous allergy to balsams allied perfumes and flavouring agents. Copenhagen: Munksgaard; 1961.

107. Veien NK, Hattel T, Justesen O, et al. Oral challenge with balsam of Peru. Contact Dermatitis 1985;12:104–7.

108. Niinimäki A. Delayed-type allergy to spices. Contact Dermatitis 1984;11:34–40.

109. Niinimäki A. Double-blind placebo-controlled peroral challenges in patients with delayed-type allergy to balsam of Peru. Contact Dermatitis 1995;33:78–83.

110. Pfützner W, Thomas P, Niedermeier A, et al. Systemic contact dermatitis elicited by oral intake of balsam of Peru. Acta Derm Venereol 2003;83: 294–5.

111. Veien NK, Hattel T, Laurberg G. Can oral challenge with balsam of Peru predict possible benefit from a low-balsam diet? Am J Contact Dermatitis 1996; 7(2):84–7.

112. Hansen O, Küchler T, Lotz G-R, et al. Es juckt mich in den Fingern, aber mir sind die Hände gebunden. [My fingers itch, but my hands are bound. An exploratory psychosomatic study of patients with dyshidrosis of the hands (cheiropompholyx)] [German]. Z Psychosom Med Psychoanal 1981;27:275–90.

113. Kellum RE. Dyshidrotic hand eczema: a psychotherapeutic approach. Cutis 1973;16:875–8.

114. Kodlys KW, Meyer RP. Biofeedback training in the therapy of dyshidrosis. Cutis 1979;24:219–21.

115. Miller RM, Coger RW. Skin conductance conditioning with dyshidrotic eczema patients. Br J Dermatol 1979;101:435–40.

116. Chowdhury MM, Hedges R, Lanigan SW. Unilateral resolution of palmar eczema and hyperhidrosis complicated by Horner's syndrome following ipsilateral endoscopic cervical sympathectomy. Br J Dermatol 2000;143:645–90.

117. Man I, Ibbotson SH, Ferguson J. Photoinduced pompholyx: a report of 5 cases. J Am Acad Dermatol 2004;50:55–60.

118. van der Vleuten C, van der Valk P. Dyshidrotic eczema giving rise to painful lower leg ulceration as a result of smoking? Acta Derm Venereol 2002;82:76–8.

119. Peck SM. Epidermophytosis of the feet and epidermophytids of the hands. Arch Derm Syphilol 1930; 22:40–76.

120. Kaaman T, Torssander J. Dermatophytid—a misdiagnosed entity? Acta Derm Venereol (Stockh) 1983;63:404–8.

121. Veien NK, Hattel T, Laurberg G. Plantar *Trichophyton rubrum* infections may cause dermatophytids on the hands. Acta Derm Venereol (Stockh) 1994; 74:403–4.

122. Veien NK, Olholm Larsen P, Thestrup-Pedersen K, et al. Long-term, intermittent treatment of chronic hand eczema with mometasone furoate. Br J Dermatol 1999;140(5):882–6.

123. Belsito DV, Fowler JF Jr, Marks JG Jr, et al. Pimecrolimus cream 1%: a potential new treatment for chronic hand dermatitis. Cutis 2004;73(1):31–8.

124. Wollina U. Pompholyx: what's new? Expert Opin Investig Drugs 2008;17(6):897–904.

125. Egan CA, Rallis TM, Meadows KP. Low-dose oral methotrexate treatment for recalcitrant palmoplantar pompholyx. Am Acad Dermatol 1999;40: 612–4.

126. Scerri L. Azathioprine in dermatological practice. An overview with special emphasis on its use in non-bullous inflammatory dermatoses. Adv Exp Med Biol 1999;455:343–8.

127. Ruzicka T, Lynde CW, Jemec GBE, et al. Efficacy and safety of oral alitretinoin (9- *cis* retinoic acid) in patients with severe chronic hand eczema refractory to topical corticosteroids: results of a randomized, double-blind, placebo-controlled, multicentre trial. Br J Dermatol 2008;158:808–17.

128. Grattan CEH, Carmichael AJ, Shuttleworth GJ, et al. Comparison of topical PUVA with UVA for chronic vesicular hand eczema. Acta Derm Venereol (Stockh) 1991;71:118–22.

129. Duff M, Cruchfield CE III, Moore J, et al. Radiation therapy for chronic vesicular hand dermatitis. Dermatitis 2006;17(3):128–32.

130. Odia S, Vocks E, Rakoski J, et al. Successful treatment of dyshidrotic hand eczema using tap water iontophoresis with pulsed direct current. Acta Derm Venereol 1996;76(6):472–4.

131. Wollina U, Karamfilow T. Adjuvant botulinum toxin A in dyshidrotic hand eczema: a controlled prospective pilot study with left-right comparison. J Eur Acad Dermatol Venereol 2002;16:40–2.

Systemic Contact Dermatitis

Rajiv I. Nijhawan, MD[a], Matthew Molenda, MD[b],
Matthew J. Zirwas, MD[b], Sharon E. Jacob, MD[c],*

KEYWORDS

- Systemic contact dermatitis (SCD)
- Allergic contact dermatitis (ACD) • Allergen
- Nickel • Balsam of Peru • Metals • Patch testing

Systemic contact dermatitis (SCD) describes a cutaneous eruption in response to the systemic exposure of allergens.[1] It was first described in the literature by Jadassohn in 1895,[2] but has been referred to by many different names, such as systemic eczematous "contact-type" dermatitis medicamentosa,[3] mercury exanthema,[4] baboon syndrome,[5] and hematogenous contact eczema.[6] A recommendation has been made to use the phrase "systemic allergic dermatitis" because skin contact is not a requirement for the elicitation of a cutaneous response from a hapten; it can also occur hematogenously.[7] Regardless of name, sensitization to an allergen usually occurs first, as is seen in allergic contact dermatitis (ACD), which is a type of T-cell– mediated, delayed-type (type IV) hypersensitivity reaction.[8,9] Thereafter, varying degrees of exposure can elicit a broad spectrum of systemic symptoms. This review of SCD provides an overview of the disease with descriptions of common allergens and some insight into the possible mechanism of action seen in SCD.

WHEN TO SUSPECT SCD

There are multiple routes of exposure for the elicitation of SCD, such as transepidermal, subcutaneous, intravenous, intramuscular, inhalation, and oral ingestion.[10] Thus, SCD should be included in the differential of most eczematous eruptions. The most important factor to consider is the time course of exposure to possible allergens and development of symptoms, because SCD can have a latency period of a few hours to a few days from the systemic exposure.[7]

Clinically, SCD has a wide spectrum of presentation, from disseminated erythematous papules to deep-seated vesicles to erythema localized to the palms and fingers.[11] Additionally, SCD can present as dermatitis localized to the flexural aspects of the extremities[12] or diffuse erythema of the anogenital region, which is commonly referred to as baboon syndrome because of its distribution.[5] Erythematous axillae may also accompany the latter presentation,[5] and it has been referred to as SDRIFE or symmetric drug-related intertriginous and flexural exanthema.[13]

Often times, exposure to the allergen can cause a flare of the dermatitis in the same area where the initial episode of elicitation occurred. Memory T cells may remain at the same locations of the previous allergen contact, which likely explains the observation of re-test reactions and flares of previously exposed skin.[14] The reasons and mechanisms explaining T-cell retention have not been elucidated.

In cases of SCD, the reaction does not necessarily occur at sites of previous exposure and can occur anywhere, including a previous patch test site. Other individuals present with exfoliative erythroderma, and some patients may even experience systemic symptoms such as nausea, vomiting, diarrhea, fever, malaise, headaches, and arthralgia.[7,15]

PATHOGENESIS

ACD is commonly defined by 2 phases: a sensitization phase (also known as the afferent phase), in which the patient remains asymptomatic, and an elicitation phase, in which cutaneous inflammation

[a] 5 Darcy Drive, Branchburg, NJ 08876, USA
[b] Ohio State University, Columbus, Ohio, USA
[c] Rady Children's Hospital, 8010 Frost Street, Suite 602, San Diego, CA 92124, USA
* Corresponding author.
E-mail address: sjacob@contactderm.net (S.E. Jacob).

Dermatol Clin 27 (2009) 355–364
doi:10.1016/j.det.2009.05.005

occurs mediated by the immune system.[16] In the sensitization phase, which lasts 10 to 15 days, a hapten penetrates the lipophilic stratum corneum and binds to 1 of a wide array of extracellular and cell membrane–associated proteins, but it does not have dedicated cellular receptors.[17,18] These haptens have antigenic properties and are taken up by the skin dendritic cells, mainly Langerhans cells (LHCs), which are the major antigen presenting cells (APCs) of the skin. After taking up and processing the antigen, LHCs present it in association with a major histocompatibility complex type II (MHCII) on the cell surface. These APCs then migrate through the lymphatic system to the paracortical areas of regional lymph nodes where the antigen/MHC molecule complexes are presented to naïve T cells. When a naïve CD4+ T cell that has a complementary T-cell receptor encounters the MHC/antigen complex and has appropriate costimulatory signals, it undergoes clonal expansion, and these clones enter the systemic circulation as memory T cells. Additionally, this immune system priming and amplification requires the role of resident cells, such as keratinocytes, mast cells, endothelial cells, and natural killer cells.[19–21] The thresholds for sensitization vary among all individuals, and susceptibility factors play a role in the development of ACD, such as age, T-cell repertoire, and type and duration of allergen exposure.[22]

The elicitation phase (also known as the efferent phase) defines the second part of ACD, which occurs after reexposure to the antigen, taking approximately 24 to 72 hours to clinically manifest after exposure. In elicitation, the skin is exposed to an antigen to which sensitization has already occurred; the antigen is once again taken up by APCs and presented to the antigen-specific memory-effector T cells, which become activated. These activated T cells produce type 1 cytokines (interferon-γ), and the other cells in the skin react by releasing other cytokines and chemokines.[16] The inflammatory reaction resulting from this release resolves in a course of several days to a few weeks, likely secondary to down-regulatory mechanisms. It has also been suggested that a type III response is involved in SCD, with the deposition of antigen-antibody complexes in the skin that leads to inflammation clinically seen.[23] Hapten-antibody complexes have been identified in serum of patients with cutaneous symptoms.[24] Resolution and prevention of the ACD occur with sustained allergen avoidance.

PROTEIN CONTACT DERMATITIS

Hjorth and Roed-Petersen first described "protein contact dermatitis" in 1976 and postulated that type I (immediate IgE-mediated) and type IV (delayed-type hypersensitivity) reactions were involved in the pathogenesis.[25] The proteins involved in this subset of dermatitis are grouped into 4 subsets: (1) fruits, vegetables, spices, and plants; (2) animal proteins; (3) grains; and (4) enzymes.[26] Clinically, patients with protein contact dermatitis present similarly to ACD; however, they have negative patch test reactions but positive skin-prick and scratch test reactions and often also have positive atopy patch tests.[27] Although the pathogenesis is not completely understood, there is some thought that it may be caused by IgE-bearing LHCs similar to atopic dermatitis.[27]

THE ALLERGENS AND MANAGEMENT OF SCD

Various metals, medicaments, foods, botanicals, and chemicals have been implicated as the causative agents of SCD. Metals that are electrophilic have the ability to ionize and react with proteins, and these complexes can be recognized by dendritic cells that allow for sensitization to occur.[28] In general, the allergen type, duration, environment, and patient susceptibility are all factors in the development of SCD. The authors focus on 2 of the most common allergens that elicit SCD, nickel and balsam of Peru (BOP), while also briefly touching on some other causative agents.

Nickel

Nickel allergy is 1 of the most common causes of ACD, and its incidence is thought to be increasing. Sensitized individuals who are exposed to nickel on their skin or mucosal surfaces generally have a predictable localized response, including erythema, vesicles, scaling, and pruritus. However, systemic reactions such as flare-ups of a previous patch test site/contact dermatitis site, flare-ups of hand dermatitis, or generalized dermatitis can also occur with exposure to the nickel antigen.[29] Still, whether dietary nickel can induce localized or generalized eruptions continues to be a matter of debate. A review of the literature suggests that dietary nickel can cause cutaneous eruptions consistent with ACD.

Dietary nickel causes dermatitis

ACD flares caused by dietary nickel have been demonstrated. Jensen and colleagues[30] showed a dose-dependent relationship between ingestion and flare-up. Their study determined that 0.3, 1, and 4 mg of nickel sulfate hexahydrate produced cutaneous reactions in 40%, 40%, and 70% of nickel-sensitive participants, respectively. 10% of the placebo group had cutaneous reactions in sites of previous dermatitis. Of note, 60% of the participants receiving 4 mg of nickel sulfate hexa-hydrate had widespread cutaneous reactions, whereas the rate in the placebo group was 0%. Although the study only had 10 patients in each dosage group, these data show that ingesting a single dose of 4 mg or more of nickel sulfate hexahydrate causes a cutaneous reaction in most nickel allergic patients.[30]

Although a study by Santucci and colleagues[31] provides additional evidence that sudden large doses of dietary nickel can elicit cutaneous flare-ups, it also asserts that nickel-allergic patients can adapt to gradual increases in dietary nickel. Out of 25 nickel-allergic patients, 22 had cuta-neous reactions to a $NiSO_4$ 10 mg oral challenge at the beginning of the study. However, upon gradual increase in oral dose of $NiSO_4$ (3 mg for 1 month, 6 mg for 1 month, and 10 mg for 1 month), only 3 out of 25 patients had to withdraw from the study because of intense worsening of cutaneous symptoms. Out of the 25 patients, 14 had no associated flare-up at all with the gradually increasing doses.[31] This study suggests that a tolerance to increasing nickel in the diet may be achieved if exposure is gradually and consis-tently increased. However, because individuals often have varied diets, and it would be difficult to justify supplementing nickel in a long-term diet plan without additional studies, the initial challenge is the most important part of this study in the opinion of the investigators.

Specific studies on hand dermatitis in relation to ingested nickel have also been done. Menné and Thorboe[32] correlated flare-ups in dishydrotic eczema with increased levels of nickel in the urine. They postulated that increased urine levels were a result of dietary bursts of high nickel content. However, it should be noted that most dietary nickel is eliminated in the feces, and a measurable amount is also excreted in sweat. Renal, cardiac, and hepatic diseases have also been shown to increase urinary nickel.[33] Nielsen and colleagues[34] also demonstrated flares of hand eczema with high nickel intake in 10 out of 12 patients. In a compli-mentary study, Sharma used a nickel chelator (di-sulfuram) and a low-nickel diet that demonstrated complete healing of hand eczema in 10 out of 11 patients in the treatment group.[35]

Avoidance of dietary nickel has also been shown to improve SCD, which gives further support that nickel ingestion plays a role in its pathogenesis. That is, a low-nickel diet and nickel chelators have been shown to improve recalcitrant dermatitis (hand or otherwise) in nickel-sensitized individuals. Scattered case reports and studies have linked clinical improvement of eczema in nickel-sensi-tized individuals who adhere to a low-nickel diet.[36–38] Veien and colleagues[37] showed clinical improvement of dermatitis in 58 out of 90 nickel-sensitive patients in the short term (4 weeks) with a low-nickel diet. Follow-up questionnaires sent to the improved patients 1 to 2 years later demon-strated that 40 out of 55 respondents reported long-term improvement from the low-nickel diet. Disulfuram, a nickel chelator, has also been shown to be an effective initial adjunct to clearing persis-tent dermatitis and an effective monotherapy in placebo controlled trials.[35,39] In the monotherapy trial, it should be noted that 3 out of 11 patients who received disulfuram at gradually increasing doses from 50 to 200 mg showed signs of hepatic toxicity over the 6-week treatment period.[39] In the opinion of the investigators, this adverse potential drug effect is not acceptable because dietary modification can be considered as an alternative benign treatment.

Nickel ingestion has also been shown to cause detectable changes in the immune system. For example, individuals whose dermatitis flared after in-gesting nickel were shown to have a decrease in CD8+ CD45RO+ CLA+ blood lymphocytes. This decrease correlates with migration of CD8+ memory T cells into tissues, which is consistent with contact dermatitis.Ingestion of nickel by nickel-sensitive patients has also been shown to increase serum levels of interleukin (IL)-5. Although contact derma-titis is classically thought of as a type IV hypersensi-tivity reaction with cytotoxic T cells (Th1 response), IL-5 is a Th2 cytokine. IL-5 enhances proliferation of eosinophils and may explain why eosinophils can be seen on biopsy of ACD.[40]

The elicitation studies, avoidance studies, and immunologic assays, above all, provide evidence to support the hypothesis that dietary nickel can induce SCD. Because dietary nickel avoidance in nickel-sensitized individuals has demonstrated improvement in patients with recalcitrant derma-titis, and because proper dietary modification should do no harm to patients, the investigators assert that counseling on ways to minimize nickel exposure should be given to patients with confirmed nickel sensitivity. Sources of dietary nickel and treatments are further discussed in the next section.

Dietary nickel

The normal daily intake of nickel has been esti-mated to be between 0.3 and 0.6 mg.[33] Although the normal dietary amount of nickel is lower than the ingested amounts producing the most convincing results in the studiesdiscussed earlier, individual diets may vary. For example, an individual might consume the following on 1 day: Breakfast, a bowl of oatmeal (0.22 mg), 1 banana (0.02 mg), 1 apple (0.005 mg); lunch, 2 slices of whole wheat bread (0.01 mg) with 2 slices of bacon (0.01 mg), a piece of lettuce (0.001 mg), a tomato slice (0.002 mg), and a chocolate (Hershey) bar (0.015 mg); dinner, a serving of broccoli (0.023 mg), a baked potato (0.015 mg), and a pork-chop (0.005 mg); snack, a half cup of peanuts (0.218 mg); drinks, 2 cups of coffee (0.003 mg).[41] Total nickel intake for the day would be 0.547 mg, which is well within the range of doses shown to cause flares. Additionally, one cannot assume that dietary nickel is insignificant at amounts as low as 0.3 mg because this dose was still shown to cause reactions in 40% of patients in an elicitation study.[40] Furthermore, the observation that chronic hand dermatitis responded to reduction of nickel intake and/or nickel chelators provides reasonable evidence that oral nickel may play a role in its pathogenesis. For these reasons, when a nickel-sensitized individual has chronic or frequently relapsing dermatitis that cannot be explained by contact exposure, the authors suggest counseling on how to minimize oral nickel intake.

Nickel can naturally occur in food or can be inadvertently added by processing, cooking, or storage. Foods that consistently contain relatively high amounts of nickel per serving include seafood (especially shellfish), chocolate, legumes, grains, and nuts.[33] There are technical difficulties in labeling other foods as "high-nickel." For example, plant foods may contain trace nickel or high nickel depending on the soil/region they are grown in. Another example is that processing foods with metal equipment (ie, flour mills) may emit nickel into the food.[41] Yet another example is nickel in tap water, especially hot water, which can leach nickel into the stagnant water within the plumbing pipes or faucet fixtures.[42] One additional source that can introduce nickel into the diet is stainless steel cookware or utensils, especially with high cooking temperatures and acidic foods.[43] The release of significant amounts of nickel from stainless steel cookware was refuted by a French study that cooked foods typical in a French diet.[44] However, the foods they tested with their cookware were admittedly nonacidic. These examples illustrate the complex sources that make it difficult to avoid ingested nickel. However, some practical recommendations in achieving a low-nickel diet can be made from the information available.

Treatment of SCD caused by nickel
Because the goal for physicians is first to do no harm, the authors feel that recommending a low-nickel diet and external nickel avoidance is the most appropriate first step in treating recalcitrant dermatitis in nickel-sensitive patients. This treatment has been shown to be effective, and there is no evidence of adverse effects occurring from these recommendations. Although supplementing nickel in gradually increased dosages may produce tolerance, long-term supplementation has not been studied and is therefore not advised.[31] Because of the potential for hepatotoxicity in patients taking disulfuram for its nickel chelating properties, this medication should be used cautiously, if at all. An alternative way to decrease dietary nickel absorption (and promote fecal excretion) is to recommend addition of iron-rich foods to the diet in clinically appropriate scenarios. Iron and nickel are absorbed by way of the same gastrointestinal transport system, but iron is the preferred cation. Less nickel is absorbed when competing with iron-rich foods.[41]

From a practical perspective, the low-nickel diet must be explained in a simple achievable way to maximize patient compliance. The low-nickel diet requires slightly more patient education than simply recommending avoidance of seafood (especially shellfish), chocolate, legumes, grains, and nuts. Although nickel content varies in foods and water due to the numerous reasons listed earlier, a nickel-sensitive patient may find improvement in their dermatitis if some basic principles are followed.

In 2007, Sharma[45] proposed 9 points important in achieving a low-nickel diet. Using Sharma's points and the available literature as a guide, the authors of this review agree with the following simplified recommendations:[41] (1) avoid or moderate high-nickel foods (listed earlier), canned foods, leafy green vegetables, vitamin supplements/drinks with nickel, and margarine; (2) eat animal meats (other than shellfish), eggs, dairy, polished rice/refined wheat/corn cereal, nongreen vegetables, citrus fruits, high vitamin C- and high iron-containing foods; (3) run tap water for a few seconds before washing, drinking, or cooking to flush out nickel that may have leaked from pipes or fixtures; (4) avoid stainless steel cookware and utensils, especially with acidic foods. Glass or ceramic cookware are good alternatives.

Motivated patients may request additional information on a nickel diet and a more comprehensive list of nickel content in foods.[46] *Managing Food Allergy & Intolerance: A Practical Guide* has a list of nickel levels in common foods.[41] Before directing a patient to additional resources, however, it is important to emphasize the variability of nickel content in foods grown in different soils.

In summary, there is significant evidence that dietary nickel can cause SCD. The most conservative and safe treatment, dietary modification, has been shown to be effective, but it requires significant patient education and compliance.

Balsam of Peru and Related Chemicals

Contact allergy to (BOP) or *Myroxilon pereirae* is commonly evidenced with positive patch test reactions.[47] Coreactivity to fragrance mix, cinnamic aldehyde, and balsam of tolu is also commonly seen.[48] After first being described by Bonnevie in 1939,[49] Hjorth[50] recognized the association of allergy to BOP to allergy to spices and flavorings, such as cinnamon, vanilla, and cloves. This relationship presents the possibility of the occurrence of SCD to orally ingested agents that contain substances related to or contained in BOP. Cross reactions are also seen with cinnamon, cinnamic aldehyde, clove, orange peel, and eugenol.[51]

BOP is a fairly specific marker for an allergy to spice, although it is not very sensitive.[52] It is also believed that topical products containing BOP, including cosmetics, sensitize patients predisposing them to SCD with oral ingestion.[53] Studies have evidenced the clinical improvement of balsal allergic patients who avoid foods that are balsam related,[48,54–56] demonstrating the importance of educating these patients regarding dietary avoidance.[48] Oral challenge with BOP has not proven to be a predictor of which patients might benefit from these diet restrictions.[57,58] A study also showed that 41% of patients with a positive patch test reaction to BOP also reacted to spices.[59] For patients with BOP allergy, the authors recommend a strict avoidance of BOP products and foods and BOP-related products, such as flavorings and spices.

Other Common Metal Allergens

Cobalt

Cobalt is a metal that is more commonly reported to cause SCD, and its prevalence is clinically relevant because it is the main component of vitamin B12 (**Box 1**).[28] Fisher[60] described a patient who had a recall reaction at the site of a previous vitamin B12 injection after oral ingestion of cobalt. An allergy to either cobalt or nickel can increase one's sensitivity to the other metal. In 1987, Veien and colleagues[61] described 7 out of 13 patients who were sensitive to cobalt but not to nickel, as having a flare of their dermatitis with oral challenge of 1 mg cobalt sulfate. In another study, Veien and colleagues[62] reported that out of 9 patients who had positive patch test reactions to cobalt and not nickel, 6 experienced flares of their dermatitis after

Box 1
Metals that cause SCD

Metals
Aluminum
Chromium
Cobalt
Copper
Gold
Mercury
Nickel
Zinc

a placebo-controlled oral challenge of 1 mg of cobalt. When dietary restriction of cobalt was initiated, 4 of these 6 patients had an improvement of their dermatitis. Cross-sensitization has been seen in cobalt allergic patients with nickel and palladium.[63] Palladium is seen increasingly in dental appliances, jewelry, and electrical appliances,[28] and avoidance can be imperative for the management of these patients.

Mercury

Mercury is 1 of the earlier recognized metals to cause SCD, usually as a result of inhalation of mercury vapors from a broken thermometer, commonly after previous sensitization to other mercury compounds, such as thimerosal, merbromin (Mercurochrome), topical disinfectants,[64] ophthalmologic preparations,[65] and antiparasitic powders.[66] SCD from mercury can also be caused by amalgam dental restorations.[67,68] Mercury has also been reported to induce acute generalized exanthematous pustulosis.[64] Although systemically absorbed mercury may lead to lymphocytic proliferation, its excretion through sweat may also attract and concentrate T cells in the flexural areas, which may explain the common clinical presentation of mercury-related SCD.[64,69]

Gold

Gold, which has commonly been used as a restoration material in dentistry and as an intramuscular injection as an antiinflammatory for the treatment of rheumatoid arthritis, has emerged as a significant metal allergen.[70] Diagnosing gold allergy traditionally through patch testing has proven to be challenging if late leads are not performed 7 days or later, and thus it is recommended to follow up patients with suspected gold allergy for 3 weeks, in case a late reaction presents.[70] Intramuscular injection with gold sodium thiosulfate has shown to flare patients' previous dermatitis and/or patch test reaction in addition to increasing these patients' body temperature.[71]

Copper

Although copper has been less commonly reported to induce SCD, it is an allergen to consider. Copper has been used in dental devices, with evidence of delayed-type stomatitis.[72] Copper-sensitive women have also experienced SCD from intrauterine contraceptive devices that happened to contain copper.[73,74]

Medications

SCD from medications has been reported from a broad spectrum of drugs (**Box 2**). It is suspected that SCD from drugs is different from other drug eruptions because sensitization is required and the mechanism is likely different.[7] It is believed that a patient's intrinsic sensitivity to the drug and the size of drug dosage is related to the severity of the cutaneous inflammation.[75]

Oral drugs

Some of the most convincing evidence of the existence of SCD is due to the cutaneous reactions seen with a well-observed temporal relationship in medications that are available for topical and oral use.[10] Reports of SCD to the following have been evidenced in the literature: miconazole,[76] gentamycin,[77,78] methyl salicylate,[12] erythromycin,[79] corticosteroids,[80] such as prednisone[81] and dexamethasone,[82] mesalazine (5-aminosalicylic acid or 5-ASA),[83] ethylenediamine,[84] and clobazam.[85] A delayed-type reaction with a cutaneous eruption similar to toxic epidermal necrolysis has also been reported to ampicillin.[86] Many of these drugs are important for the management of patients' other medical conditions, thus alternative drug classes or chemical structures may be substituted, such as switching dexamethasone for prednisone or vice versa.[82]

Botanicals/Foods

There is significant evidence that foods and botanic products can also cause allergic reactions that present as SCD (**Box 3**). An increasing number of people are using herbal remedies and alternative therapies, which often contain plant extracts. Additionally, these items have also been introduced in cosmetics, providing multiple ways for sensitization.

In terms of foods, although allergic and irritant contact dermatitis is a common cause of hand

---

Box 2
Medications that cause SCD

5-Fluorouracil

Allopurinol

Aminopenicillins

Ampicillin

Bacitracin

Benzocaine

Cinchocaine

Clobazam

Corticosteroids (inhaled)

Corticosteroids (systemic)

Erythromycin

Ethylenediamine

Gentamycin

Hydroxyzine

Intravenous immune globulin (0.4 g/kg)

Mesalazine (5-aminosalicylic acid or 5-ASA)

Methyl salicylate

Miconazole

Mitomycin C

Naproxen

Neomycin

Oxycodone

Penicillin

Psuedoephedrine

Streptomycin

Suxamethonium

Terbinafine

Tetracaine

Box 3
Plants that cause SCD

Arnica

Balsam of Peru

Chamomile

Cinnamon oil

Compositae (daisy family)

Echinacea

Feverfew

Marigold

Mugwort

Parthenium

Ragweed

Vanilla oil

dermatitis in food handlers,[87] there have been a few published reports on SCD from diet other than the nickel- and BOP-related foods, but this entity may be underreported and underdiagnosed.[88,89]

Compositae (Asteraceae)

Botanicals from the family Compositae (Asteraceae), commonly referred to as the 'daisy family', are increasingly being used for alternative remedies.[90] This broad family also includes flowers, herbs, vegetables, and weeds (eg, ragweed, chamomile, *Tanacetum vulgare*, *Arnica montana*, parthenolide, *Achillea millefolium*, marigold, mugwort, and *Echinacea*).[28,87] Additionally, extracts from this family are found in many different cosmetics and personal hygiene products. The main allergens in these plants are sesquiterpene lactones, which are the main inducers of both ACD and SCD. Wintzen and colleagues[91] reported recalcitrant atopic dermatitis in Compositae-sensitive patients, secondary to their food intake. Chamomile, commonly found in tea, has also been evidenced to cause severe SCD with just minimal amounts of sesquiterpene lactones.[90]

Parthenium hysterophorus ("parthenium weed")

Parthenium hysterophorus, a common weed allergen in India,[92] has been shown to sensitize 56% of those occupationally exposed to it.[93] Other than a cutaneous eruption occurring from airborne exposure, it is suspected that an eczematous reaction may also occur by inhalation or ingestion.[92] To determine whether a patient had SCD to parthenium from inhalation or cutaneous exposure, Mahajan and colleagues asked the patient to inhale from a polythene bag containing parthenium without any direct or airborne contact with the weed. About 8 to 10 hours later, the patient's dermatitis flared.[92] When researchers tried to hyposensitize patients with parthenium sensitivity, 30% had flares of their dermatitis.[94]

Garlic and onions

Garlic and onions are 2 food items commonly recognized as inducers of allergy.[95] A case report details the development of hand dermatitis after the ingestion of garlic tablets.[96] Allergens seen in garlic include diallyl disulfide, allyl-propyl sulfur, and allicine.[97,98]

Other Common Chemicals

Propylene glycol

Propylene glycol, used for many purposes, including as a solvent, emulsifier, vehicle, antifreeze, and humectants,[87] has been implicated to cause systemic reactions in previously sensitized individuals. Its properties also allow for its use as a thickening agent in many foods, including cake mixes, salad dressings, popcorn, and soda drinks.[87] It is also found in topical corticosteroids and other medicaments, cosmetics, and fragrances.[99] Experimentally, researchers have shown that the ingestion of propylene glycol flares patients sensitive to this chemical.[100] Fisher[101] also reported a case in which a patient developed SCD after being administered intravenous valium, in which propylene glycol was used as a solvent.[101]

Formaldehyde

Formaldehyde has been implicated in systemic reactions that include migraine headaches, asthma, and generalized eczema.[102] Aspartame, a synthetic sweetener commonly found in children's chewable vitamins, diet drinks, and low-calorie food-items, is metabolized to methanol and later into formic acid, and it can be associated with SCD in formaldehyde-sensitive patients.[103] For sensitized individuals, avoidance of products and foods that contain formaldehyde, aspartame, or other formaldehyde releasers is recommended.

SUMMARY

SCD describes a cutaneous eruption in response to systemic exposure to an allergen. The exact pathologic mechanism remains uncertain. The broad spectrum of presentations that are often nonspecific can make it difficult for the clinician to suspect this disease, but it is an important diagnosis to consider in cases of recalcitrant, widespread, or recurrent dermatitis, in which patch testing reveals allergy to nickel or BOP. Diagnosis and appropriate management can be life-altering for affected patients.

REFERENCES

1. Fisher AA. Contact dermatitis. Philadelphia: Lea & Febiger; 1973. p. 293–305.
2. Jadassohn J. Zur Kenntnis der medikamentösen Dermatosen. Verhandlungen der Deutschen Dermatologischen Gesellschaft. Fünfter Kongress, Raz, 1895. Vienna: Braunmüller; 1896. p. 106 [in German].
3. Fisher AA. Systemic eczematous "contact-type" dermatitis medicamentosa. Ann Allergy 1966; 24(8):406–20.
4. Nakayama H, Niki F, Shono M, et al. Mercury exanthema. Contact Dermatitis 1983;9:411–7.
5. Andersen KE, Hjorth N, Menné T. The baboon syndrome: systemically-induced allergic contact dermatitis. Contact Dermatitis 1984;10(2):97–100.
6. Klaschka F, Ring J. Systemically induced (hematogenous) contact eczema. Semin Dermatol 1990; 9(3):210–5.

7. Thyssen JP, Maibach HI. Drug-elicited systemic allergic (contact) dermatitis–update and possible pathomechanisms. Contact Dermatitis 2008;59(4): 195–202.

8. Grabbe S, Schwarz T. Immunoregulatory mechanisms involved in elicitation of allergic contact hypersensitivity. Immunol Today 1998;19:37–44.

9. Rustemeyer T, van Hoogstraten IMW, Scheper RJ, et al. Mechanisms in allergic contact dermatitis. In: Rycroft RJG, Menne T, Frosch PJ, editors. Textbook of contact dermatitis. 3rd edition. Berlin: Springer-Verlag; 2001. p. 13–58.

10. Veien NK. Ingested food in systemic allergic contact dermatitis. Clin Dermatol 1997;15(4):547–55.

11. Menne T, Weismann K. [Hematogenous contact eczema following oral administration of neomycin]. Hautarzt 1984;35:319–20.

12. Hindson C. Contact eczema from methyl salicylate reproduced by oral aspirin (acetyl salicylic acid). Contact Dermatitis 1977;3(6):348–9.

13. Hausermann P, Harr TH, Bircher AJ. Baboon syndrome resulting from systemic drugs: is there strife between SDRIFE and allergic contact dermatitis syndrome? Contact Dermatitis 2004;51: 297–310.

14. Scheper RJ, von Blomberg M, Boerrigter GH, et al. Induction of immunological memory in the skin. Role of local T cell retention. Clin Exp Immunol 1983;51(1):141–8.

15. Menne T, Hjorth N. Reactions from systemic exposure to contact allergens. Semin Dermatol 1982;1: 15–24.

16. Saint-Mezard P, Berard F, Dubois B, et al. The role of CD4+ and CD8+ T cells in contact hypersensitivity and allergic contact dermatitis. Eur J Dermatol 2004;14(3):131–8.

17. Divkovic M, Pease CK, Gerberick GF, et al. Hapten-protein binding: from theory to practical application in the in vitro prediction of skin sensitization. Contact Dermatitis 2005;53(4):189–200.

18. Cavani A, De Pita O, Girolomoni G. New aspects of the molecular basis of contact allergy. Curr Opin Allergy Clin Immunol 2007;7:404–8.

19. Albanesi C, Scarponi C, Giustizieri ML, et al. Keratinocytes in inflammatory skin diseases. Curr Drug Targets Inflamm Allergy 2005;4(3):329–34.

20. Biedermann T, Kneilling M, Mailhammer R, et al. Mast cells control neutrophil recruitment during T cell-mediated delayed-type hypersensitivity reactions through tumor necrosis factor and macrophage inflammatory protein 2. J Exp Med 2000; 192(10):1441–52.

21. O'Leary JG, Goodarzi M, Drayton DL, et al. T cell- and B cell-independent adaptive immunity mediated by natural killer cells. Nat Immunol 2006;7(5):507–16.

22. Zug KA, McGinley-Smith D, Warshaw EM, et al. Contact allergy in children referred for patch testing: North American contact dermatitis group data, 2001–2004. Arch Dermatol 2008;144(10): 1329–36.

23. Veien N, Menne T. Systemic contact dermatitis. In: Frosh PJ, Menne T, Lepoittevin JP, editors. Contact dermatitis. Berlin-Heidelberg: Springer; 2006. p. 295–307.

24. Veien NK, Christiansen AH, Svejgaard E, et al. Antibodies against nickel-albumin in rabbits and man. Contact Dermatitis 1979;5(6):378–82.

25. Hjorth N, Roed-Petersen J. Occupational protein contact dermatitis in food handlers. Contact Dermatitis 1976;2(1):28–42.

26. Janssens V, Morren M, Dooms-Goossens A, et al. Protein contact dermatitis: myth or reality? Br J Dermatol 1995;132(1):1–6.

27. Levin C, Warshaw E. Protein contact dermatitis: allergens, pathogenesis, and management. Dermatitis 2008;19(5):241–51.

28. Jacob SE, Zapolanski T. Systemic contact dermatitis. Dermatitis 2008;19(1):9–15.

29. Mowad CM, Marks JG. Allergic contact dermatitis. In: Bolognia JL, Jorizzo JL, Rapini RP, editors. Dermatology. 2nd edition. Spain: Mosby Elsevier; 2008. p. 209–21.

30. Jensen CS, Menné T, Lisby S, et al. Experimental systemic contact dermatitis from nickel: a dose-response study. Contact Dermatitis 2003;49(3): 124–32.

31. Santucci B, Cristaudo A, Cannistraci C, et al. Nickel sensitivity: effects of prolonged oral intake of the element. Contact Dermatitis 1988;19(3):202–5.

32. Menné T, Thorboe A. Nickel dermatitis–nickel excretion. Contact Dermatitis 1976;2(6):353–4.

33. Rietschel RL, Fowler JF. Contact dermatitis and other reactions to metals. In: Rietschel RL, Fowler JF, editors. Fisher's contact dermatitis. 5th edition. Philadelphia: Lippincott Williams & Wilkins; 2001. p. 638–40.

34. Nielsen GD, Jepsen LV, Jørgensen PJ, et al. Nickel-sensitive patients with vesicular hand eczema: oral challenge with a diet naturally high in nickel. Br J Dermatol 1990;122(3):299–308.

35. Sharma AD. Disulfiram and low nickel diet in the management of hand eczema: a clinical study. Indian J Dermatol Venereol Leprol 2006;72(2): 113–8.

36. Gawkrodger DJ, Shuttler IL, Delves HT. Nickel dermatitis and diet: clinical improvement and a reduction in blood and urine nickel levels with a low-nickel diet. Acta Derm Venereol 1988;68(5):453–5.

37. Veien NK, Hattel T, Laurberg G. Low nickel diet: an open, prospective trial. J Am Acad Dermatol 1993; 29(6):1002–7.

38. Veien NK, Hattel T, Justesen O, et al. Dietary restrictions in the treatment of adult patients with eczema. Contact Dermatitis 1987;17(4):223–8.

39. Kaaber K, Menné T, Veien N, et al. Treatment of nickel dermatitis with antabuse; a double blind study. Contact Dermatitis 1983;9(4):297–9.

40. Jensen CS, Lisby S, Larsen JK, et al. Characterization of lymphocyte subpopulations and cytokine profiles in peripheral blood of nickel-sensitive individuals with systemic contact dermatitis after oral nickel exposure. Contact Dermatitis 2004;50(1):31–8.

41. Joneja JM. Section III: specific food restrictions nickel allergy. In: Joneja JM, editor. Managing food allergy & intolerance: a practical guide. Port Coquitlam (BC): J.A. Hall Publications; 1995. p. 247–62.

42. Andersen KE, Nielsen GD, Flyvholm MA, et al. Nickel in tap water. Contact Dermatitis 1983;9(2):140–3.

43. Kuligowski J, Halperin KM. Stainless steel cookware as a significant source of nickel, chromium, and iron. Arch Environ Contam Toxicol 1992;23(2):211–5.

44. Accominotti M, Bost M, Haudrechy P, et al. Contribution to chromium and nickel enrichment during cooking of foods in stainless steel utensils. Contact Dermatitis 1998;38(6):305–10.

45. Sharma AD. Relationship between nickel allergy and diet. Indian J Dermatol Venereol Leprol 2007;73:307–12.

46. Scheman A, Jacob S, Zirwas M, et al. Contact allergy: alternatives for the 2007 North American contact dermatitis group (NACDG) Standard Screening Tray. Dis Mon 2008;54(1–2):7–156.

47. Warshaw EM, Belsito DV, DeLeo VA, et al. North American contact dermatitis group patch-test results, 2003–2004 study period. Dermatitis 2008;19(3):129–36.

48. Salam TN, Fowler JF Jr. Balsam-related systemic contact dermatitis. J Am Acad Dermatol 2001;45(3):377–81.

49. Bonnevie P. Aetiologie und pathogenese der eckzemkrankheiten. Copenhagen: Busck; 1939 [in Danish].

50. Hjorth N. Eczematous allergy to balsams, allied perfumes, and flavouring agents [thesis]. Copenhagen; 1961.

51. Fisher AA, Mitchell JC. Toxicodendron plants and spices. In: Reitschel RL, Fowler JF, editors. Fisher's contact dermatitis. Baltimore (MD): Williams & Wilkins; 1995. p. 461–523.

52. Kanerva L, Estlander T, Jolanki R. Occupational allergic contact dermatitis from spices. Contact Dermatitis 1996;35(3):157–62.

53. Bedello PG, Goitre M, Cane D. Contact dermatitis and flare from food flavouring agents. Contact Dermatitis 1982;8(2):143–4.

54. Veien NK, Hattel T, Justesen O, et al. Oral challenge with balsam of Peru in patients with eczema: a preliminary study. Contact Dermatitis 1983;9(1):75–6.

55. Veien NK, Hattel T, Justesen O, et al. Oral challenge with balsam of Peru. Contact Dermatitis 1985;12(2):104–7.

56. Veien NK, Hattel T, Justesen O, et al. Reduction of intake of balsams in patients sensitive to balsam of Peru. Contact Dermatitis 1985;12(5):270–3.

57. Veien NK, Hattel T, Laurberg G. Can oral challenge with balsam of Peru predict possible benefit from a low-balsam diet? Am J Contact Dermatitis 1996;7(2):84–7.

58. Niinimäki A. Double-blind placebo-controlled peroral challenges in patients with delayed-type allergy to balsam of Peru. Contact Dermatitis 1995;33(2):78–83.

59. Niinimäki A. Delayed-type allergy to spices. Contact Dermatitis 1984;11(1):34–40.

60. Fisher AA. Contact dermatitis at home and abroad. Cutis 1972;10:719.

61. Veien NK, Hattel T, Justesen O, et al. Oral challenge with nickel and cobalt in patients with positive patch tests to nickel and/or cobalt. Acta Derm Venereol 1987;67(4):321–5.

62. Veien NK, Hattel T, Laurberg G. Placebo-controlled oral challenge with cobalt in patients with positive patch tests to cobalt. Contact Dermatitis 1995;33(1):54–5.

63. Hindsen M, Spiren A, Bruze M. Cross-reactivity between nickel and palladium demonstrated by systemic administration of nickel. Contact Dermatitis 2005;53:2–8.

64. Lerch M, Bircher AJ. Systemically induced allergic exanthema from mercury. Contact Dermatitis 2004;50:349–53.

65. Barrazza V, Meunier P, Escande JP. Acute contact dermatitis and exanthematous pustulosis due to mercury. Contact Dermatitis 1998;38:361.

66. Vena GA, Foti C, Grandolfo M, et al. Mercury exanthema. Contact Dermatitis 1994;31:214–6.

67. White IR, Smith BG. Dental amalgam dermatitis. Braz Dent J 1984;156(7):259–60.

68. Veien NK. Stomatitis and systemic dermatitis from mercury in amalgam dental restorations. Dermatol Clin 1990;8(1):157–60.

69. Cederbrant K, Hultman P. Characterization of mercuric mercury (Hg2+)-induced lymphoblasts from patients with mercury allergy and from healthy subjects. Clin Exp Immunol 2000;121(1):23–30.

70. Hostýnek JJ. Gold: an allergen of growing significance. Food Chem Toxicol 1997;35(8):839–44.

71. Möller H, Björkner B, Bruze M. Clinical reactions to systemic provocation with gold sodium thiomalate in patients with contact allergy to gold. Br J Dermatol 1996;135(3):423–7.

72. Hostynek JJ. Metals. In: Maibach HI, editor. Toxicology of the skin. Philadelphia: Taylor and Francis; 2001. p. 345–56.

73. Barranco VP. Eczematous dermatitis caused by internal exposure to copper. Arch Dermatol 1972; 106(3):386–7.

74. Zabel M, Lindscheid KR, Mark H. Copper sulfate allergy with special reference to internal exposure. Z Hautkr 1990;65(5):481–2, 485–6.

75. Park RG. Cutaneous hypersensitivity to sulphonamides. Br Med J 1943;2:69–72.

76. Fernandez L, Maquiera E, Rodriguez F, et al. Systemic contact dermatitis from miconazole. Contact Dermatitis 1996;34(3):217.

77. Ghadially R, Ramsay CA. Gentamicin: systemic exposure to a contact allergen. J Am Acad Dermatol 1988;19(2 Pt 2):428–30.

78. Guin JD, Phillips D. Erythroderma from systemic contact dermatitis: a complication of systemic gentamicin in a patient with contact allergy to neomycin. Cutis 1989;43(6):564–7.

79. Fernandez Redondo V, Casas L, Taboada M, et al. Systemic contact dermatitis from erythromycin. Contact Dermatitis 1994;30(5):311.

80. Whitmore SE. Delayed systemic allergic reactions to corticosteroids. Contact Dermatitis 1995;32(4): 193–8.

81. Quirce S, Alvarez MJ, Olaguibel JM, et al. Systemic contact dermatitis from oral prednisone. Contact Dermatitis 1994;30(1):53–4.

82. Nucera E, Buonomo A, Pollastrini E, et al. A case of cutaneous delayed-type allergy to oral dexamethasone and to betamethasone. Dermatology 2002; 204(3):248–50.

83. Gallo R, Parodi A. Baboon syndrome from 5-aminosalicylic acid. Contact Dermatitis 2002;46(2):110.

84. Guin JD, Fields P, Thomas KL. Baboon syndrome from i.v. aminophylline in a patient allergic to ethylenediamine. Contact Dermatitis 1999;40(3):170–1.

85. Machet L, Vaillant L, Dardaine V, et al. Patch testing with clobazam: relapse of generalized drug eruption. Contact Dermatitis 1992;26(5):347–8.

86. Tagami H, Tatsuta K, Iwatski K, et al. Delayed hypersensitivity in ampicillin-induced toxic epidermal necrolysis. Arch Dermatol 1983; 119(11):910–3.

87. Warshaw EM, Botto NC, Zug KA, et al. Contact dermatitis associated with food: retrospective cross-sectional analysis of North American Contact Dermatitis Group data, 2001–2004. Dermatitis 2008;19(5):252–60.

88. Chan EF, Mowad C. Contact dermatitis to foods and spices. Am J Contact Dermatitis 1998;9(2):71–9.

89. Brancaccio RR, Alvarez MS. Contact allergy to food. Dermatol Ther 2004;17(4):302–13.

90. Paulsen E. Contact sensitization from compositae-containing herbal remedies and cosmetics. Contact Dermatitis 2002;47(4):189–98.

91. Wintzen M, Donker AS, van Zuuren EJ. Recalcitrant atopic dermatitis due to allergy to compositae. Contact Dermatitis 2003;48(2):87–8.

92. Mahajan VK, Sharma NL, Sharma RC. Parthenium dermatitis: is it a systemic contact dermatitis or an airborne contact dermatitis? Contact Dermatitis 2004;51(5–6):231–4.

93. Rao PV, Mangala A, Rao BS, et al. Clinical and immunological studies on persons exposed to *Parthenium hysterophorus* L. Experientia 1977;33(10): 1387–8.

94. Handa S, Sahoo B, Sharma VK. Oral hyposensitization in patients with contact dermatitis from *Parthenium hysterophorus*. Contact Dermatitis 2001; 44(5):279–82.

95. Sinha SM, Pasricha JS, Sharma R, et al. Vegetables responsible for contact dermatitis of the hands. Arch Dermatol 1977;113(6):776–9.

96. Burden AD, Wilkinson SM, Beck MH, et al. Garlic-induced systemic contact dermatitis. Contact Dermatitis 1994;30(5):299–300.

97. Papageorgiou C, Corbet JP, Menezes-Brandao F, et al. Allergic contact dermatitis to garlic (*Allium sativum* L). Identification of the allergens: the role of mono-, di-, and trisulfides present in garlic. A comparative study in man and animal (guinea-pig). Arch Dermatol Res 1983;275(4):229–34.

98. Lembo G, Balato N, Patruno C, et al. Allergic contact dermatitis due to garlic (*Allium sativum*). Contact Dermatitis 1991;25(5):330–1.

99. Lowther A, McCormick T, Nedorost S. Systemic contact dermatitis from propylene glycol. Dermatitis 2008;19(2):105–8.

100. Hannuksela M, Förström L. Reactions to peroral propylene glycol. Contact Dermatitis 1978;4(1): 41–5.

101. Fisher AA. Systemic contact dermatitis to intravenous valium in a person sensitive to propylene glycol. Cutis 1995;55:327.

102. Jacob SE, Stechschulte S. Formaldehyde, aspartame, and migraines: a possible connection. Dermatitis 2008;19(3):E10–1.

103. Hill AM, Belsito DV. Systemic contact dermatitis of the eyelids caused by formaldehyde derived from aspartame? Contact Dermatitis 2003;49(5):258–9.

Management of Occupational Dermatitis

Shane C. Clark, BA, Matthew J. Zirwas, MD*

KEYWORDS

- Contact dermatitis • Occupational contact dermatitis
- Occupational skin disease • Management
- Allergic contact dermatitis

Contact dermatitis is the most common occupational skin disorder, responsible for up to 30% of all cases of occupational disease in industrialized nations.[1] Epidemiologic data suggest that contact dermatitis accounts for 90% to 95% of all cases of occupational skin disease,[2–4] imposing considerable social and economic implications. Occupational contact dermatitis (OCD) is broadly classified into allergic and irritant subtypes. Irritant contact dermatitis (ICD) is widely quoted in the literature to account for 80% of OCD cases, with allergic cases held responsible for the remaining 20%.[5,6] However, as reviewed by Holness,[7] numerous studies have shown wide variation in the distribution of cases of ICD versus ACD. As discussed by Belsito[8] ICD accounts for 71% to 32% of OCD cases, whereas ACD is responsible for 60% to 34%.[9–14] The incidence rate of OCD is suggested by epidemiologic studies to be approximately 0.5 to 1.9 cases per 1000 full-time workers per year[1] with a 1-year prevalence estimate of 10% and lifetime prevalence of approximately 20%.[15,16] Mild cases of OCD are rarely registered, leading to underestimation of incidence by perhaps 20 to 50 times.[17] In the occupational setting, the hands are the most commonly affected area, with involvement in 80% to 90% of cases.[18] However, true epidemiologic data regarding OCD are lacking, secondary to a lack of standardization of case definitions and methods.

The economic, social, and psychologic repercussions of OCD defy understatement. The Bureau of Labor Statistics estimated 41,800 cases of OCD in the United States in 2000.[19] However, as a result of underreporting of mild cases, Lushniak has suggested the true number could approach 400,000 to 2 million cases per year.[20] Mathias had estimated the total annual costs in 1985 to be between $222 million and $1 billion in the United States alone.[21] A survey of reported cases of occupational hand eczema (HE) established that in 1 year, 19.9% to 23% of cases experienced prolonged sick leave and job loss respectively.[22] Showing the socioeconomic toll of OCD, in a 12-year Swedish questionnaire and phone interview study following 517 patients who reported OCD to the Social Insurance Office, 82% of HE patients reported having changed their work situation and 48% declared taking sick leave for at least 1 period of 7 days secondary to HE. In culmination, 15% of HE patients were excluded from the occupational workforce through unemployment or disability pension.[23]

One of the often overlooked burdens of occupational dermatitis, like any visible skin disease, is the concomitant social stigmata. As discussed by Diepgen and colleagues,[24] the importance of the hands as tools for communication and expression is manifested by the major psychosocial problems (eg, anxiety, depression, social phobia) affected individuals suffer. A lower quality of life, comparable to generalized eczema or psoriasis is reported in severely affected cases.[25,26]

CLINICAL FEATURES

Traditionally, the mechanisms underlying ICD and ACD were divided into nonimmunologic and immunologic pathways respectively. However, recent studies suggest significant pathophysiologic overlap between the entities. Likewise

Department of Internal Medicine, Division of Dermatology, Ohio State University College of Medicine, 5965 E Broad Street, Suite 290, Columbus, OH 43213, USA

* Corresponding author.

E-mail address: matt.zirwas@osumc.edu (M. Zirwas).

Dermatol Clin 27 (2009) 365–383
doi:10.1016/j.det.2009.05.002

many, if not most, substances do not exclusively induce irritant or allergic reactions; instead being able to induce both.

Irritant Contact Dermatitis

Overview

ICD results from failure of the barrier function of the stratum corneum with the consequential release of inflammatory mediators from keratinocytes. In contrast to ACD, ICD is not a singular entity, but rather encompasses a spectrum of abnormal skin changes.[27] The lack of a standard definition of ICD results commonly in the misclassification of ICD and hence attendant over or underestimation of the disease frequency. Irritants are physical or chemical agents exerting a cytotoxic effect, which after single or repeated exposure elicits a non-allergic inflammatory host response. Irritants do not require sensitization (unlike ACD) and highly irritating substances such as alkalis, acids, and strong oxidizing and reducing agents may cause dermatitis with the first exposure.[28] Most cases, however, result from chronic cumulative exposure to 1 or multiple low grade irritants. ICD requires a threshold concentration (which may vary from person to person) above which the responsible chemicals cause dermatitis and below which they do not.

Risk factors

The development of ICD is dependent on exogenous and endogenous risk factors. Repeated exposure with nearly any chemical can result in ICD. The irritating potential of a substance is dependent on its physical properties, concentration, duration of exposure, and vehicle. Molecular size, ionization state, and fat solubility affect penetration through the skin.[29] As reviewed by Slodownik and colleagues,[29] physical, mechanical, and environmental factors significantly contribute to the onset of ICD; a fact which is unfortunately often overlooked.[30] Low humidity enhances irritability by decreasing ceramide levels in the stratum corneum[31] which can lead to cracking or fissuring. Heat or occlusion with gloves may precipitate ICD through increased exposure to sweat which is more irritating than water.[32] Common skin irritants include water, detergents, solvents, rubber, fiberglass, cutting fluids, and food products. Identifying a single substance causing ICD is inefficient at best, and often impossible, as ICD is usually multifactorial.[29] The most commonly implicated exogenous factor in ICD is "wet work".[33] Wet work includes wearing occlusive gloves for more than 2 hours per day, exposure of the skin to liquid for more than 2 hours per day, or frequent hand washing.[34]

Endogenous factors including sex, age, atopy and other skin disease, and anatomic site influence vulnerability to ICD.[35] Occupational ICD affects women nearly twice as often as men, in contrast to other occupational disorders which more frequently affect men. Although the picture remains cloudy, it has been suggested that the increased incidence in females is secondary to the disproportionate role women occupy in housecleaning, hair styling, and childcare. An atopic diathesis increases the susceptibility to skin irritants[36] and atopics should therefore be cautioned regarding professions with significant irritant exposure. Anatomic site further influences the propensity to develop ICD. The thickness of the protective stratum corneum varies considerably depending on location. It is thickest on the palms of the hands. Consequently, hand dermatitis often occurs on the dorsal hand and finger web spaces where the stratum corneum is thinner.

Presentation

Classically the dermatitis affects the dorsum of the hand and the finger webs where the protective stratum corneum is thinnest. Patients typically complain of pain, irritation, burning, and/or itching. Itching is typically less intense than what is seen in ACD. Two major forms of ICD are recognized: acute and cumulative. Cumulative ICD is more common than acute. Acute ICD can develop rapidly, within minutes after exposure to highly irritating substances, especially powerful acids and alkalis, and strong oxidizing and reducing agents. Typically, such exposure produces rapid development of burning and pruritus with coincident erythema, blistering, and swelling. The rash does not extend beyond the area of contact and typically resolves within a few weeks with removal of further insult. In contrast, weak irritants produce cumulative ICD, which may require months of continual exposure before the repair capacity of the skin is overwhelmed and ICD clinically manifests. Repeated exposure to mild irritants such as soap, water, greases, and solvents causes chronic cumulative irritant dermatitis. The chronic lesions of cumulative ICD appear lichenified with fissuring, hyperkeratosis, excoriations, and scaling and can take considerably longer to resolve than acute irritant dermatitis.

Pathogenesis

Historically, ICD was considered to be a nonimmunologic process. Conversely, current theories suggest that the immune system plays a central role in the pathogenesis of ICD. Irritants may be physical or chemical in nature. Either can initiate ICD if skin is subjected to exposure for a sufficient duration at an adequate concentration and/or force. Repeated exposure with nearly any chemical may elicit ICD. Irritants may damage the skin by way of a multitude of effects, including, but not limited to: direct cytotoxicity, lipid-barrier removal, cell membrane damage, and denaturation of keratins.[37] Despite varying mechanisms, the final common pathway is executed with the release of inflammatory mediators from damaged and viable keratinocytes. Keratinocytes are essential in the propagation of ICD, releasing cytokines upon penetration of irritants through the stratum corneum, up-regulating cell adhesion molecules, and up-regulating MHC class II antigens.[38] A plethora of cytokines are liberated during propagation of ICD, but perhaps the most important is TNF-α. Research suggests that TNF-α may be the major mediator of inflammation, notably shown by a study in which mice administered anti–TNF-α antibodies failed to develop ICD.[39]

As reviewed by Slodownik and colleagues,[29] the chronicity of ICD which is observed in some patients has 2 probable explanations. First, prolonged inflammation exposes the immune system to immunogenic skin peptides resulting in persistent recruitment of inflammatory mediators. Second, TNF-α is regulated in an autocrine manner and thus engaged in the maintenance of inflammation.[40]

Allergic Contact Dermatitis

Overview
ACD is a classic, type IV, delayed, T-cell mediated, hypersensitivity reaction, the pathophysiology of which has been extensively reviewed in standard texts and articles; to which the interested reader is referred. The trademark of an allergy is its specificity; a discrete, predictable, and reproducible inflammatory reaction occurring exclusively in sensitized individuals only after rechallenge with a specific allergen. Hypersensitivity to an allergen usually lasts indefinitely.

Risk factors
Environmental factors such as friction, heat exposure, humidity, and pressure[41] have been implicated in ACD likely through embarrassment of the skin's barrier function; and have previously and succinctly been reviewed by Belsito.[8] Specifically, maceration effected by wet work and repetitious cycles of wetting and drying (ie, hand washing) provoke fissuring and cracking, enhancing cutaneous penetrance of allergens and irritants. Similarly, decreased ambient humidity results in desiccation and epidermal barrier disruption. In contrast, humid and/or hot environments promote perspiration, into which

soluble contactants are dissolved, enhancing cutaneous penetration.[8] Finally, persistent friction likewise incites barrier disruption with an attendant increased risk for sensitization.[42]

Beyond host and environmental factors, specific occupations are associated with relatively greater rates of ACD including hairdressers, printers, cement workers, painters, mechanics, animal handlers, food processors, florists, chefs, builders, pharmaceutical factory workers, and laundry workers.[43–45] As a collective, the features shared by the majority of the above occupations are an excessive exposure to water, solvents, and/or micro trauma. More extensive allergen lists and occupational exposures are available in reference books.[6,46]

Presentation
Reexposure to an allergen after sensitization evokes the elicitation phase, which normally presents between 12 and 48 hours after exposure; this is the obligatory time for allergen to be processed, presented, and for lymphocytes to be recruited. However, clinically evident ACD may require months to years of exposure to low levels of an allergen (eg, chromate dermatitis in cement workers) before manifesting. After contact, sensitized individuals develop an eczematous rash with significant pruritus, erythema, and edema, thereafter accompanied by vesicles, papules, bullae, and scaling. Subsequently, lesions evolve with crusting and weeping with associated risk for infection. Chronic ACD appears lichenified with scaling and often fissured. The lesions of ACD are initially sharply demarcated; occurring only at the site of contact, but with time can potentially become more generalized and less strikingly delineated. The lesions of ACD after a singular encounter with an allergen typically resolve in 7 to 21 days but continual exposure inducing chronic ACD may persist for weeks or months after antigen removal.[27]

DIAGNOSIS OF OCCUPATIONAL CONTACT DERMATITIS

The diagnosis of OCD is dependent on patient history, exposure history, dermatitis pattern, and patch testing (if indicated). Differentiation between ICD and ACD requires a methodical and fastidious approach and hence an attendant time obligation. If OCD is suspected as the cause of dermatitis, criteria proposed by Mathias[47] or the operational definition propounded by Marrakchi and colleagues[48,49] will assist in both the diagnosis of OCD as well as subsequent workers' compensation (WC) claims.[48] The 7 criteria (**Table 1**)

Table 1
Summary of the Mathias criteria for assessing occupational causation and/or aggravation of contact dermatitis

Criterion 1:	Is the clinical appearance consistent with contact dermatitis?
Criterion 2:	Are there workplace exposures to potential cutaneous irritants or allergens?
Criterion 3:	Is the anatomic distribution of dermatitis consistent with cutaneous exposure in relation to the job task?
Criterion 4:	Is the temporal relationship between exposure and onset consistent with contact dermatitis?
Criterion 5:	Are non-occupational exposures excluded as probable causes?
Criterion 6:	Does dermatitis improve away from work exposure to the suspected irritant or allergen?
Criterion 7:	Do patch or provocation tests identify a probable causal agent?

Data from Mathias CG. Contact dermatitis and workers' compensation: criteria for establishing occupational causation and aggravation. J Am Acad Dermatol 1989;20(5 Pt 1):842–8.

proposed by Mathias should be used to assess probability for workplace causality. Answering "yes" to at least 4 of the questions leads to a presumption of a greater than 50% probability of occupational causation, which implies a "reasonable degree of medical certainty" that the dermatitis is the result of occupational activities. The diagnosis of ACD rests on proper diagnostic patch testing and determination of relevance. The diagnosis of ICD unfortunately remains one of exclusion. A maxim which must be appreciated is that contact dermatitis, especially of the hand is often the collective consequence of irritant, allergic, endogenous, and climactic factors; and therefore may be nonoccupational, partially occupational, or wholly occupational.[50]

History of the Dermatitis

A detailed history of the dermatitis by the patient remains paramount to the workup of OCD. The date of onset, site of onset, description, evolution of the dermatitis, and accompanying symptoms may suggest ACD or ICD or even a causative factor. For example, erythema, burning, and stinging immediately after contact implies an irritant reaction whereas the abrupt appearance of hives suggests contact urticaria. Moreover, intense pruritus may support ACD. A previous history of atopic eczema, psoriasis, or other dermatitis should be elicited, as many cases of possible OCD are complicated by secondary diagnoses and the disease course of atopic individuals may be protracted.[51] The time course of the dermatitis, one of the Mathias criteria, is often highly relevant. ACD may be precipitated by as few as 2 exposures or require years of persistent contact. The rapidity of developing OCD after

exposure varies greatly between professions and even among individuals with similar exposures. For example, apprentice hairdressers have a propensity to develop irritant OCD within the first year. ACD to chromates in cement is not influenced by exposure time and may take years before induction. In stark contrast, a delayed type IV sensitivity to epoxy may be elicited by a single contact. Furthermore, observations of improvement away from work, (or lack thereof) and response to therapy are noteworthy. Patients must be questioned specifically regarding the topical application of all medicaments (eg, topical antibiotics, topical steroids) and home remedies, as any may contain ingredients capable of provoking a superimposed irritant and/or allergic dermatitis which may perpetuate or mask the underlying etiology.

Despite the importance of thorough elicitation of history, a Canadian survey of dermatologists revealed that occupational history taking was poor, as only 5% of dermatologists queried about exposures and only 3% asked patients to bring material safety data sheets (MSDSs) from their workplace.[52]

Occupational History and Workplace Surveys

Investigation of the possibility of OCD requires that the physician gain extensive knowledge of a patient's occupational activities. It is not sufficient to know what their job title is; the physician must know what they actually do. Relevant information includes past and previous jobs, (including length of employment in that job) chemical exposures, and workplace environment. The patient should be queried regarding dermatitis at any previous jobs and if any WC was received. The duration and frequency of contact with chemicals, both irritants and potential allergens, should be documented. The patient should be questioned regarding exposure to and duration of wet work, which itself can cause ICD or predispose to ICD or ACD from other sources. Likewise, the physical environment of the workplace including humidity, temperature, airflow, and control measures (if any, such as encapsulation), cleansing agents, frequency of hand washing, and use of barrier creams may elucidate precipitating factors which predispose the skin to dermatitis. MSDSs may reveal significant exposures, but they have shortcomings, which are discussed later. The physician should request information regarding the use of personal protective equipment such as gloves (including the material, thickness, frequency with which they are exchanged for new pairs, donning technique, duration of daily wear, presence of cuffs), and safety training received (if any). ACD is typically sporadic whereas ICD may affect groups of workers; therefore inquire if any other employees have dermatitis. Knowledge of the patient's hobbies and exposures away from work may reveal competing etiologies of dermatitis such as gardening, painting, or woodwork.

Physicians must be aware that the identification of the offending agent is principally dependent on the history and thus the patient's interpretation of details. Therefore, if clinical history, physical examination, and patch test results remain inconclusive, a workplace survey may be required. Such visits by a physician may reveal inadvertent or previously unrecognized exposures, the degree and duration of exposures to irritants, possible allergens, and environmental factors such as humidity, heat, and cold. If ACD is suspected, the relevance (or irrelevance) of positive patch test/s may (possibly) be established. The reader is referred to **Box 1** for a summary of important questions critical to the diagnosis and management of OCD.

Physical Examination

The examination should focus on the areas of suspected OCD, but inspection of the entire integument should follow with an emphasis on evidence of competing diagnoses such as extensive psoriasis, flexural eczema, or dermatophyte infection. The cause of dermatitis can only rarely be determined by anatomical location or morphology of lesions alone, but specific patterns may narrow the possibilities, suggest an exposure, or aid in ruling out competing diagnoses such as tinea or psoriasis. There are no pathognomonic features that distinguish irritant from allergic contact dermatitis, although vesicles are more

---

Box 1
Integral components in the initial evaluation of suspected OCD

History of the dermatitis

○ Date and initial anatomic location of onset, progression of lesion/s, and description (including rapidity of evolution)
○ Relative severity of symptoms (especially itch versus pain/stinging/burning)
○ Course of the dermatitis as related to work exposures, vacations, and weekends
○ Response to and/or use of prescribed medications, over-the-counters, and home remedies

Medical History

○ Previous history of skin disease especially contact dermatitis, atopic dermatitis, psoriasis

Occupational history and exposures

○ List of previous and present occupations with dates of employment
○ Potential exposures to irritants and allergens, including duration and frequency
○ Duration and exposure to wet work
○ Previous history of OCD, receipt of previous WC benefits
○ Job title and description of work (be specific and detailed) including length of time in current position, recent job change/s, and time spent on specific work activities
○ General work conditions including ambient humidity, temperature, airflow; and control measures (if any) including ventilation and encapsulation
○ Occupational hygiene including number of times hands are washed/day, cleanser used, and water temperature; use of moisturizers and barrier creams
○ Use of personal protective equipment including glove material, thickness, changing schedule, donning and removal technique, and safety training received (if any)
○ Coworker – are any other workers affected?

Hobbies and extracurricular activities

○ Hobbies, including their relation to the dermatitis, duration of exposures, recent changes
○ House work, including all personal care products, detergents and soaps, and personal protective equipment used; and any recent changes in the aforementioned products

likely in ACD. Historically, involvement of the dorsal skin of the hands was suggestive of contact dermatitis according to some investigators, whereas palmar or lateral digit dermatitis connotes atopic eczema or dyshidrotic eczema.[53] Studies refute this theory, proposing that there is no correlation between location of dermatitis and the etiological diagnosis of ACD or ICD[54,55] with the exception that central palmar dermatitis is correlated with endogenous etiology, that is, atopic dermatitis.[54,56] Therefore, any attempt to distinguish ACD from ICD solely on the basis of appearance is perilous and fraught with pitfalls. It is important to keep in mind, though, that distinguishing between ACD and ICD is irrelevant to determining occupational causation, as both are commonly caused by occupational exposures, but distinguishing between the 2 can be vital for determining proper management.

Diagnostic Testing

Patch testing is essential to the workup of skin disease and remains the foundation of the diagnosis of ACD. As reviewed by Slodownik and colleagues,[29] follow-up studies have shown beneficial effects in the long-term outcomes for patients even when results are negative.[57–59] Further, the absence of patch testing correlates with a concomitant increase in morbidity as well as adverse financial implications for patients, health services providers, and the state.[50] The patch test attempts to reproduce a contact dermatitis under uniform conditions but remains imperfect, for it is incapable of replicating the exact conditions (ie, friction, sweating, humidity, duration or concentration of exposure) which precipitated the dermatitis. With a sensitivity and specificity of 70% to 80%[60] patch testing is cost-effective if patients meet 2 conditions:[61]

1. There is a strong clinical suspicion of allergy.
2. Patients are tested with chemicals relevant to exposures.

Post-patch test probabilities do not justify testing with random selections of chemicals, as noted by Bruze.[62]

The patch testing process used to investigate potential OCD is identical to the standard patch testing procedure which has been reviewed extensively in many manuscripts and textbooks[6] to which the interested reader is referred. The only significant difference when investigating potential OCD as compared with non-OCD is in the allergens selected for testing. In addition to the standard panel that is applied to all patients being investigated for contact dermatitis, additional allergens must be specially selected based on the occupational exposures of the patient. Several occupations with a high risk for contact dermatitis, such as hairdressing, metalworking, and dentistry, have standard patch tests series which are commercially available. Testing with additional allergens depending on exposure and specific occupation of each individual patient significantly increases the probability of detecting relevant allergens.[63] As discussed by Slodownik and colleagues,[29] patch testing that is performed in a dedicated patch-test clinic enhances the identification of relevant allergens,[64,65] which is attributable to the increased number of patch tests applied, the testing of patient's own products, and to the interpretation of results.[66]

Job Interruption

Prescribing a leave of absence from the workplace can be diagnostic and therapeutic. However, a number of practical issues, unrelated to the potential occupational dermatitis demand consideration.

Regarding the diagnostic value of prescribing work leave, several issues must be considered. First, when a patient is given a medical work excuse, but continues to report to perform alternative "light duty," the patient may still be exposed to workplace irritants or allergens; the most common example being the soap in the bathroom. In this situation, if a patient's dermatitis does not clear, it does not necessarily indicate that factors outside of work are causing persistence. Second, when a patient is medically proscribed completely for diagnostic purposes, it should be for a sufficient period of time to see clear improvement in the dermatitis, typically at least 2 weeks. Care must be taken to make sure that aggressive therapy does not lead to a mistaken assumption of improvement while off work, for example if a patient is put on a 2 week prednisone taper for the concurrent 2 weeks of work leave, because of the prednisone the dermatitis will improve during the leave and flare upon the return to work as the prednisone is tapered.

For removal from work to have a significant therapeutic effect, 2 points should be considered. First, the exposure or activity that caused the dermatitis cannot be resumed upon return to work, or the dermatitis will quickly recur. Second, the barrier function of the skin recovers more slowly than the clinical appearance of the skin, so to allow the barrier function to recover, the patient should be kept off work for additional time after the dermatitis has resolved, although exactly how long it takes for the barrier function to recover will vary from patient to patient.

Practical considerations regarding options for removing the patient from the work environment must be taken into account. The patient may be able to take paid sick time off from work, they may be able to take paid Family Medical Leave Act (FMLA) time off from work, or they may be able to take paid vacation time off from work. However, depending on the policies of their employer they may not be paid while taking time off by any of these routes (sick time, FMLA time, or vacation time), and many patients are unable to afford the loss of income associated with a prolonged (2 week) period of lost wages. Another possible option is that they may be able to take time off by short term disability if it is offered as a benefit by their employer. Short term disability usually applies to the first 6 weeks to 90 days of time off of work, if it is offered by their employer. With any of these methods of getting a worker time off from work, the physician who recommends the time off should be prepared to complete significant amounts of paperwork on the patient's behalf to justify the leave.

By law, all workers can use the FMLA if they need time off of work as a result of illness or injury, and the law states that they cannot lose their job for taking time off for this purpose. However, employers do not have to pay employees while they are off work under the FMLA. Although it is unethical to do so, employers can often find creative reasons to justify discharging the employee if the employee takes time off from work.

Material Safety Data Sheets: Functions and Limitations

MSDSs play a fundamental role in the evaluation of suspected occupational dermatitis. Regulations protecting workers were first established in 1970 through passing of the Occupational Safety and Health Act by Congress. Subsequent legislation founded the Occupational Safety and Health Administration (OSHA). In 1986 OSHA instituted the Hazard Communication Standard (HCS) which included the origination of MSDSs . MSDSs must include at least the minimum following requirements:

1. Chemical and common (trade) names of all hazardous ingredients
2. Physical and chemical characteristics of the agent or agents
3. Physical hazards such as flammability or explosive reactivity
4. Medical symptoms, signs, or known diseases that can be caused or aggravated by exposure

5. Primary route or routes of entry
6. Legal time-weighted exposure limits and toxicity information established by OSHA
7. Carcinogenicity
8. Precautions for safe handling and use, including appropriate hygienic practices, personal protective equipment, and procedures for clean up of spills and leaks
9. Engineering control requirements
10. Emergency and first-aid measures
11. Dates of MSDS preparation, edits, and updates
12. Manufacturer contact information

Use of MSDSs in the workup of occupational dermatitis is crippled by serious handicaps. According to Bernstein[67] there are 4 major limitations to MSDSs. First, vital information is often omitted regarding generic names and formulas of hazardous chemicals because OSHA permits exclusion of such information if the manufacturer deems said information a trade secret or the chemical not hazardous. Second, potential respiratory or skin sensitizing chemicals (ie, known contact allergens) are generally not considered toxic or hazardous. Third is a deficiency to update the most current permissible exposure levels.[68,69] The fourth limitation stems from neglect to require documented clinical information with respect to specific occupational cutaneous diseases which have been correlated with a particular agent. In addition, it should be noted that the definition of a hazardous chemical is relatively vague in the OSHA guidelines, meaning that manufacturers and importers have significant leeway in deciding which chemicals to list on an MSDS.

If MSDSs are not readily accessible, the internet provides several major MSDS sites (eg, the Cornell MSDS web site).[67] When reviewing MSDSs, a summation of constituents totaling less than 100% should forewarn that a manufacturer may have omitted agents they deemed nonhazardous or a trade secret. A suspected omission should prompt a telephone conversation by way of the required contact information provided on the MSDS. Furthermore, an emergency obligates the release of proprietary information by the manufacturer per OSHA.

In summary, under current OSHA guidelines, most known contact allergens do not need to be listed on MSDSs, which relegates the utility of MSDSs to nearly useless as an aid in the evaluation of the patient with suspected OCD. MSDSs do typically contain information regarding the skin irritancy potential of a substance, and this information can be used to help determine if it is possible or advisable to patch test the patient with the substance. In most situations, the most important, and possibly the only useful, information on an MSDS is the name and contact information of the manufacturer of the substance.

WORKERS' COMPENSATION AND DISABILITY

Workers' compensation and disability insurance are explicit entities and must be considered separately. WC is a form of insurance that all employers must carry. When an injury or illness occurs to an employee when at work, this insurance pays for the medical care of the injured worker and, if the worker is unable to work, the insurance will also pay the worker a fraction of their normal wages. It does not matter if the worker caused the injury or disease through personal negligence, if the injury or disease was caused by employer negligence, or if the injury or disease was purely accidental and unforeseeable. The only requirement for coverage by WC is that the injury or illness occurs when the person is working.

Workers who receive WC are required to continue working if a job is available which they are able to perform, given the restrictions imposed upon their activities by the disease or illness. Physicians are often asked to list what tasks a worker with an occupational injury or illness is able to perform and what tasks they are not able to perform. A "Work Abilities Form" is frequently used to report these limitations. The physician should be aware that the more restrictions they place on the worker, the less likely the worker will be able to return to work, but if inadequate restrictions are instituted, the worker may continue to suffer from the illness or injury because of repeated exacerbations.

The details of WC laws vary significantly from state to state in several ways. Examples of interstate differences include the percentage of the employee's salary which is covered by WC and the duration the worker is entitled to WC benefits. It must be noted that in many cases the employer will dispute whether or not the worker's illness or injury truly was the result of workplace activities. The method of resolution of these disputes also shows interstate variance. As a result of these issues, it is often advisable to recommend that a worker pursuing WC retain an attorney. In most cases there is no upfront cost to the worker and the attorney is compensated through the receipt of a percentage of any WC benefits awarded.

Conversely, disability insurance, similar to health insurance, is purchased by individuals for themselves, is provided to individuals by the government Social Security Disability Insurance (SSDI), or is purchased for an individual by their employer.

Unlike WC, disability is independent of where, when, or how an individual is injured or acquires an illness. All that matters is how severely the function of the individual is affected. If the individual is deemed unable to partake in gainful employment of any type, they are considered totally disabled. If they are deemed to able to partake in at least some type of gainful employment, then they are considered partially disabled. In the case of SSDI, a judge makes the decision if the individual is totally, partially, or not disabled. In the case of disability insurance, the insurance company responsible for the policy determines if the worker is disabled based on the details of the policy.

To summarize, the key question of WC regards if the injury or illness was caused by the individual's job – the type or severity of injury is irrelevant until after occupational causality is established. In the case of disability, the key question is if the injury or illness is severe enough to limit the individual's ability to be gainfully employed – independent of how or where the injury occurred. Several examples to illustrate these points are in **Box 2**.

The concept of impairment should be understood by physicians dealing with potential OCD. According to the fifth edition of the *AMA Guides to the Evaluation of Permanent Impairment*,[70] impairment is defined as "a loss, loss of use, or derangement of any body part, organ system, or organ function." In disability cases, the physician evaluates the degree of impairment (judged by anatomical or functional loss) and provides an assessment of impairment to disability raters, judges, hearing officers, or commissioners.[46] Subsequently, these non-medical personnel judge an individual's disability. Again, impairment is a medical assessment determined by health care personnel whereas disability is a non-medical pronouncement concluded by WC boards or by way of litigation.[8]

Unlike impairment, disability is dependent on a specific job and the ability to compete in the open market. Impairment does not necessarily imply disability and the 2 must be considered separately. For instance, and individual with loss of the distal phalanx of the second digit results in the same impairment rating in a roofer and concert violinist, yet the rated disability is much greater for the musician.[46] A physician requested to perform an evaluation of impairment should employ the most current edition of *AMA Guides to the Evaluation of Permanent Impairment*.[71]

Preparing a Letter and/or Report

Subsequent to patient evaluation and initiation of treatment, a letter should be prepared and

Example 1: An individual who works as a dishwasher develops irritant hand dermatitis because of chronic exposure to soap and water at work. He is able to keep working but requires physician visits and prescription steroids. He would qualify for WC compensation which would pay for the physician visits and prescriptions. He would not qualify for disability since he is able to work.

Example 2: An individual develops severe palmoplantar psoriasis that is recalcitrant to therapy. It is so severe that it is intensely painful to walk and she cannot use her hands. She is no longer able to perform her job as a janitor, nor is she able to perform any other jobs. She would qualify for disability but not for WC.

Example 3: An individual develops severe vesicular hand dermatitis when working as a machinist. She is found to be allergic to nickel. The hand dermatitis is sufficiently severe that she is unable to work. She stops working, but the hand dermatitis develops into an endogenous chronic vesicular hand dermatitis which is sufficiently severe to prevent her from engaging in gainful employment. She qualifies for WC because the nickel allergy and hand dermatitis developed while she was working as a machinist. Because the condition persists permanently and prevents gainful employment, she would also qualify for disability.

formatted. In general, the report should be formatted as a letter to a referring physician, but is distinguished by the necessity to include language which is comprehensible by non-physicians. This letter will need to be intelligible by the worker, worker's employer, and/or professional disability rating personnel. Beyond inclusion of the patient's occupational history, patch test results, and physical examination, the report should also contain the following: (1) a brief overview of the Mathias criteria for establishing occupational causation or aggravation; (2) a declaration of which of the 7 Mathias criteria are satisfied and attendant justification for each criterion; (3) acknowledgment that since 4 or more of the 7 criteria have been fulfilled, occupational causation is established to "a reasonable degree of medical certainty"; (4) if needed, the letter should include specific instructions regarding treatment, future prevention (eg, workplace hygiene), and rehabilitation, as well as projected length of illness and prognosis.

Preparing a report that maximizes the chances for a good medical and occupational outcome for the patient can be exceptionally difficult. Appropriate accuracy (or vagueness) and detail are paramount. Although it is often medically appropriate to indicate that a certain degree of uncertainty remains in opinions regarding diagnosis, prognosis, and causality, noting this uncertainty in the report can lead to significant misinterpretation and misrepresentation by biased attorneys and biased disability insurance reviewers. Alternatively, if opinions regarding diagnosis, prognosis, future course, or activity restrictions are presented with excessive certainty, it can present difficulties if any additional information comes to light that in any way refutes these opinions. Sensitivity to the patient's occupational status may require communication with the employee and/or their employer before any final conclusions are drawn to diminish unintended consequences.[6]

MANAGEMENT: PREVENTION AND THERAPY

The initial treatment of OCD focuses on the avoidance of possible sources of antigens and/or irritants and control of the disease process. The symptoms of OCD can be acute or chronic, allergic or irritant; each of which requires a modified approach. In any case, implementation of lifestyle changes is often necessary but difficult, resulting in reduced patient compliance. An acute allergic reaction involving a limited amount of skin should respond well to potent topical steroids applied 2 to 3 times daily. Widespread involvement and/or severe symptoms may necessitate a systemic steroid taper. Typically, a starting dose of 40 to 80 mg/day of prednisone tapered over 3 weeks is adequate to control acute symptoms, but unless exposure ceases, a severe flare of dermatitis will almost certainly follow the taper.

The cornerstones of symptomatic, short term management of occupational hand dermatitis are avoidance of potential irritants and allergens, frequent moisturization, and proper hand cleansing (ie, avoid harsh/abrasive soaps, solvents). All patients should receive instruction to suspend the application of all topical medicaments and personal care products to the affected areas except those products with little-to-no potential for irritancy or allergy, such as petrolatum or desoximetasone ointment.

Acute lesions of OCD may benefit from soaks with cool water or Burrows solution. Topical steroids can provide symptomatic relief. Note, though, that applying a steroid which contains an ingredient to which the individual is allergic is akin to "tossing gasoline on the fire." Suspicion of steroid allergy should precipitate the use of hypo-allergenic products, such as desoximetasone ointment or tacrolimus ointment. As stated previously, severe cases may require systemic steroids, but said therapy will necessarily delay patch testing.

Long-term management of occupational hand dermatitis revolves around first establishing an accurate diagnosis, then individualizing the appropriate recommendations.

Education of Worker

Roughly half of all cases of OCD was reported to occur in the first 2 years of employment[72] perhaps accounted for by a lack of awareness of any probable health hazards, leading to complacency and poor occupational skin hygiene. As reviewed by Brown,[73] multiple studies have investigated the effect of education on the prevalence of OCD in various industries and proved them effective. These studies included wet work employees,[74] bakers' apprentices,[75,76] caterers,[77] hairdressers,[78,79] student auxiliary nurses,[80] manufacturers of fine chemicals,[81] and individuals in the metal working industry.[82] Ideally, job training should be instituted before placement and resultant exposure to sensitizing and irritant chemicals, and employees should receive periodic retraining. Education during training or apprenticeship is likely most important.[83,84] As stated by Brown,[73] studies have shown education to be cost-effective,[82] as well as efficacious in primary (trainee), secondary (worker), and tertiary (afflicted individual) prevention. Educational initiatives should stress the proper use of personal protective equipment, personal and environmental hygiene, and recognition of early signs and symptoms of OCD.[73]

Public Health Interventions

Recognition, elimination, substitution, and/or avoidance of hazardous materials are paramount to the prevention of OCD. Ideally, contactants with inherent strong sensitizing or irritating capacity will be identified before introduction to the workplace and every effort should be made to find a suitable substitute or to use engineering measures to eliminate the possibility of worker exposure. Passive methods to eliminate exposure (ie, methods that do not require any action or effort on the part of the worker) are much more effective than are methods involving use of personal protective equipment or other actions to be taken by workers. Examples of successful interventions include the addition of ferrous sulfate to cement in Scandinavian countries to inhibit chromate

sensitization[85–87] and the substitution of ethylene glycol with zinc borate in cooling towers.[88] Likewise, recognizing that protracted wet work contributes to the vast majority of OCD cases, Germany conceived legislation regulating wet work.

Barrier Creams and Moisturizers

Barrier creams are intended to operate as a protective layer, shielding the skin from hazardous chemicals. They are typically oil-based creams formulated to repel oils, paints, grease or solvents, or silicone-based creams intended to be efficacious against water-based products such as acids, alkalis, and metalworking fluids.[73] Barrier creams should only be applied to normal skin as they may potentiate secondary aggravation of dermatitis with application to inflamed skin. Substances to which barrier creams have proven effective are beyond the scope of this article but have been succinctly reviewed by Brown.[73] Barrier creams have been shown to aid in the prevention of hand irritation in occupations which includes health care workers,[89] textile-dyeing and printing plant workers, hairdressers, and workers in the food processing industry. Despite experimental evidence supporting the use of barrier creams, experts remain skeptical. In a survey of international experts in OCD, 98% believed barrier creams to be no more effective than bland emollients in the prevention of hand dermatitis.[90] There is also doubt concerning the translation of experimental efficacy to clinical benefits as barrier creams must be applied frequently, and in adequate amounts to be effective to all skin areas needing protection. Barrier creams may give workers a false sense of security, leading to laxity in adherence to other methods to reduce cutaneous exposure.

Beyond barrier creams, emollients are purported to prevent OCD of the irritant type, despite a scarcity of evidence.[1] The water content of the stratum corneum in healthy skin is 10% to 20%.[91] If the water content falls below 10%, the barrier capacity of the skin is impaired with concomitant increased susceptibility to irritants. As reviewed by Chew and Maibach,[91] moisturizers hydrate the stratum corneum (eg, humectants such as glycerin or urea) or reduce transepidermal water loss (eg, lipids such as petrolatum); consequently preserving barrier function and reducing the risk of irritation. Therefore, therapeutic moisturizers are of relatively greater importance in the treatment and/or prevention of ICD versus ACD. Moisturizers can prevent the development of experimentally-induced ICD and enhance the rate of healing of damaged skin.[92] Habitual application of moisturizers may prove to be an integral component in the secondary prevention of OCD.[93] Ointments or creams with the fewest possible sensitizing agents possible are recommended, including plain petrolatum, Eucerin Plus Intensive Repair Hand Cream (Beiersdorf AG, Hamburg, Germany), and Neutrogena Norwegian Formula Hand Cream (Neutrogena Corp., Los Angeles, CA.).[94] Patients should avoid moisturizers with fragrances or other potential sensitizers as well as lotions which are primarily water and ineffective because of their low lipid content.

The efficacy of barrier creams versus moisturizers is controversial and remains hotly debated. As discussed by Chew and Maibach,[91] trials with repetitive hand washing and repetitive irritation have shown contradictory conclusions, with studies concluding barrier creams to be more effective,[95] equally effective,[96,97] or less effective than moisturizers.[95] Further clouding the debate, specific barrier creams may prove efficacious against only a restricted range of irritants.[98] Notably, no known barrier cream is effective against a wide spectrum of irritants. Consequently, only barrier creams with proven efficacy against the specific exposures relevant to the patient should be recommended to prevent irritation by the agent in question. It is important to recognize that barrier creams themselves can induce ACD or ICD.[99]

Hygiene and Cleansers

Cleanliness is an important consideration in the prevention of OCD and should always be addressed. There are several fundamental requirements for an efficient skin cleanser in the prevention of OCD. As reviewed by English,[100] the cleanser should be soluble in hard, soft, cold, or hot water; it should remove foreign matter with minimal damage to the skin; should avoid defatting the skin; should be stable during storage, be easily dispensable, and not clog plumbing. Punctual rinsing of the skin or washing with a mild soap is often adequate to remove most allergens and irritants but more abrasive soaps may be required in specific situations. Wet work including frequent hand washing especially with hot water and harsh soaps contributes to the pathogenesis of ICD or causes ICD directly. Therefore, patients with active ICD of the hands should wash the hands as infrequently as possible using a mild soap and warm, not hot water, followed by application of a moisturizer. Moisturizing non-lathering cleansers such as Cetaphil Cleanser (Galderma Laboratories, Fort Worth, TX) or CeraVe Cleanser (Coria Laboratories, Dallas, TX) provide viable alternative if the hands are not extremely soiled. Workers should also maintain hygiene by regularly washing contaminated clothing, as excessive soiling often results in inadvertent skin contact when clothing is donned or removed.[101] Alcohol-based waterless hand sanitizers have been repeatedly shown to cause less irritation than washing with soap and water, even though they often sting when applied to hands with ongoing irritant dermatitis. These products should be recommended as a replacement for hand washing in appropriate occupations, especially in the health care field, as recommended by the Centers for Disease Control and Prevention. Ideally, products with an added emollient are preferred.

Gloves

Considering hand dermatitis constitutes 80% of cases of OCD, proper glove use is paramount for sufficient hand protection. Industry provides a large number of permutations of glove materials, thicknesses, and designs. The physician should have a knowledge of the basic physical and chemical properties of the glove materials available and of the job that is to be performed, including which chemical, physical, and biologic exposures are present and must be protected against. Leather and textile gloves can be used to prevent irritation from mechanical friction, as well as environmental hazards such as cold and heat.[6] Plastic and rubber gloves are used for protection from most chemical and biologic substances. As reviewed by Chew and Maibach,[91] the selection of an appropriate glove is dependent on the nature and extent of the dermal hazards,[102] as well as impermeability to chemicals, resistance to cuts, tears, abrasions, and tensile strength.[103] Further considerations include ergonomics[91] (eg, pliability, tactile sense, and gripping qualities), and cost.[102,103] Finally, the worker's individual characteristics need be examined including allergy (eg, sensitivity to latex, natural rubber, glove powder, or rubber additives), irritability, and magnitude of perspiration.[103] Excellent resources assisting in proper glove selection for the chemical in question include the "Quick Selection Guide to Chemical Protective Clothing"[104] and World Wide Web sites of glove manufacturers that provide technical support, including search engines which provide glove recommendations after a chemical exposure is entered (www.ansellpro.com, www.bestglove.com/site/chemrest/, www.northsafety.com). Finally, proper glove use, including donning and removal techniques, frequency of glove replacement and glove storage are crucially important, as the perfect glove is worthless if not used correctly.

To an extend all glove materials are permeable to some chemicals; there is no universal material affording protection from all chemicals. **Table 2** lists the general characteristics and chemical resistance of various glove materials. For some jobs and certain chemicals, there is no glove capable of furnishing a significant barrier.[6] If sweating and maceration are a significant problem, light textile gloves should be worn beneath polymer gloves.[6] Although effective in the prevention of OCD;[101,105,106] gloves can increase the risk for OCD[1] if not used properly. Mechanisms include: irritation from sweat entrapment and/or friction, accidental occlusion of irritants and allergens beneath the glove enhancing cutaneous absorption, and contact sensitivity to glove additives (especially accelerators).[73] Glove failure may occur secondary to improper selection and/or inappropriate use. Kwon and colleagues[107] reviewed 3 primary mechanisms by which gloved hands can be exposed to chemicals: permeation (ie, substance diffuses through glove at molecular level), penetration (ie, substance passes through physical hole in glove), and contamination (ie, hands are contaminated before glove donning and substance is transferred to interior glove surface).

It is exceedingly important that the selected gloves be changed at appropriate intervals to minimize permeation. Likewise, the longer a given pair of gloves is used, the more likely they undergo degradation. Degradation is defined as a change in the physical properties of a glove as a result of exposure to chemicals and it begins as soon as the glove is first exposed to a causative chemical. The most common chemicals causing degradation of rubber gloves (latex, nitrile, and neoprene) are organic solvents and petrochemicals. Gloves that have undergone degradation are much more susceptible to permeation and physical damage, leading to severely compromised gloves. The sign of advanced degradation is a loss of elasticity or an increase in the stiffness of the glove material. Finally, employee education should emphasize proper donning and removal technique to minimize contamination.[107] The employee must be instructed to never don a glove when their hands are contaminated with any irritants or allergens.

Although proper selection and use of gloves is absolutely necessary to prevent OCD, practitioners should not rely excessively on gloves as a solution for occupational hand dermatitis, especially occupational ACD. It was the senior author's experience that even with selection of the correct glove and training on proper use; it is distinctly uncommon for workers to be able to completely eliminate exposure to a chemical by using gloves. This is usually because of an inability to complete their work in a timely fashion when wearing gloves or because of other practical issues in the workplace.

Steroids

Topical corticosteroids remain the keystone in the first-line intervention of acute OCD. Corticosteroids exhibit broad mechanisms of action including suppression of the production and effects of humoral factors involved in the inflammatory response; inhibition of leukocyte migration to areas of inflammation; and interference with the functions of endothelial cells, granulocytes, mast cells, and fibroblasts.[108] The effectiveness of topical corticosteroids in the symptomatic treatment of ACD is well documented in the literature. In a double-blinded study of female volunteers ($n = 20$) with documented nickel allergy, 0.05% fluticasone propionate was effective in reducing nickel-induced contact dermatitis.[109] Other studies have upheld the benefits of topical steroids in ACD,[110] however their efficacy in ICD remains disputable. Treatment of ICD with steroids can offer rapid relief of symptoms, but has yielded conflicting results when considering overall effects. Recent studies support the traditional use of topical steroids to treat the inflammation of ICD.[111–113] Contradictorily, Levin and colleagues[114] concluded corticosteroids to be ineffective in the therapy of surfactant-induced irritant dermatitis when compared with the vehicle and the untreated control. Evidence suggests that repeated use of steroids impairs skin barrier function by decreasing the production of intercellular stratum corneum lipids and through a decrease in thickness of the epidermis; and these effects would be expected to delay recovery from ICD and to increase susceptibility to repeated exposures. In summary, corticosteroids appear clearly beneficial in ACD and to be effective for acute control of the symptoms of ICD. Conflicting conclusions in the chronic therapy of ICD warrant further investigation.

In choosing a steroid, the physician should consider: the site and frequency of application, the vehicle and associated advantages and disadvantages of ointment, cream, gel, lotion, solution, or foam, and amount to be dispensed.[115] In general, steroid ointments are preferred to other vehicles secondary to fewer preservatives and additives and greater lipid content. This is especially true considering that patients with ICD and ACD have an elevated risk for developing

Table 2
Summary of general characteristics of glove materials

Material	Chemical Protection		Biologic Protection	Puncture and Tear Resistance	Dexterity	Price	Allergy
	Good	Poor					
Latex	Water	Most chemicals	Excellent	Good	Excellent	Low	Type I Type IV
Nitrile	Water, most organic solvents, most hydrocarbons, oils, greases, selected acids and bases	Ketones, aromatics, chlorinated hydrocarbons, esters, some acids	Good	Good	Good	Low	Type IV
Vinyl	Acids, bases, oils, greases, peroxides, amines	Organic or petroleum based solvents, aldehydes	Poor	Poor	Poor	Low	Rare
Neoprene	Alcohols, phenols, peroxides, acids, hydrocarbons, bases	Halogenated and aromatic hydrocarbons	Good	Good	Good	Med	Type IV
Multilayer laminates	All classes	Isolated small molecule solvents	N/A	Medium	Very poor	High	Rare

Material	Chemical Protection	Biologic Protection	Dexterity	Durability	Price	Allergy
Latex	Poor	Best	Best	Good	Low	Type I Type IV
Nitrile	Good	Good	Good	Good	Low	Type IV
Vinyl	Fair	Poor	Poor	Poor	Low	None
Neoprene	Good	Good	Good	Good	High	Uncommon

sensitivity to any potential allergens that are applied to the inflamed skin. Caution is necessary in the prescription of protracted therapy with topical steroids as long-term use can result in well known local effects including permanent skin atrophy, striae, and telangiectasia.[108]

Topical Calcineurin Inhibitors

In the therapy of contact dermatitis, topical steroids have long been a cornerstone in the dermatologists' armamentarium. Recent studies suggest that topical calcineurin inhibitors (TCIs) may provide an appropriate therapeutic alternative. TCIs are often prescribed as a component of a rotational regimen with both topical steroids and moisturizers. In a double-blind, intraindividual (both medications were compared in the same patient) study of 28 individuals, topical 0.1% tacrolimus under occlusion proved as effective as 0.1% mometasone in petrolatum in the suppression of ACD elicited by nickel.[116] The most common side effects reported with TCIs are transient skin burning or sensation of warmth.[117,118] TCIs do not induce skin atrophy, telangiectasia, or tachyphylaxis.[119,120] Such characteristics of TCIs are particularly appealing for use in sensitive skin areas such as the neck, face, and groin. As a result of its increased efficacy and lower allergenicity of its vehicle, the author's strong preference in TCIs is to use only tacrolimus 0.1% ointment in the treatment of OCD.

As reviewed in the third edition of *Contact and Occupational Dermatology;*[6] when therapeutic intervention and preventative measures fail, chronic skin impairment and disability may ensue. Such scenarios demand the institution of rehabilitation to restore vocational abilities and economic success for the patient. Often, such restoration can be realized by changing jobs within the workplace. Recalcitrant cases may require temporary removal from the workplace environment and subsequent vocational retraining in a different occupation. Such rehabilitation interventions can be coordinated through insurance carriers or by way of WC agencies. Comparatively speaking, rehabilitation, although expensive, remains much more fiscally responsible than disability benefits.

PROGNOSIS

As reviewed by Cahill and colleagues[121] the prognosis of OCD remains difficult to quantify and compare between studies secondary to a lack of standardization. With these limitations the prognosis of OCD is generally considered to be poor but highly variable; some patients exhibit a self-limited disease with no or infrequent exacerbations, others evolve a chronic disabling process. Recent studies show the recalcitrance of HE. An 8-year follow-up study reported that 67.6% of patients were still experiencing episodes of HE 8 years after diagnosis.[122] Likewise, a 12-year follow-up on farmers showed that 12 years after diagnosis 40% had persistent disease in the last 12 months.[123] A 12-year follow-up study on OCD showed 70% with symptoms in the last year;[23] and a 15-year population-based study estimated that 44% had symptoms in the last year.[124] Recent studies show that 78% to 84% of patients with OCD improve when appropriately treated.[14,125] In marked contrast, as reviewed by Hogan, Dannaker, and Maibach,[126] studies before 1990 noted improvement in only 30% to 50% of patients. Goh[127] proposes that the improved prognosis of OCD may be secondary to superior diagnostic procedures, increased education and preventative efforts, and enhanced accuracy in identification of contactants.

Studies comparing the prognosis of ACD versus ICD have failed to reach a consensus with outcomes suggesting that ACD has a better, equal, or worse prognosis than ICD.[126] Future comparisons will face similar formidable pitfalls secondary to the difficulty of definitively distinguishing cases of ACD and ICD and the widely varying prevalence of the offending agents. The corollary is that pervasive and difficult to avoid contact allergens such as formaldehyde, nickel, and chromate have a poor prognosis; their ubiquity often leads to a chronic and protracted course.[126] In contrast, epoxy resin is easily avoided outside of specific occupational settings and carries a more favorable disease course.[127] The prognosis of ICD is similarly varied. Dermatitis secondary to acids or alkalis typically clears after withdrawal from exposure, whereas chronic cumulative ICD to cutting fluids, solvents, or wet work routinely incites recalcitrant disease. Regarding both ICD and ACD, the duration of exposure is positively correlated with chronicity, meaning that the longer the patient has active ACD or ICD before the etiology is removed, the more likely they are to have protracted disease even after the etiology is removed.[125] Chronic cumulative ICD is associated with a worse prognosis than ACD or acute ICD.[14,90,128]

A variety of predictive factors for persistent dermatitis have been proposed in the literature including duration of disease, sex, inability to avoid causative agent, age, patient knowledge, job change, morphology, area or extent of disease, and history of positive patch test. The duration of symptoms before diagnosis is correlated with a poor prognosis and recalcitrant disease.[9,125,129–131]

Increased patient knowledge was associated with improved prognosis in studies by Holness and Nethercott[132] and Kalimo and colleagues.[133] The extent of the disease correlates with a negative prognosis[124,134,135] as can the morphology[136] and an inability to avoid the causative agent.[137] Atopic patients are more susceptible to irritant factors, are more likely to develop OCD and have a worse prognosis[51] and are more likely to have persistent dermatitis.[135] A history of childhood eczema contributed to a less favorable prognosis as did a history of a positive patch test.[135] The influence of sex has yielded inconclusive and mixed results.[14,123] Likewise, the literature regarding the effect of age on prognosis is varied,[14,125,138–141] but Meding and colleagues[135] observed that a younger age at onset correlated with a poorer prognosis. Literature examining occupation change on OCD prognosis yields dissenting results. As reviewed by Cahill and colleagues the majority of studies advance that a change does not significantly alter prognosis.[2,138,140–144] In contrast some authors purport prognosis is improved by a change in occupation.[123,145–147] Notably, a study by Halbert and colleagues[130] compared chromate sensitive individuals whose dermatitis resolved after a change in occupation to a group lacking any post-occupational amelioration; the only significant difference that predicted post-job change course was the duration of the disease before job change.

Occupation changes are not always associated with improvement in OCD, and the dermatologic community lacks a consensus opinion. As discussed by Meding and colleagues,[124] there is no literature supporting a guarantee to clear the dermatitis with occupation change but an improvement may be expected. Therefore, before a job change is recommended, every attempt should be made to continue the current job by taking all practical steps to limit exposure and improve patient and employer education. Furthermore, the decision to change jobs can have unforeseen consequences. For example, older workers may experience difficulty finding employment[125,126,148] or suffer a reduction in income.

REFERENCES

1. Diepgen TL, Coenraads PJ. The epidemiology of occupational contact dermatitis. Int Arch Occup Environ Health 1999;72(8):496–506.
2. Fregert S. Occupational dermatitis in a 10-year material. Contact Dermatitis 1975;1(2):96–107.
3. Keil JE, Shmunes E. The epidemiology of work-related skin disease in South Carolina. Arch Dermatol 1983;119(8):650–4.
4. Mathias CG. Occupational dermatoses. J Am Acad Dermatol 1988;19(6):1107–14.
5. Goh CL. An epidemiological comparison between occupational and non-occupational hand eczema. Br J Dermatol 1989;120(1):77–82.
6. Marks JG, Elsner P, DeLeo VA. Contact & occupational dermatology. 3rd ed. St. Louis, (MO): Mosby; 2002. p. 431.
7. Holness DL. Characteristic features of occupational dermatitis: epidemiologic studies of occupational skin disease reported by contact dermatitis clinics. Occup Med 1994;9(1):45–52.
8. Belsito DV. Occupational contact dermatitis: etiology, prevalence, and resultant impairment/disability. J Am Acad Dermatol 2005;53(2):303–13.
9. Wall LM, Gebauer KA. Occupational skin disease in Western Australia. Contact Dermatitis 1991;24(2):101–9.
10. Goh CL, Soh SD. Occupational dermatoses in Singapore. Contact Dermatitis 1984;11(5):288–93.
11. Kanerva L, Estlander T, Jolanki R. Occupational skin disease in Finland. An analysis of 10 years of statistics from an occupational dermatology clinic. Int Arch Occup Environ Health 1988;60(2):89–94.
12. Sertoli A, Gola M, Martinelli C, et al. Epidemiology of contact dermatitis. Semin Dermatol 1989;8(2):120–6.
13. Rietschel RL, Mathias CG, Fowler JF Jr, et al. Relationship of occupation to contact dermatitis: evaluation in patients tested from 1998 to 2000. Am J Contact Dermatitis 2002;13(4):170–6.
14. Nethercott JR, Holness DL. Disease outcome in workers with occupational skin disease. J Am Acad Dermatol 1994;30(4):569–74.
15. Meding B, Swanbeck G. Prevalence of hand eczema in an industrial city. Br J Dermatol 1987;116(5):627–34.
16. Bryld LE, Agner T, Kyvik KO, et al. Hand eczema in twins: a questionnaire investigation. Br J Dermatol 2000;142(2):298–305.
17. Mathias CG, Morrison JH. Occupational skin diseases, United States. Results from the Bureau of Labor Statistics Annual Survey of Occupational Injuries and Illnesses, 1973 through 1984. Arch Dermatol 1988;124(10):1519–24.
18. Koch P. Occupational contact dermatitis. Recognition and management. Am J Clin Dermatol 2001; 2(6):353–65.
19. Bureau of Labor Statistics. Occupational Injuries and illnesses in the United States. [WWW document.] Available at: http://www.bls.gov/iif. Accessed December 2009.
20. Lushniak BD. Occupational contact dermatitis. Dermatol Ther 2004;17(3):272–7.
21. Mathias CG. The cost of occupational skin disease. Arch Dermatol 1985;121(3):332–4.
22. Cvetkovski RS, Rothman KJ, Olsen J, et al. Relation between diagnoses on severity, sick leave, and

loss of job among patients with occupational hand eczema. Br J Dermatol 2005;152(1):93–8.

23. Meding B, Lantto R, Lindahl G, et al. Occupational skin disease in Sweden–a 12-year follow-up. Contact Dermatitis 2005;53(6):308–13.

24. Diepgen TL, Agner T, Aberer W, et al. Management of chronic hand eczema. Contact Dermatitis 2007; 57(4):203–10.

25. Skoet R, Zachariae R, Agner T. Contact dermatitis and quality of life: a structured review of the literature. Br J Dermatol 2003;149(3):452–6.

26. Cvetkovski RS, Zachariae R, Jensen H, et al. Quality of life and depression in a population of occupational hand eczema patients. Contact Dermatitis 2006;54(2):106–11.

27. Beltrani VS. Occupational dermatoses. Ann Allergy Asthma Immunol 1999;83(6 Pt 2):607–13.

28. Basketter DA. Chemistry of contact allergens and irritants. Am J Contact Dermatitis 1998;9(2): 119–24.

29. Slodownik D, Lee A, Nixon R. Irritant contact dermatitis: a review. Australas J Dermatol 2008; 49(1):1–9, quiz 10–1.

30. Heinemann C, Paschold C, Fluhr J, et al. Induction of a hardening phenomenon by repeated application of SLS: analysis of lipid changes in the stratum corneum. Acta Derm Venereol 2005;85(4):290–5.

31. Yoshikawa N, Imokawa G, Akimoto K, et al. Regional analysis of ceramides within the stratum corneum in relation to seasonal changes. Dermatology 1994;188(3):207–14.

32. Hu CH. Sweat-related dermatoses: old concept and new scenario. Dermatologica 1991;182(2):73–6.

33. Dickel H, Kuss O, Schmidt A, et al. Importance of irritant contact dermatitis in occupational skin disease. Am J Clin Dermatol 2002;3(4):283–9.

34. Jungbauer FH, Lensen GJ, Groothoff JW, et al. Exposure of the hands to wet work in nurses. Contact Dermatitis 2004;50(4):225–9.

35. Berardesca E, Distante F. The modulation of skin irritation. Contact Dermatitis 1994;31(5):281–7.

36. Tupker RA, Pinnagoda J, Coenraads PJ, et al. The influence of repeated exposure to surfactants on the human skin as determined by transepidermal water loss and visual scoring. Contact Dermatitis 1989;20(2):108–14.

37. Rietschel RL. Mechanisms in irritant contact dermatitis. Clin Dermatol 1997;15(4):557–9.

38. Effendy I, Loffler H, Maibach HI. Epidermal cytokines in murine cutaneous irritant responses. J Appl Toxicol 2000;20(4):335–41.

39. Piguet PF, Grau GE, Hauser C, et al. Tumor necrosis factor is a critical mediator in hapten induced irritant and contact hypersensitivity reactions. J Exp Med 1991;173(3):673–9.

40. Lisby S. Mechanisms of irritant contact dermatitis. In: Menne T, Frosch PJ, Lepoittevin JP, editors. Contact dermatitis. Berlin: Springer; 2006. p. 69–80.

41. Gaspari AA. The role of keratinocytes in the pathophysiology of contact dermatitis. Contact Dermatitis 1997;17:377–405.

42. Pigatto PD, Legori A, Bigardi AS. Occupational dermatitis from physical causes. Clin Dermatol 1992;10(2):231–43.

43. Ingber A, Merims S. The validity of the Mathias criteria for establishing occupational causation and aggravation of contact dermatitis. Contact Dermatitis 2004;51(1):9–12.

44. Templet JT, Hall S, Belsito DV. Etiology of hand dermatitis among patients referred for patch testing. Dermatitis 2004;15(1):25–32.

45. Warshaw E, Lee G, Storrs FJ. Hand dermatitis: a review of clinical features, therapeutic options, and long-term outcomes. Am J Contact Dermatitis 2003;14(3):119–37.

46. Adams RM. Occupational skin disease. 3rd ed. Philadelphia: Saunders; 1999. p. 792.

47. Mathias CG. Contact dermatitis and workers' compensation: criteria for establishing occupational causation and aggravation. J Am Acad Dermatol 1989;20(5 Pt 1):842–8.

48. Marrakchi S, Maibach HI. What is occupational contact dermatitis? An operational definition. Dermatol Clin 1994;12(3):477–84.

49. Kanerva L. Handbook of occupational dermatology. New York: Springer; 2000. p. 1300.

50. Rietschel RL. Human and economic impact of allergic contact dermatitis and the role of patch testing. J Am Acad Dermatol 1995;33(5 Pt 1):812–5.

51. Shmunes E, Keil J. The role of atopy in occupational dermatoses. Contact Dermatitis 1984;11(3): 174–8.

52. Holness DL. Health care services use by workers with work-related contact dermatitis. Dermatitis 2004;15(1):18–24.

53. Marks JG Jr. Occupational skin disease in hairdressers. Occup Med 1986;1(2):273–84.

54. Veien NK, Hattel T, Laurberg G. Hand eczema: causes, course, and prognosis I. Contact Dermatitis 2008;58(6):330–4.

55. Magina S, Barros MA, Ferreira JA, et al. Atopy, nickel sensitivity, occupation, and clinical patterns in different types of hand dermatitis. Am J Contact Dermatitis 2003;14(2):63–8.

56. Cronin E. Clinical patterns of hand eczema in women. Contact Dermatitis 1985;13(3):153–61.

57. Paul MA, Fleischer AB Jr, Scherertz EF. Patients' benefit from contact dermatitis evaluation: Results of a follow-up study. Am J Contact Dermatitis 1995;6(2):63–6.

58. Lewis FM, Cork MJ, McDonagh AJ, et al. An audit of the value of patch testing: the patient's perspective. Contact Dermatitis 1994;30(4):214–6.

59. Rajagopalan R, Anderson R. Impact of patch testing on dermatology-specific quality of life in patients with allergic contact dermatitis. Am J Contact Dermatitis 1997;8(4):215–21.

60. Nethercott J. The positive predictive accuracy of patch tests. Immunol Allergy Clin North Am 1989; 9:549–53.

61. van der Valk PG, Devos SA, Coenraads PJ. Evidence-based diagnosis in patch testing. Contact Dermatitis 2003;48(3):121–5.

62. Bruze M. What is a relevant contact allergy? Contact Dermatitis 1990;23(4):224–5.

63. Menńe T, Dooms-Goossens A, Wahlberg JE, et al. How large a proportion of contact sensitivities are diagnosed with the European standard series? Contact Dermatitis 1992;26(3):201–2.

64. Ormond P, Hazelwood E, Bourke B, et al. The importance of a dedicated patch test clinic. Br J Dermatol 2002;146(2):304–7.

65. Goulden V, Wilkinson SM. Evaluation of a contact allergy clinic. Clin Exp Dermatol 2000;25(1):67–70.

66. Soni BP, Sherertz EF. Evaluation of previously patch-tested patients referred to a contact dermatitis clinic. Am J Contact Dermatitis 1997;8(1):10–4.

67. Bernstein JA. Material safety data sheets: are they reliable in identifying human hazards? J Allergy Clin Immunol 2002;110(1):35–8.

68. Hazard Communication Standard. [WWW document.] Available at: http://chemlabs.uoregon.edu/safety/hazcom.html. Accessed February 2009.

69. Côté R, Davis H, Dimock C, et al. The evaluation and hazard classification of toxicological information for workplace hazardous materials information system material safety data sheets. Regul Toxicol Pharmacol 1998;27(1 Pt 1):61–74.

70. Cocchiarella L, Andersson G, American Medical Association. Guides to the evaluation of permanent impairment. 5th ed. Chicago: American Medical Association; 2001. p. 613.

71. Rondinelli RD, Genovese E, Katz RT, et al. Guides to the evaluation of permanent impairment. 6th ed. Chicago: American Medical Association; 2008. p. 634.

72. Dickel H, Kuss O, Blesius CR, et al. Occupational skin diseases in Northern Bavaria between 1990 and 1999: a population-based study. Br J Dermatol 2001;145(3):453–62.

73. Brown T. Strategies for prevention: occupational contact dermatitis. Occup Med (Lond) 2004; 54(7):450–7.

74. Held E, Mygind K, Wolff C, et al. Prevention of work related skin problems: an intervention study in wet work employees. Occup Environ Med 2002;59(8): 556–61.

75. Bauer A, Kelterer D, Bartsch R, et al. Prevention of hand dermatitis in bakers' apprentices: different efficacy of skin protection measures and UVB hardening. Int Arch Occup Environ Health 2002; 75(7):491–9.

76. Bauer A, Kelterer D, Bartsch R, et al. Skin protection in bakers' apprentices. Contact Dermatitis 2002;46(2):81–5.

77. Bauer A, Kelterer D, Stadeler M, et al. The prevention of occupational hand dermatitis in bakers, confectioners and employees in the catering trades. Preliminary results of a skin prevention program. Contact Dermatitis 2001;44(2):85–8.

78. Uter W, Pfahlberg A, Gefeller O, et al. Hand dermatitis in a prospectively-followed cohort of hairdressing apprentices: final results of the POSH study. Prevention of occupational skin disease in hairdressers. Contact Dermatitis 1999;41(5):280–6.

79. van der Walle HB. Dermatitis in hairdressers (II). Management and prevention. Contact Dermatitis 1994;30(5):265–70.

80. Held E, Wolff C, Gyntelberg F, et al. Prevention of work-related skin problems in student auxiliary nurses: an intervention study. Contact Dermatitis 2001;44(5):297–303.

81. Heron RJ. Worker education in the primary prevention of occupational dermatoses. Occup Med (Lond) 1997;47(7):407–10.

82. Salinas AM, Villarreal E, Nuńez GM, et al. Health interventions for the metal working industry: which is the most cost-effective? A study from a developing country. Occup Med (Lond) 2002;52(3): 129–35.

83. Itschner L, Hinnen U, Elsner P. Prevention of hand eczema in the metal-working industry: risk awareness and behavior of metal worker apprentices. Dermatology 1996;193(3):226–9.

84. Rustemeyer T, Frosch PJ. Occupational skin diseases in dental laboratory technicians. (I). Clinical picture and causative factors. Contact Dermatitis 1996;34(2):125–33.

85. Goh CL, Gan SL. Change in cement manufacturing process, a cause for decline in chromate allergy? Contact Dermatitis 1996;34(1):51–4.

86. Avnstorp C. Cement eczema. An epidemiological intervention study. Acta Derm Venereol Suppl (Stockh) 1992;179:1–22.

87. Fregert S, Gruvberger B, Sandahl E. Reduction of chromate in cement by iron sulfate. Contact Dermatitis 1979;5(1):39–42.

88. Adams RM, Fisher AA. Contact allergen alternatives: 1986. J Am Acad Dermatol 1986;14(6): 951–69.

89. McCormick RD, Buchman TL, Maki DG. Double-blind, randomized trial of scheduled use of a novel barrier cream and an oil-containing lotion for protecting the hands of health care workers. Am J Infect Control 2000;28(4):302–10.

90. Hogan DJ, Dannaker CJ, Lal S, et al. An international survey on the prognosis of occupational

contact dermatitis of the hands. Derm Beruf Umwelt 1990;38(5):143–7.

91. Chew AL, Maibach HI. Occupational issues of irritant contact dermatitis. Int Arch Occup Environ Health 2003;76(5):339–46.

92. Zhai H, Maibach HI. Moisturizers in preventing irritant contact dermatitis: an overview. Contact Dermatitis 1998;38(5):241–4.

93. Schwanitz HJ, Uter W. Interdigital dermatitis: sentinel skin damage in hairdressers. Br J Dermatol 2000;142(5):1011–2.

94. Antezana M, Parker F. Occupational contact dermatitis. Immunol Allergy Clin North Am 2003; 23(2):269–90, vii.

95. de Fine Olivarius F, Hansen AB, Karlsmark T, et al. Water protective effect of barrier creams and moisturizing creams: a new in vivo test method. Contact Dermatitis 1996;35(4):219–25.

96. Berndt U, Wigger-Alberti W, Gabard B, et al. Efficacy of a barrier cream and its vehicle as protective measures against occupational irritant contact dermatitis. Contact Dermatitis 2000;42(2): 77–80.

97. Nouaigui H, Antoine JL, Masmoudi ML, et al. [Invasive and non-invasive studies of the protective action of a silicon-containing cream and its excipient in skin irritation induced by sodium laurylsulfate]. Ann Dermatol Venereol 1989;116(5): 389–98 [in French].

98. Frosch PJ, Kurte A, Pilz B. Efficacy of skin barrier creams (III). The repetitive irritation test (RIT) in humans. Contact Dermatitis 1993;29(3):113–8.

99. Wigger-Alberti W, Elsner P. Do barrier creams and gloves prevent or provoke contact dermatitis? Am J Contact Dermatitis 1998;9(2):100–6.

100. English JS. Current concepts of irritant contact dermatitis. Occup Environ Med 2004;61(8):722–6, 674.

101. Mathias CG. Prevention of occupational contact dermatitis. J Am Acad Dermatol 1990;23(4 Pt 1): 742–8.

102. Mansdorf SZ. Guidelines for the selection of gloves for the workplace. NIOSH. Dermatol Clin 1994; 12(3):597–600.

103. Estlander T, Jolanki R. How to protect the hands. Dermatol Clin 1988;6(1):105–14.

104. Forsberg K, Mansdorf S.Z. Quick selection guide to chemical protective clothing. 5th ed. Hoboken (NJ): Wiley-Interscience; 2007. p. 203

105. Mellstrom G. Protective effect of gloves–compiled in a data base. Contact Dermatitis 1985;13(3):162–5.

106. Berardinelli SP. Prevention of occupational skin disease through use of chemical protective gloves. Dermatol Clin 1988;6(1):115–9.

107. Kwon S, Campbell LS, Zirwas MJ. Role of protective gloves in the causation and treatment of occupational irritant contact dermatitis. J Am Acad Dermatol 2006;55(5):891–6.

108. Brazzini B, Pimpinelli N. New and established topical corticosteroids in dermatology: clinical pharmacology and therapeutic use. Am J Clin Dermatol 2002;3(1):47–58.

109. Hachem JP, De Paepe K, Vanpée E, et al. Efficacy of topical corticosteroids in nickel-induced contact allergy. Clin Exp Dermatol 2002;27(1):47–50.

110. Queille-Roussel C, Duteil L, Padilla JM, et al. Objective assessment of topical anti-inflammatory drug activity on experimentally induced nickel contact dermatitis: comparison between visual scoring, colorimetry, laser Doppler velocimetry, and transepidermal water loss. Skin Pharmacol 1990;3(4):248–55.

111. Ramsing DW, Agner T. Efficacy of topical corticosteroids on irritant skin reactions. Contact Dermatitis 1995;32(5):293–7.

112. Le TK, De Mon P, Schalkwijk J, et al. Effect of a topical corticosteroid, a retinoid, and a vitamin D3 derivative on sodium dodecyl sulphate induced skin irritation. Contact Dermatitis 1997; 37(1):19–26.

113. Kucharekova M, Hornix M, Ashikaga T, et al. The effect of the PDE-4 inhibitor (cipamfylline) in two human models of irritant contact dermatitis. Arch Dermatol Res 2003;295(1):29–32.

114. Levin C, Zhai H, Bashir S, et al. Efficacy of corticosteroids in acute experimental irritant contact dermatitis? Skin Res Technol 2001;7(4):214–8.

115. Cohen DE, Heidary N. Treatment of irritant and allergic contact dermatitis. Dermatol Ther 2004; 17(4):334–40.

116. Alomar A, Puig L, Gallardo CM, et al. Topical tacrolimus 0.1% ointment (protopic) reverses nickel contact dermatitis elicited by allergen challenge to a similar degree to mometasone furoate 0.1% with greater suppression of late erythema. Contact Dermatitis 2003;49(4):185–8.

117. Kang S, Lucky AW, Pariser D, et al. Long-term safety and efficacy of tacrolimus ointment for the treatment of atopic dermatitis in children. J Am Acad Dermatol 2001;44(1 Suppl):S58–64.

118. Luger T, Van Leent EJ, Graeber M, et al. SDZ ASM 981: an emerging safe and effective treatment for atopic dermatitis. Br J Dermatol 2001;144(4): 788–94.

119. Reitamo S, Rissanen J, Remitz A, et al. Tacrolimus ointment does not affect collagen synthesis: results of a single-center randomized trial. J Invest Dermatol 1998;111(3):396–8.

120. Queille-Roussel C, Paul C, Duteil L, et al. The new topical ascomycin derivative SDZ ASM 981 does not induce skin atrophy when applied to normal skin for 4 weeks: a randomized, double-blind

controlled study. Br J Dermatol 2001;144(3): 507–13.

121. Cahill J, Keegel T, Nixon R. The prognosis of occupational contact dermatitis in 2004. Contact Dermatitis 2004;51(5–6):219–26.

122. Lerbaek A, Kyvik KO, Ravn H, et al. Clinical characteristics and consequences of hand eczema: an 8-year follow-up study of a population-based twin cohort. Contact Dermatitis 2008; 58(4):210–6.

123. Susitaival P, Hannuksela M. The 12-year prognosis of hand dermatosis in 896 Finnish farmers. Contact Dermatitis 1995;32(4):233–7.

124. Meding B, Wrangsjo K, Jarvholm B. Fifteen-year follow-up of hand eczema: persistence and consequences. Br J Dermatol 2005;152(5):975–80.

125. Adisesh A, Meyer JD, Cherry NM. Prognosis and work absence due to occupational contact dermatitis. Contact Dermatitis 2002;46(5):273–9.

126. Hogan DJ, Dannaker CJ, Maibach HI. The prognosis of contact dermatitis. J Am Acad Dermatol 1990;23(2 Pt 1):300–7.

127. Goh CL. Prognosis of contact and occupational dermatitis. Clin Dermatol 1997;15(4):655–9.

128. Jungbauer FH, van der Vleuten P, Groothoff JW, et al. Irritant hand dermatitis: severity of disease, occupational exposure to skin irritants, and preventive measures 5 years after initial diagnosis. Contact Dermatitis 2004;50(4):245–51.

129. Wall LM, Gebauer KA. A follow-up study of occupational skin disease in Western Australia. Contact Dermatitis 1991;24(4):241–3.

130. Halbert AR, Gebauer KA, Wall LM. Prognosis of occupational chromate dermatitis. Contact Dermatitis 1992;27(4):214–9.

131. Hogan DJ. The prognosis of occupational contact dermatitis. Occup Med 1994;9(1):53–8.

132. Holness DL, Nethercott JR. Is a worker's understanding of their diagnosis an important determinant of outcome in occupational contact dermatitis? Contact Dermatitis 1991;25(5): 296–301.

133. Kalimo K, Kautiainen H, Niskanen T, et al. 'Eczema school' to improve compliance in an occupational dermatology clinic. Contact Dermatitis 1999;41(6): 315–9.

134. Veien NK, Hattel T, Laurberg G. Hand eczema: causes, course, and prognosis II. Contact Dermatitis 2008;58(6):335–9.

135. Meding B, Wrangsjo K, Jarvholm B. Fifteen–year follow-up of hand eczema: predictive factors. J Invest Dermatol 2005;124(5):893–7.

136. Meding B, Wrangsjo K, Jarvholm B. Hand eczema extent and morphology–association and influence on long-term prognosis. J Invest Dermatol 2007; 127(9):2147–51.

137. Lips R, Rast H, Elsner P. Outcome of job change in patients with occupational chromate dermatitis. Contact Dermatitis 1996;34(4):268–71.

138. Hellier FF. The prognosis in industrial dermatitis. Br Med J 1958;1(5064):196–8.

139. Burrows D. Prognosis in industrial dermatitis. Br J Dermatol 1972;87(2):145–8.

140. Pryce DW, White J, White JS, et al. Soluble oil dermatitis: a review. J Soc Occup Med 1989;39(3):93–8.

141. Holness DL, Nethercott JR. Work outcome in workers with occupational skin disease. Am J Ind Med 1995;27(6):807–15.

142. Keczkes K, Bhate SM, Wyatt EH. The outcome of primary irritant hand dermatitis. Br J Dermatol 1983;109(6):665–8.

143. Shah M, Lewis FM, Gawkrodger DJ. Prognosis of occupational hand dermatitis in metalworkers. Contact Dermatitis 1996;34(1):27–30.

144. Fitzgerald DA, English JS. The long-term prognosis in irritant contact hand dermatitis. Curr Probl Dermatol 1995;23:73–6.

145. Rosen RH, Freeman S. Prognosis of occupational contact dermatitis in New South Wales, Australia. Contact Dermatitis 1993;29(2):88–93.

146. Rystedt I. Atopic background in patients with occupational hand eczema. Contact Dermatitis 1985; 12(5):247–54.

147. Nielsen J. The occurrence and course of skin symptoms on the hands among female cleaners. Contact Dermatitis 1996;34(4):284–91.

148. Freeman S. Occupational skin disease. Curr Probl Dermatol 1995;22:80–5.

Impact of Regulation on Contact Dermatitis

Daniel Hogan, MD[a], Johnathan J. Ledet, MD[b],*

KEYWORDS

- Contact dermatitis • Regulation • European Union
- Metals • Occupational contact dermatitis

Contact dermatitis is an inflammation of the skin as a result of contact with 1 or more substances. This localized inflammation can be triggered by various metals, ingredients in cosmetics, plants, detergents, and many other materials people come into contact with frequently or occasionally. Contact dermatitis can be subdivided into three types: irritant, allergic, and photo.[1] Inflammation in all forms of contact dermatitis is primarily in the epidermis and outer dermis. Acute signs and symptoms often include: erythematous papules and plaques, weeping vesicles, burning (irritant contact dermatitis [ICD]), and pruritus. These signs and symptoms may take days to weeks to heal after the offending exposure is terminated and may evolve through stages of subacute, chronic, and lichenified dermatitis.[2]

Contact dermatitis is a serious public health and dermatologic concern. The prevalence of contact dermatitis in the United States was estimated to be 13.6 per 1000 population according to the National Health and Nutritional Examination Survey using physical examinations by dermatologists of a selected sample of Americans.[3] The American Medical Care Survey estimated that for all American physicians dermatitis is the second most common dermatologic diagnosis proffered. Dermatitis accounts for 9% of visits to dermatologists.

Allergic contact dermatitis (ACD) is the cutaneous manifestation of the allergic response to an allergen. ACD is a type IV delayed hypersensitivity reaction that involves a cell-mediated response that has both an induction stage in which the immune system is sensitized and an elicitation stage whereby the allergic response is triggered.[2] Allergy to a substance may develop at any age in life. Allergy is long lasting whereby subsequent contact with the allergen will usually produce an inflammatory reaction.

ICD results in inflammation after the release of proinflammatory cytokines by skin cells (mainly keratinocytes). Irritants may be chemical or physical with inflammation intensifying after repeated or prolonged exposure to the offending substance. Epidermal cellular changes, skin barrier disruption, and the release of cytokines are the 3 main pathophysiologic changes seen.[2]

Photo contact dermatitis (PCD) occurs only when skin together with the offending substance is exposed to ultraviolet or visible light. PCD can further be divided into photoallergic and phototoxic from exposure to a topical allergen and irritant respectively.[1]

Distinguishing between the various types of contact dermatitis can be a daunting task; history and patch testing aid in this distinction. Substances may act as both an irritant and an allergen.

BUREAUCRACY AND LEGISLATION

This article does not review workers' compensation or regulation of clinical trials but instead focuses on other issues of regulation in the field of ACD.[4,5]

Bureaucracy is often thought as "endless red tape malevolently contrived by petty, self-serving, and small minded bureaucrats."[6] The bureaucratic perspective ignores the wider social environment and tends to protect its internal activities from public scrutiny and control.[7]

A bureaucracy should be efficient because it benefits from economies of scale and avoids duplication of effort while maintaining standards of

[a] NOVA Southeastern University, Largo, FL, USA
[b] Louisiana State University Health Sciences Center, Shreveport, LA, USA
* Corresponding author.
E-mail address: jledet27@yahoo.com (J.J. Ledet).

Dermatol Clin 27 (2009) 385–394
doi:10.1016/j.det.2009.05.006

quality. Bureaucracies exist for want of a better method to provide large scale delivery of services.[6]

Rules reduce variability and set patterns of behavior.[6] People tend to complain about either a lack of rules or too many rules. Workers tend to apply or ignore rules arbitrarily because of rule inflation, whereby they do not know which rules are operational and which are historical.[6] There is also the concept that those at the top of the bureaucracy think, whereas those beneath follow orders or procedures.[6] In a bureaucracy no one takes responsibility for a decision unless forced to. Problems that require decisions are forced up a long chain of command. One part of the bureaucracy may have the authority but another part has responsibility to address a problem.[6] Bureaucracies typically take a long time to make a decision, with the process itself being sacrosanct. The myriad regulations seem unapproachable for those not part of the bureaucracy.[8]

Dermatologists crossing the Atlantic may think they have entered a strange new world when they arrive at their destination. American dermatologists going to the European Society of Contact Dermatitis meetings hear dermatologists frequently advocate more government regulation particularly of allergens in consumer products in a continent where patch test allergens are abundantly available. European dermatologists coming to the American Contact Dermatitis Society meetings will find only 29 allergens that are Food and Drug Administration (FDA) approved to help dermatologists diagnose complex cases of ACD. European dermatologists quickly learn that CLIA (the Clinical Laboratory Improvement Amendments) and HIPAA (the Health Insurance Portability and Accountability Act) do not facilitate the clinical practice of medicine and that honest dermatologists live in fear of a Medicare auditor coming to their office and telling them, "I'm from the government and I'm here to help." In 1986 President Ronald Reagan called this phrase "the nine most terrifying words in the English language." This article will review governmental regulations—some helpful for patients and workers and some not helpful for dermatologists in their quest to assist patients with contact dermatitis.

REGULATION OF ALLERGENS

It should be fundamental that dermatologists who are the experts in contact dermatitis provide their clinical knowledge for the most useful legislation for patients and consumers.

Regulation has been useful in reducing nickel allergy in Europe. It is less certain that regulation has reduced ACD to chromate, thiurams,

methylchloroisothiazolinone/methylisothiazolinone (MCI/MI), and methyldibromo glutaronitrile (MDBGN).

The European Union (EU) Dangerous Substances Directive has specific concentration limits on strong skin sensitizers such as formaldehyde, glutaraldehyde, acrylates, and isocyanates. The Directive requires that allergens present in concentrations of more than 0.1% be labeled.[9]

CHROMATE

For nearly 20 years the Nordic countries have had legislation limiting hexavalent chromium in cement to fewer than 2 ppm. Danish legislation has required that iron sulfate be added to cement manufactured there to produce this low concentration. This resulted in a reported decrease in the prevalence of chromium allergy among construction workers in Denmark. A similar reduction in chromate dermatitis has been reported in Singapore, attributed to a change in the manufactured constituents of cement which also resulted in a reduction of hexavalent chromate levels without legislation.[10]

COSMETICS AND PRESERVATIVES

The United States was the first country with compulsory cosmetic labeling except for professional products used by beauticians. Europe currently has the most highly developed set of legislation regarding contact dermatitis.[11–17]

The FDA regulates the labeling of cosmetics and requires safety and efficacy data on new products that are claimed to have preventive or health benefits. The FDA maintains a voluntary registration program whereby cosmetic manufacturers may register their finished products and ingredients with the FDA. The Office of Cosmetics and Colors also contains a database on cosmetic complaints that it receives in its Cosmetic Adverse Reaction Monitoring Program. Under the Fair Packaging and Labeling Act and Federal Food, Drug, and Cosmetic Act all cosmetics and over-the-counter (OTC) drugs must be accurately labeled with regard to the net quantity of contents. Cosmetic ingredients must be named in descending order of predominance. Fragrances do not have to be specified. Active ingredients must be listed in alphabetical order separately from the inactive ingredients for OTC drug products. A manufacturer may petition the FDA to allow the listing of an ingredient as "other ingredients" if it believes that the ingredient is a trade secret. This status is not routinely granted.[18]

Cosmetics are to some extent legislated through the Federal Food, Drug, and Cosmetic Act issued by the FDA and US Department of Health and Human Services.[18] All preservatives for cosmetic use are evaluated by the Cosmetic Ingredient Review, which has representatives from industry, the FDA, and consumers.[18] In the United States, the Personal Care Products Council (formerly called the Cosmetic, Toiletry and Fragrance Association [CTFA]) reviews existing literature on ingredients and makes voluntary recommendations to the industry.

Cosmetics and preservatives are regulated by the EU's Cosmetic Directive.[18] It is expected that many companies will follow the same regulations for all countries and will follow the EU's Cosmetic Directive. Canada has said that it will follow this directive. The International Nomenclature for Cosmetic Ingredients (INCI) is based on the CTFA nomenclature used in the United States and must be used in the EU. The Scientific Committee on Consumer Products (SCCP) makes recommendations to the EU commission.[18]

PRESERVATIVES

MDBGN was originally restricted to a maximum concentration of 0.1% in both leave-on and rinse-off products in 1986 by the EU Scientific Committee on Cosmetology, but in view of increasing frequency of ACD to MDBGN in the next 2 decades, the EU Cosmetics Directive restricted its use to 0.1% in rinse-off products only since 2005 and then prohibited it from rinse-off products as well in 2007.[19] A significant decrease in positive patch reactions to this allergen has been seen in the EU since this legislation along with a significant decrease in the proportion of patients for whom a positive patch reaction to this allergen is of current relevance.[18] It took 4 years and 4 different opinions from the SCCP to ban this preservative followed by a period of time for the industry to change to alternative preservatives and a total of 6 years to remove this allergen.[18]

The EU Cosmetics Directive prohibits the use of Kathon CG/Euxyl K100 (MCI/MI = 3:1) in concentrations above 15 ppm. The chemical industry then began to produce MI separately without MCI in different concentrations or in combination with other preservatives. MI has recently been approved for use in cosmetic products.[18] MI may elicit and possibly induce ACD. The Personal Care Products Council recommends a concentration of no more than 7.5 ppm in cosmetic leave-on products and 15 ppm for cosmetic rinse-off products.[18]

PRESERVATIVE LABELING

Even in highly educated unilingual countries, half the population has difficulty reading cosmetic labels because of the small size of the letters and the long chemical names.[20] Poorly educated patients and consumers have more trouble reading labels.[20] Patients found it easier to identify fragrance on labels than formaldehyde or MDBGN. The SCCP advisory to the EU commission has expressed concern regarding very long and difficult INCI names assigned to well known allergens. They suggested that more easily recognized names might be of assistance to consumers.

Preservatives may be mislabeled in up to half of consumer products.[21] Some products do not contain labeled preservatives, but more commonly unlabeled preservatives may be found in products. A preservative may be found in the fragrance added to a product. Unlabeled formaldehyde is a concern.[22] Manufacturers state that formaldehyde may be produced via post-formulation reactions, may occur as contamination in the early stage of formulation, and may occur in urea or glycerin used in the formulation of products.[21]

FRAGRANCE

Fragrance is the most common cosmetic allergy found when patients with dermatitis are patch tested in the United States and many other parts of the world.[23,24] Fragrance chemicals are ubiquitous in our environment and can be found in a wide rage of products including household, industrial, and cosmetic. Widespread use is a major contributing factor in the role of fragrance in ACD.

Fragrance mix I (FM I), and Myroxylon pereirae (MP) are 2 of the main screening chemicals used in standard patch test series. The 8 chemicals that compose FM I are: isoeugenol, hydroxycitronellal, cinnamal, cinnamic alcohol, eugenol, α-amyl cinnamal, geraniol and oak moss absolute (Evernia prunastri). Patch testing with FM I has been reported to detect up to 70% to 80% patients who are allergic to fragrance. Fragrance allergy correlates with exposure to products containing FM I constituents.[25] MP is also known as balsam of Peru and is a complex mixture of natural fragrance resins with more than 250 constituents.[26] MP has a patch testing sensitivity of up to 50% in patients with fragrance allergy. A second fragrance mix (FM II) was developed as a result of large multisite studies to further aid in the diagnosis of fragrance allergy. FM II contains the following additional 6 compounds: hydroxyisohexyl 3-cyclohexene carboxaldehyde (HICC or Lyral), α-hexyl cinnamal, citral, citronellol, coumarin, and farnesol.[27,28]

Over 4000 different chemicals are used in artificial fragrance products, yet most of these have never been tested for human toxicity.[29]

Sensitization to fragrance is thought to occur primarily in non-occupational settings, commonly after the use of cosmetic products both scented and unscented. A frequent primary site of dermatitis in patients with fragrance allergy is the hands; this possibly reflects the diminished barrier function of skin after exposure to irritants allowing penetration and sensitization to occur.[30] Occupations reported to have ACD and ICD to fragrance include hairdressers, aromatherapists, bakers, confectioners, coal miners, and workers in the cosmetic manufacturing industry.[30,31] Buckley and colleagues[31] concluded that health care workers also have an increased risk for fragrance allergy because of frequent hand washing with soaps and antiseptic solutions. Buckley and colleagues also found that retired individuals have the highest overall risk for fragrance allergy. This risk was exaggerated even more in health care workers with advanced age, suggesting that factors from their workplace environment contributed to potential sensitization. Students with a median age of 21.3 in the Buckley study had lesser prevalence of fragrance allergy, thought to be because of their younger age and less cumulative exposure to fragrance containing products.

Almost all fragrance allergic patients have non-occupational exposure, regardless of their occupation. Assessing occupational exposure is a difficult process. The International Fragrance Association has set advisory limits on the nature and concentration of sensitizing fragrance chemicals added to cosmetics. Household chemicals are still a concern for sensitization of individuals. Employers should make an attempt to provide employees with products that are fragrance free.

Fragrance composition in cosmetics may be indicated simply by the word *parfum* even in the EU, but 26 fragrance allergens must be identified in the EU if 1 of the fragrance substances is present at more than 10 ppm for leave-on products and more than 100 ppm for rinse-off products, even though some of these fragrances may be of little or no importance as contact allergens.[9] It remains to be seen how quickly regulations will be updated to reflect updated data on current and emerging contact allergens.[32]

PARAPHENYLENEDIAMINE

Contact dermatitis to hair dye is a widely recognized clinical problem. Aromatic amines such as paraphenylenediamine (PPD) and paratoluenediamine are common causes of allergic contact sensitization leading to severe dermatitis with facial edema. PPD and other phenylenediamines

in cosmetic products are for application to hair only and not to skin.

A review of the literature suggests that contact allergy to PPD may occur in 0.1% to 2.3% of the general population.[33] Sosted and colleagues[34] conducted an interview-based study of 4000 Danish adults, with a median age of 16 years at first exposure and found that 74.9% of female respondents had dyed their hair at some time compared with 18.4% of male respondents. In this study 5.3% of individuals reported an adverse skin reaction consistent with that of an allergic reaction to the dyes.

Another cohort study of 2545 individuals from Thailand's general populous concluded that 2.3% had an allergic reaction to PPD on patch testing. Five hundred nine patch-test negative individuals who then used hair dye for 6 months were compared with a control group of 514 who did not use hair dye during this same 6 month interval; the study found that 1% of individuals who used the dye reacted to PPD.[34]

Data from these various studies highlight the importance of phenylenediamines as a contact allergen globally and affirm that it should continue to be included among standard series of contact allergens.

Hairdressers are commonly affected by occupational skin diseases (OSD) as a result of their repetitive exposure to water, shampoos, hair dyes, and other allergens. In hairdressers ICD predominates over ACD. Hand dermatitis is endemic among workers, hairdressing ranking in the top 5 occupations associated with OSDs in some European studies. Though the actual prevalence of OSDs is difficult to determine some estimates are as high as 50% with skin pathology beginning as early as the first year in this profession. Studies show that apprentices are disproportionately affected. An Australian study showed 97% of hair dressers affected with OSDs were apprentices; a study preformed in London showed that 30 of 33 junior hairdressers had hand dermatitis. This disproportionality is thought to reflect the large amount of wet work done by apprentices. OSDs are considered "part of the job" for hair dressers.[35] With regard to skin changes, irritant changes tended to occur early, whereas sensitization had a tendency to occur later in their careers. Cutaneous adverse effects to PPD are significantly more prevalent in hairdressers than in the general population.

PPD was prohibited in Germany in 1906 and in the middle of the century in Sweden and France. The EU Cosmetics Directive allows PPD in hair dye products with a concentration limit of 6%.[36] Hair dye allergy remains a problem in Europe.

In 1933, more than a dozen women were blinded and 1 woman died after using permanent mascara–Lash Lure which contained PPD. This was the first product seized under FDA authority. The FDA Act of 1938 prohibited marketing of hair dyes for eyelash and eyebrow tinting. An eyelash dye containing PPD is still marketed in Europe.[18,37]

Dermatologists have advocated that PPD in black henna tattoos be regulated in the United States particularly for children. The American Contact Dermatitis Society, The Society of Pediatric Dermatology and the Advisory Board of the American Academy of Dermatology advocate against the use of PPD in these tattoos.[38]

METALS

Metals and metal salts are a frequent cause of ACD because of the repeated and sometimes constant contact with the skin. Metals may also cause urticaria and an acute hypersensitivity with respiratory symptoms.

Metals such as nickel (Ni) and mercury (Hg) have long been a recognized cause of ACD. Chromium (Cr) and cobalt (Co) are also widely known causes of ACD. Recently gold (Au) and palladium (Pd) have become more accepted as patch test allergens.[39] Many metals produce in vitro production of both Th1 and Th2 type cytokines in peripheral blood mononuclear cells in patients with patch test reactivity to the same metal.[40]

Hg-induced ACD was report as early as 1895. Hg compounds are readily absorbed through the skin when applied topically and accumulate in the body.[41] FDA regulation of Hg compounds in cosmetics limits them to cosmetics applied to the eye area, at a concentration which cannot exceed 65 ppm.[41] Use of Hg compounds is only permitted when no alternative is available.[41] Chemical forms of Hg that are known to cause sensitization include phenyl mercuric salts, Hg from broken thermometers, and organic forms such as thimerosal and merbromin. Cross-reactions between inorganic and organic forms have been reported. Thimerosal is the most common form of Hg that causes ACD. Thimerosal can be found in numerous topical medications, cosmetics, and is a declining preservative in vaccines. Dental amalgams also contain Hg, occasionally leading to localized oral lichenoid reactions.[42] Although patch test reactions to thimerosal are frequently encountered, a careful history will often show that the positive result is not related to the current dermatitis of the patient.[39]

Cobalt (Co) is essential to animal life; it is the main component of vitamin B12. Co is abundant in the environment. Industrially it is used in an alloy with Ni, chromium, and iron. Additionally its oxidized form is found in many paints and pigments. Exposure to Co is mainly found in those who wear costume jewelry and individuals who have occupations such as cement working and bricklaying.[39] Many patients with an allergy to Co are also allergic to Ni; it is thought that this is co-sensitization. As a result of this cosensitization, allergy to either metal will be heightened if a patient is sensitized to the other.[43]

Pd is becoming an increasingly popular metal in the jewelry industry; in part because of the popularity of white gold which may contain up to 20% Pd. Pd is also used in dental alloys, telecommunications products, and temperature solders. In metal patch testing series Pd is tested as palladium chloride 1% in petrolatum. Allergy to palladium chloride has been documented but in almost all cases patients reacted to another metal, causing most authors to feel that the initial positive result is a cross-reaction.[44] Although the incidence of patients reacting to Pd is increasing, it is difficult to discern the relevance of Pd sensitization.

Metal-induced ACD can be reduced through stricter government regulations, avoidance, and patient education.

Nickel

Ni is the most common cause of metal-induced ACD. Ni is a component of many different types of metals including white gold, Ni plating, gold plating, Monel solder, and stainless steel, making Ni extremely difficult to avoid.

The North American Contact Dermatitis Group consistently ranks Ni the most frequent allergen causing positive patch test reactions. Ongoing efforts to diminish the amount of Ni in products that are in direct and prolonged contact with skin have led to an increase in the use of other metals in alloys used in jewelry, dentistry, and orthopedics.[40] This effort may lead to an increase in ACD to other metals.[40]

The incidence of Ni allergy is more in women; this is attributed to increased prevalence of ear piercing and the donning of jewelry.[45] Allergy to Ni may predispose individuals to hand dermatitis. One literature review stated "previous or concomitant Ni sensitivity also appears to worsen the prognosis somewhat" of hand dermatitis.[9] ACD to Ni is a significant dermatologic problem in most of the world.

The Nickel Directive was adopted by the EU in 1994, prohibiting trade with products that released more than 0.5 µg per cm^2 per week of Ni. Denmark and Sweden limited Ni in objects in contact with the skin in 1989. Reduced sensitization to Ni among Danish children and German women younger than 30 years has been reported subsequent to these regulations[4,46,47] In contrast, 6% of children's clothing fasteners still contain Ni in the United States and may be a source of sensitization to Ni for young children.[48]

Latex

In 1989 the FDA was alerted to adverse reactions to natural latex medical devices.[49] Two years later the FDA issued a Medical Alert to the medical community on the problem of natural latex allergy. The agency issued guidance for protein content labeling for medical gloves in 1995. The FDA has yet to approve a latex skin testing reagent, so in vitro tests remained important for the diagnosis of latex allergy in the United States. Latex skin testing reagents have been available in Europe for years and are regarded as the preferred method to diagnose latex allergy.[50] In 2000 the European commission recommended that the contact of proteins in rubber latex gloves be reduced mainly by leaching.[50] Manufacturers were also encouraged to reduce the content and use of thiurams, which are considered to be the most frequent contact sensitizers in rubber gloves. Subsequently the frequency of sensitization to thiurams has declined in Denmark from 1995 to 2004.[50]

PATCH TESTING

The only FDA approved patch test system in the United States is the Thin Layer Rapid Use Epicutaneous Test which consists of 29 allergens. The lack of other FDA approved antigens for patch testing is a concern for American but not European physicians performing patch testing.[51–53] The rationale for the stringent requirements of the FDA for patch testing allergens is obscure[54,55] and may lessen the enthusiasm of American dermatologists for more regulations related to contact dermatitis testing.

The FDA "Guidance for Industry: On the Content and Format of Chemistry, Manufacturing and Controls Information and Establishment Description Information for an Allergenic Extract or Allergen Patch Test" provides guidance to applicants on the content and format of the chemistry, manufacturing, and controls. "Application to Market a New Drug, Biologic, or an Antibiotic Drug for Human Use" (revised Form FDA 356h) is required for an allergenic extract or allergen patch test. This action is part of FDA's continuing effort to achieve the objectives of the President's "Reinventing Government" initiatives and the FDA Modernization Act of 1997, and is intended to

"reduce unnecessary burdens for industry without diminishing public health protection." As part of the application for patch test allergens the manufacturer must provide a manufacturing flow chart, floor diagram of the general layout of the facilities, and a comprehensive list of all additional products that are manufactured or manipulated in the areas used to produce the drug substance that is the subject of the application.

OCCUPATIONAL SKIN DISEASES

There are at least 14 federal regulations and 3 agencies that are involved in the regulation of occupational skin exposures in the United States. The Environmental Protection Agency (EPA) requires reporting of health effects information on chemicals. The Toxic Substances Control Act requires manufacturers and distributors to provide toxicity data to the EPA. The EPA maintains a chemical substance inventory of thousands of chemicals employed in commerce. The employer is required to provide on the material safety data sheets (MSDSs) or alternate form of warning the measures such as protective clothing that are required to control worker exposure. The EPA has the authority to ban hazardous chemicals for certain uses. The EPA is mandated to control the use of pesticides, including use of personal protective equipment and safe use of pesticides.

The Occupational Safety and Health Administration (OSHA) is part of the Department of Labor and has the most direct contact with workplaces in the field through its field inspection compliance activity which is directed at the reduction of workplace injuries and illnesses.

OCCUPATIONAL CONTACT DERMATITIS

OSDs may be caused by biologic, chemical, and physical insults. The most common manifestations of OSDs are ICD and ACD. The dermatologist's role includes not only diagnosis and treatment, but also determination of the etiologic agent and prevention of future occurrences. The National Institute for Occupational Safety and Health (NIOSH) offers an occupational dermatoses program and photo library for physicians on its Web site: http://www.cdc.gov/ocderm.html.[56]

Epidemiologic data show that contact dermatitis is the most common OSD, making up 90% to 95% of all reported cases. The US Bureau of Labor Statistics conducts approximately 160,000 annual surveys of employers from private industries in the United States and tabulates all occupational skin disorders.[57,58] In 2006 the incidence of skin diseases was reported to be 4.5 per 10,000 full-time workers. Questions that can assist in the diagnosis related to occupation include: (1) Are there workplace exposures to potential cutaneous irritants or allergens? (2) Is the clinical appearance consistent with contact dermatitis? (3) Is the anatomic distribution of dermatitis consistent with cutaneous exposure in relation to the job task? (4) Is the temporal relationship between exposure and onset consistent with contact dermatitis? (5) Does the dermatitis improve away from exposure to the suspected irritant or allergen? (6) Are non-occupational exposures excluded as probable causes? (7) Do patch tests or provocation tests identify a probable causal agent?[59]

Avoiding future contact with offending substances is an important aspect in preventing OCD. Other strategies in prevention include identifying irritants and allergens, subsequently substituting chemicals that are less irritating or allergenic, and using protective equipment. Additional methods to assist in prevention include emphasizing both personal and occupational hygiene, and increased awareness of potential irritants or allergens in the workplace.[60]

The goal of the US Public Health Service for 2010 is to reduce national OSDs to an incidence of less than 46 per 100,000 full-time workers. This goal has been established in *Healthy People 2010: National Health Promotion and Disease Prevention Objectives*. Both ACD and ICD are considered priority research by NIOSH.[61] OSDs have an important public health impact because they are frequent, often have a poor prognosis, and have a significant economic impact when affected individuals cannot continue their chosen vocation.

MATERIAL SAFETY DATA SHEETS

MSDSs are widely used across North America, Europe, and increasingly in other parts of the world to catalog information on chemical compounds and mixtures. MSDSs serve to communicate potential hazards in workplaces. They are produced by chemical suppliers and are disturbed to employers who are required by law in most parts of the world to inform and train employees. MSDSs help to identify hazardous ingredients in products and their specific toxicologic properties. MSDSs provide information such as handling procedures, health effects, chemical reactivity, and first aid that helps both employees and emergency personnel to handle these products in a safe manner.

MSDSs were developed after Congress passed the Occupational Safety and Health Act in 1970 which also led to the development of OSHA. The first major regulatory document released by OSHA was the Hazard Communication Standard (HCS). In addition to MSDS, HCS contained 5 other sections including: (1) chemical labeling, (2) hazard determination, (3) trade secrets, (4) employee training, and (5) written implementation program. Despite these regulations MSDSs have often been criticized in the medical literature over their effectiveness as a tool for workplace hazard and health communication.[62] OSHA permits exclusion of information deemed solely by the manufacturer as not hazardous or protected as a trade secret.[62]

American workers are more aware of MSDSs then workers in other countries where MSDSs were not regulated until more recently.[62] The preparer of MSDSs is required to update the MSDS if he/she becomes newly aware of any significant information but there is no requirement to actively review the literature for new information on health effects of ingredients.[63]

In Australia, sensitizers present at a concentration of more than1% and irritants present at a concentration of more than 20% must be listed on the MSDSs.[64] A study of MSDSs for cases of OCD in Australia found that irritants were often correctly listed but that allergens were correctly listed less than half of the time following these Australian regulations.

Sensitizers may be important causes of ACD at concentrations of less than 1% and would not be listed on American MSDSs. Data about skin sensitization are required for Canadian MSDSs. EU legislation requires that sensitizers present at a concentration of more than 0.1% be listed. Not all metal working fluid ingredients known to cause ACD are classified as sensitizers in the EU and their declaration is not required in these fluids.[65]

Though research suggests that MSDS are inaccurate and usually incomplete, they are still considered vital to employee health and safety. Lack of enforcement by employers coupled with inaccurateness, incompleteness, and incomprehensibility make MSDSs inadequate as a prevention tool. Many MSDSs are written with highly technical language which many employees do not understand. In 2002 Bernstein cited 4 major limitations of MSDSs as: (1) omission of vital information regarding generic chemical names, (2) omission of potential respiratory and skin sensitizing agents that are known to induce reactions through a specific immune response, (3) failure to update current permissible exposure levels (PELs) for 212 agents that are higher than the PELs set by OSHA in 1989, and (4) failure to require documented clinical information regarding specific occupational lung or cutaneous diseases associated with a specific agent.[66] Health care professionals and safety personnel should be aware of the multitude of problems that plague MSDSs.[63]

When updated and properly constructed MSDSs have the potential to play an important role in evaluating patients with dermatitis that is potentially related to his or her occupation. Guidelines set forth by the US federal government do not require certain information that may be vital for the correct diagnosis. Health care professionals must be able to correctly interpret MSDSs to better treat patients with occupationally derived dermatitis.

The Globally Harmonized System for the Classification and Labeling of Chemicals (GHS) is a combined system of Safety Data Sheets and labeling that will supersede the MSDS. The GHS was established to provide an internationally agreed system for hazard classification of chemical products.[67] Hazards for chemical products are also communicated through this system to those involved with the transport of dangerous goods, consumers, emergency personnel, and employees.[67,68] Chemicals are classified according to their physical, environmental, and toxicologic hazards. Toxicologic endpoints used include: acute toxicity, irritation, corrosivity, sensitization, carcinogenicity, mutagenicity, reproductive toxicity, and chronic or repeat dose toxicity. Goals of the GHS are to enhance protection to both mankind and the environment. Methods used in the GHS include: (1) providing an internationally comprehensible system for hazard communication, (2) providing a recognized framework for countries without an existing system, (3) facilitating international trade in chemicals whose hazards have been properly identified and assessed on an international basis, and (4) reducing the need for testing and evaluation of chemicals.[67] The GHS was formally adopted by the UN Committee of Experts for the Transport of Dangerous Goods in December of 2002. The first and second revised editions of the GHS document were published in 2005 and 2007 respectively.[68] The GHS lists sensitizers present at a concentration of more than 0.1%.[67] To date the GHS has been implemented in 65 countries.[68]

ROLE OF AMERICAN ACADEMY OF DERMATOLOGY AND AMERICAN CONTACT DERMATITIS SOCIETY

The American Contact Dermatitis Society (ACDS) was born from the American Academy of Dermatology's (AAD's) Committee on Contact Dermatitis. The ACDS is a professional organization of dermatologists, allergists, researchers, and other health care professionals dedicated to improving patient care, with regard to contact dermatitis and OSDs. Patient care is improved by promoting investigative research, stimulating and gathering information on contact dermatitis and related topics. ACDS also provides a forum to facilitate the exchange of information among health care professionals, and encourages physician courses at national scientific meetings and regional dermatology training centers.

Since its inception in 1989 the ACDS has focused on meeting the challenges of its mission through education, research and teaching, and service. A joint effort between ACDS and the Mayo Foundation is Contact Allergen Replacement Database to enhance patient education. This database allows ACDS members to customize cross-reactivity of chemical groups and compose patient specific lists that are free of the patient's allergens. Dermatitis, the official journal of the ACDS highlights scholarly research and presentations from semiannual meetings. The ACDS Web site also has a wealth of information including lectures on patch testing, self-assessment questions from past issues of Dermatitis, and documentation on the diagnosis and importance of inflammatory skin diseases.

ACDS works together with the AAD to increase the awareness of contact dermatitis and OSDs. The American Academy of Dermatology Association has a legislative team to monitor and lobby on issues that specifically affect dermatology. The focus of this legislative team is on patient safety, research, Medicare reform, and scope of practice. Together the ACDS and AAD strive to improve health care policy on both a state and national level.

SUMMARY

It is essential that government, industry, and dermatologists work together to enhance regulatory methods to control and prevent contact allergy epidemics. Increased knowledge and awareness of OSDs by dermatologists and other health care professionals will assist in achieving national public health goals.

REFERENCES

1. Bourke J, Coulson I, English J. Guidelines for care of contact dermatitis. Br J Dermatol 2001;145(6):877–85.
2. Rietschel RL. Mechanisms in irritant contact dermatitis. Clin Dermatol 1997;15(4):557–9.

3. Cohen DE. Contact dermatitis: a quarter century perspective. J Am Acad Dermatol 2004;51(Suppl 1): S60–3.

4. Frosch PJ, Aberer W, August PJ, et al. International comparison of legal aspects of worker compensation for occupational contact dermatitis. In: Frosch PJ, Menne T, Lepoittevin J-P, editors. Contact dermatitis. 4th edition. Berlin: Springer; 2006. p. 875–92.

5. Feinsod M, Chambers WA. Trials and tribulations: a primer on successfully navigating the waters of the Food and Drug Administration. Ophthalmology 2004;111(10):1801–6.

6. Ballé M. Making bureaucracy work. J Manag Med 1999;13(2–3):190–200.

7. Bolon DS. Bureaucracy, institutional theory and institutionaucracy: applications to the hospital industry. J Health Hum Serv Adm 1998;21(1):70–9.

8. Boeniger MF, Ahlers HW. Federal government regulation of occupational skin exposure in the USA. Int Arch Occup Environ Health 2003;76(5):387–99.

9. Lidén C. Legislative and preventive measures related to contact dermatitis. Contact Dermatitis 2001;44:65–9.

10. Goh CL, Gan SL. Change in cement manufacturing process a cause for decline in chromate allergy. Contact Dermatitis 1996;34:51–4.

11. Larsen WG. Why is the USA the only country with compulsory cosmetic labeling? Contact Dermatitis 1989;20(1):1–2.

12. Snijders-Keilholz A, Trimbos JB. A preliminary report on new efforts to decrease radiotherapy related small bowel toxicity. Radiother Oncol 1991;22(3): 206–8.

13. Schapiro M. New power for "Old Europe". Int J Health Serv 2005;35(3):551–60.

14. Lindenschmidt RC, Anastasia FB, Dorta M, et al. Global cosmetic regulatory harmonization. Toxicology 2001;160(1–3):237–41.

15. Schnuch A, Uter W, Geier J, et al. Sensitization to 26 fragrances to be labeled according to current European regulation. Results of the IVDK and review of the literature. Contact Dermatitis 2007;57(1):1–10.

16. Thyssen JP, Johansen JD, Menné T. Contact allergy epidemics and their controls. Contact Dermatitis 2007;56(4):185–95.

17. White IR, Basketter D, Frosch PJ, et al. Legislation in contact dermatitis. (Editors). 4th edition. Berlin: Springer; 2006.

18. Lundow MD, Moesby L, Claus Z, et al. Contamination versus preservation of cosmetics: a review on legislation, usage, infections, and contact allergy. Contact Dermatitis 2009;60(2):70–8.

19. Johansen JD, Veien N, Laurberg G, et al. Decreasing trends in methyldibromo glutaronitrile contact allergy–following regulatory intervention. Contact Dermatitis 2008;59(1):48–51.

20. Noiesen E, Munk MD, Larsen K, et al. Difficulties in avoiding exposure to allergens in cosmetics. Contact Dermatitis 2007;57(2):105–9.

21. Rastogi SC. Analytical control of preservative labelling on skin creams. Contact Dermatitis 2000;43(6): 339–43.

22. Packham C. The problem with material safety data sheets. Occup Med (Lond) 2002;52(2):67–8.

23. Marks JG, Belsito DV, DeLeo VA, et al. North American Contact Dermatitis Group patch test results for the detection of delayed-type hypersensitivity to topical allergens. J Am Acad Dermatol 1998;38: 911–8.

24. Buckley DA, Rycroft RJ, White IR, et al. The frequency of fragrance allergy in patch-tested patients increases with their age. Br J Dermatol 2003;149:986–9.

25. Scheiman PL. Exposing covert fragrance chemicals. Am J Contact Dermat 2001;12(4):225–8.

26. Hausen BM, Simatupang T, Bruhn G, et al. Identification of new allergenic constituents and proof of evidence of coniferyl benzoate in balsam of Peru. Am J Contact Dermat 1995;6:199–208.

27. Frosch PJ, Rastogi SC, Pirker C, et al. Patch testing with a new fragrance mix-reactivity to the individual constituents and chemical detection in relevant cosmetic products. Contact Dermatitis 2005;52: 216–25.

28. Frosch PJ, Pirker C, Rastogi SC, et al. Patch testing with a new fragrance mix detects additional patients sensitive to perfumes and missed by the current fragrance mix. Contact Dermatitis 2005;52:207–15.

29. Ashford N, Miller C. Chemical exposures: low levels. New York: Von Nostrand Reinold; 1991.

30. De Groot AC, Frosch PJ. Adverse reactions to fragrances: a clinical review. Contact Dermatitis 1997;36:57–86.

31. Buckley DA, Rycroft RJG, White IR, et al. Contact allergy to individual fragrance mix constituents relation to primary site of dermatitis. Contact Dermatitis 2000;43:304–5.

32. Basketter DA. Skin sensitization: strategies for the assessment and management of risk. Br J Dermatol 2008;159(2):267–73 [Epub 2008 May 22].

33. Khumalo NP, Jessop S, Ehrlich R. Prevalence of cutaneous adverse effects of hairdressing: a systematic review. Arch Dermatol 2006;142:377–83.

34. Sosted H, Hesse U, Menne T, et al. Contact allergy to hair dyes in a Danish adult population: an interview-based study. Br J Dermatol 2005;153:132–5.

35. Buckley DA, Rycroft RJG, White IR, et al. Fragrance as an occupational allergen. Occup Med 2002; 52(1):13–6.

36. Sosted H, Rastogi SC, Andersen KE, et al. Dye contact allergy: quantitative exposure assessment of selected products and clinical cases. Contact Dermatitis 2004;50(6):344–8.

37. Teixeira M, de Wachter L, Ronsyn E, et al. Contact allergy to para-phenylenediamine in a permanent eyelash dye. Contact Dermatitis 2006;55(2):92–4.

38. Jacob SE, Zapolanski T, Chayavichitsilp P, et al. p-Phenylenediamine in black henna tattoos: a practice in need of policy in children. Arch Pediatr Adolesc Med 2008;162(8):790–2.

39. McFadden JP, Jefferies D, Jowsey I, et al. Incidence and prevalence of contact allergy to the permanent hair dye agent para-phenylenediamine – results of the Anglo-Thai study. Br J Dermatol 2006;155(Suppl 1):1–9.

40. Minang JT, Arestom M, Troye-BlombergLundeberg L, et al. Nickel, cobalt, chromium, palladium and gold induce a mixed Th1- and Th2-type cytokine response in vitro in subjects with contact allergy to the respective metals. Clin Exp Immunol 2006;146(3):417–26.

41. Food and Drug Administration, Code of Federal Regulation, Vol. 38 No. 3, January 5, 1973. p. 853–4.

42. Belsito DV. Thimerosal: contact (non)allergen of the year. Am J Contact Dermat 2002;13:1–2.

43. Laine J, Kalimo K, Happonen RP. Contact allergy to dental restorative materials in patients with oral lichenoid lesions. Contact Dermatitis 1997;36:141–6.

44. Koch P, Bahmer FA. Oral lesions and symptoms related to metals used in dental restorations: a clinical, allergological, and histologic study. J Am Acad Dermatol 1999;41:422–30.

45. Garner LA. Contact dermatitis to metals. Dermatol Ther 2004;17:321–7.

46. Schnuch A, Uter W. Decrease in nickel allergy in Germany and regulatory interventions. Contact Dermatitis 2003;49:107–8.

47. Veien NK, Hattel T, Laurberg G. Reduced nickel sensitivity in young Danish women following regulation of nickel exposure. Contact Dermatitis 2001;45:104–6.

48. Heim KE, McKean BA. Children's clothing fasteners as a potential source of exposure to releasable nickel ions. Contact Dermatitis 2009;60:100–5.

49. Farnham JJ, Tomazic-Jezic VJ, Stratmeyer ME. Regulatory initiatives for natural latex allergy: US perspectives. Methods 2002;27(1):87–92.

50. Knudsen B, Lerbaek A, Johansen JD, et al. Reduction in the frequency of sensitization to thiurams. A result of legislation? Contact Dermatitis 2006;54(3):170–1.

51. Scheman A, Jacob S, Zirwas M, et al. Contact allergy: alternatives for the 2007 North American contact dermatitis group (NACDG) Standard Screening Tray. Dis Mon 2008;54(1–2):7–156.

52. Jacob SE, Steele T. Contact dermatitis and workforce economics. Semin Cutan Med Surg 2006;25:105–9.

53. Warshaw EM, Moore JB, Nelson D. Patch-testing practices of American Contact Dermatitis Society members: a cross-sectional survey. Am J Contact Dermat 2003;14:5–11.

54. Elgart ML. Patch tests: will they die a bureaucratic death? Ann Allergy 1991;67:548–9.

55. Fisher DA. Desideratum dermatologica–wanted: an extensive menu of patch test allergens available to American dermatologists. Int J Dermatol 1998;37(6):418–20.

56. National Institute for Occupational Safety and Health (NIOSH). Proposed national strategy for the prevention of leading work-related diseases and injuries – dermatological conditions. Cincinnati (OH): US Department of Health and Human Services/DHHS Publication (NIOSH); 1988. p. 89–136.

57. Keil JE, Shmunes E. The epidemiology of work-related skin disease in South Carolina. Arch Dermatol 1983;119:650–4.

58. Mathias CGT. Occupational dermatoses. J Am Acad Dermatol 1988;16:1107–14.

59. Mathias CGT. Contact dermatitis and workers' compensation – criteria for establishing occupational causation and aggravation. J Am Acad Dermatol 1989;20:842–8.

60. Bureau of Labor Statistics. Current population survey, 2004 (microdata files) and labor force data from the current population survey. In: BLS handbook of methods. Washington, DC: US Department of Labor, Bureau of Labor Statistics; 2003. Available at. http://www.bls.gov/cps/home.htm. Accessed February 16, 2009.

61. US Department of Health and Human Services. Healthy people 2010. In: Deering MJ, Guidry M, Maise DR, et al, editors. With understanding and improving health and objectives for improving health, vol. 2. 2nd edition. Washington, DC: US Government Printing Office; November 2000.

62. Nicol AM, Hurrell AC, Wahyuni D, et al. Accuracy, comprehensibility, and use of material safety data sheets: a review. Am J Ind Med 2008;51(11):861–76.

63. Lerman SE, Kipen HM. Material safety data sheets. Caveat emptor. Arch Intern Med 1990;150(5):981–4.

64. Keegel T, Saunders H, LaMontagne AD, et al. Are material safety data sheets (MSDS) useful in the diagnosis and management of occupational contact dermatitis? Contact Dermatitis 2007;57(5):331–6.

65. Henriks-Eckerman ML, Suuronen K, Jolanki R. Analysis of allergens in metalworking fluids. Contact Dermatitis 2008;59(5):261–7.

66. Bernstein JA. Material safety data sheets: are they reliable in identifying human hazards? J Allergy Clin Immunol 2002;110(1):35–8.

67. Pratt IS. Global harmonisation of classification and labelling of hazardous chemicals. Toxicol Lett 2002;128:5–15.

68. United Nations. United Nations Committee of Experts on the Transport of Dangerous Goods (UNCETDG). Working document ST/SG/AC.10/30/Rev.2 Globally Harmonized System of Classification and Labelling of Chemicals. 2001. Available at: http://www.unece.org/trans/danger/publi/ghs/ghs_rev02/English/00e_intro.pdf.

Index

Note: Page numbers of article titles are in **boldface** type.

Dermatol Clin 27 (2009) 395–400
doi:10.1016/S0733-8635(09)00038-2
0733-8635/09/$ – see front matter © 2009 Elsevier Inc. All rights reserved.

Moving?

Make sure your subscription moves with you!

To notify us of your new address, find your **Clinics Account Number** (located on your mailing label above your name), and contact customer service at:

E-mail: elspcs@elsevier.com

800-654-2452 (subscribers in the U.S. & Canada)
314-453-7041 (subscribers outside of the U.S. & Canada)

Fax number: 314-523-5170

Elsevier Periodicals Customer Service
11830 Westline Industrial Drive
St. Louis, MO 63146

*To ensure uninterrupted delivery of your subscription, please notify us at least 4 weeks in advance of move.

Printed and bound by CPI Group (UK) Ltd, Croydon, CR0 4YY

03/10/2024

01040362-0018